Travel Medicine

Guest Editors

ALIMUDDIN ZUMLA, MD, MSc, PhD, FRCP(Lond), FRCP(Edin), FRCPATH(UK), FSB
RONALD H. BEHRENS, MB ChB, MD, FRCP(London)
ZIAD MEMISH, MD, FRCP(Can), FACP, FRCP(Edin), FRCP(Lond), FIDSA

INFECTIOUS DISEASE CLINICS OF NORTH AMERICA

www.id.theclinics.com

Consulting Editor
ROBERT C. MOELLERING Jr, MD

September 2012 • Volume 26 • Number 3

SAUNDERS an imprint of ELSEVIER, Inc.

W.B. SAUNDERS COMPANY

A Division of Elsevier Inc.

1600 John F. Kennedy Blvd., Suite 1800, Philadelphia, PA 19103-2899.

http://www.theclinics.com

INFECTIOUS DISEASE CLINICS OF NORTH AMERICA Volume 26, Number 3
September 2012 ISSN 0891-5520, ISBN-13: 978-1-4557-4898-3

Editor: Stephanie Donley
Developmental Editor: Teia Stone

Infectious Disease Clinics of North America (ISSN 0891-5520) is published in March, June, September, and December by Elsevier Inc., 360 Park Avenue South, New York, NY 10010-1710. Periodicals postage paid at New York, NY and additional mailing offices. Subscription prices are $271.00 per year for US individuals, $463.00 per year for US institutions, $134.00 per year for US students, $321.00 per year for Canadian individuals, $573.00 per year for Canadian institutions, $383.00 per year for international individuals, $573.00 per year for international institutions, and $185.00 per year for Canadian and international students. To receive student rate, orders must be accompanied by name of affiliated institution, date of term, and the *signature* of program/residency coordinator on institution letterhead. Orders will be billed at individual rate until proof of status is received. Foreign air speed delivery is included in all *Clinics* subscription prices. All prices are subject to change without notice. **POSTMASTER**: Send address changes to *Infectious Disease Clinics of North America*, Elsevier Health Sciences Division, Subcription Customer Service, 3251 Riverport Lane, Maryland Heights, MO 63043. **Customer Service: 1-800-654-2452 (US). From outside of the US and Canada, call 1-314-447-8871. Fax: 1-314-447-8029. E-mail: JournalsCustomerService-usa@elsevier.com (print support) or JournalsOnlineSupport-usa@elsevier.com (online support).**

Infectious Disease Clinics of North America is also published in Spanish by Editorial Inter-MÅdica, Junin 917, 1ᵉʳ A 1113, Buenos Aires, Argentina.

Reprints. For copies of 100 or more, of articles in this publication, please contact the Commercial Reprints Department, Elsevier Inc., 360 Park Avenue South, New York, New York 10010-1710. Tel. (212) 633-3812, Fax: (212) 462-1935, E-mail: reprints@elsevier.com.

Infectious Disease Clinics of North America is covered in *MEDLINE/PubMed (Index Medicus), Current Contents/Clinical Medicine, Science Citation Alert, SCISEARCH,* and *Research Alert.*

Printed and bound by CPI Group (UK) Ltd, Croydon, CR0 4YY

Transferred to Digital Print 2012

Contributors

CONSULTING EDITOR

ROBERT C. MOELLERING Jr, MD
Shields Warren-Mallinckrodt Professor of Medical Research, Harvard Medical School;
Department of Medicine, Beth Israel Deaconess Medical Center, Boston, Massachusetts

GUEST EDITORS

ALIMUDDIN ZUMLA, MD, MSc, PhD, FRCP(LOND), FRCP(EDIN), FRCPATH(UK), FSB
Professor of Infectious Diseases and International Health, Division of Infection and Immunity, University College London Medical School; Consultant Infectious Diseases Physician, Directorate of Infection, University College London Hospitals NHS Foundation Trust, London, United Kingdom

RONALD H. BEHRENS, MB ChB, MD, FRCP(LOND)
Consultant in Travel Medicine and Director, Travel Clinic, Hospital for Tropical Diseases, University College Hospital; Senior Lecturer, London School of Hygiene and Tropical Medicine, London, United Kingdom

ZIAD A. MEMISH, MD, FRCP(CAN), FACP, FRCP(EDIN), FRCP(LOND), FIDSA
Professor, College of Medicine, Alfaisal University, Deputy Minister for Public Health, Ministry of Health, Riyadh, Kingdom of Saudi Arabia

AUTHORS

JAFFAR A. AL-TAWFIQ, MD, FACP, FCCP
Saudi Aramco Medical Services Organization, Dhahran, Kingdom of Saudi Arabia

RONALD H. BEHRENS, MB ChB, MD, FRCP(Lond)
Consultant in Travel Medicine and Director, Travel Clinic, Hospital for Tropical Diseases, University College Hospital; Senior Lecturer, London School of Hygiene and Tropical Medicine, London, United Kingdom

SARA BIGONI, MD
Institute of Infectious and Tropical Diseases, Spedali Civili Hospital, University of Brescia, Brescia, Italy

ANDREA K. BOGGILD, MSc, MD
Tropical Disease Unit, UHN-Toronto General Hospital; Assistant Professor, Division of Infectious Diseases, Department of Medicine, University of Toronto, Toronto, Ontario, Canada

BERNADETTE CARROLL, BSc, RN
Research Nurse, Travel Clinic, Hospital for Tropical Diseases, London, United Kingdom

ANNA CRISTINA C. CARVALHO, MD, PhD
Institute of Infectious and Tropical Diseases, Spedali Civili Hospital, University of Brescia, Brescia, Italy

WILSON W. CHAN, MD
Calgary Laboratory Services; Assistant Professor, Department of Pathology and Laboratory Medicine, University of Calgary, Calgary, Alberta, Canada

PETER L. CHIODINI, MB, PhD
Professor, Hospital for Tropical Diseases; London School of Hygiene and Tropical Medicine, London, United Kingdom

VALÉRIE D'ACREMONT, MD, PhD, DTMH
Senior Lecturer of Travel/Tropical Medicine, Travel Clinic Department of Ambulatory Care and Community Medicine, University Hospital, Lausanne, Switzerland; Global Malaria Program, World Health Organization, Geneva, Switzerland

ROSEMARIE DALY, MBBS
Hospital for Tropical Diseases, London, United Kingdom

SUNDEEP DHILLON, MBE, MA, BM BCh, MRCGP, Dip IMC, RCSEd, DCh, FRGS, FAWM
Institute of Human Health and Performance, Centre for Aviation Space and Extreme Environment Medicine, University College London, London, United Kingdom

MAIA FUNK, MD
Senior Consultant, Division of Communicable Diseases, Institute of Social and Preventive Medicine, University of Zurich, Zurich, Switzerland

BLAISE GENTON, MD, PhD, DTMH
Professor of Travel/Tropical Medicine, Infectious Diseases, Department of Medicine, Travel Clinic Department of Ambulatory Care and Community Medicine, University Hospital, Lausanne, Switzerland; Swiss Tropical & Public Health Institute, University of Basel, Basel, Switzerland

CHRISTOPH F.R. HATZ, MD, DTM&H
Professor of Tropical and Travel Medicine, Swiss Tropical and Public Health Institute; University of Basel, Petersplatz, Basel, Switzerland; Professor of Epidemiology and Prevention of Communicable Diseases and Director of World Health Collaborating Center, Division of Communicable Diseases, Institute of Social and Preventive Medicine, University of Zurich, Zurich, Switzerland

JOANNA S. HERMAN, MBBS, MSc, MRCP, DTMH
Specialist Registrar in Infectious Diseases and Tropical Medicine, Hospital for Tropical Diseases, London, United Kingdom

DAVID R. HILL, MD, DTMH, FRCP, FFTM (RCPS Glasg), FASTMH
Professor of Medical Sciences and Director of Global Public Health, National Travel Health Network and Centre, London School of Hygiene and Tropical Medicine, London, United Kingdom

HERWIG KOLLARITSCH, MD
Professor, Institute of Specific Prophylaxis and Tropical Medicine, Center for Pathophysiology, Infectiology and Immunology, Medical University of Vienna, Vienna, Austria

ESTHER KUENZLI, MD, MSc
Clinical Fellow, Division of Infectious Diseases and Hospital Epidemiology, University Hospital of Basel, Basel, Switzerland

JAMES G. LOGAN, PhD, FRES
Lecturer, Department of Disease Control, London School of Hygiene and Tropical Medicine, London, United Kingdom

ALBERTO MATTEELLI, MD
Institute of Infectious and Tropical Diseases, Spedali Civili Hospital, University of Brescia, Brescia, Italy

ZIAD A. MEMISH, MD, FRCP(Can), FACP, FRCP(Edin), FRCP(Lond), FIDSA
Professor, College of Medicine, Alfaisal University, Deputy Minister for Public Health, Ministry of Health, Riyadh, Kingdom of Saudi Arabia

SARAH J. MOORE, PhD
Lecturer, Department of Disease Control, London School of Hygiene and Tropical Medicine, London, United Kingdom; Ifakara Health Institute, Bagamoyo Research and Training Centre, Bagamoyo, Tanzania

ANNE JENNIFER MORDUE (LUNTZ), PhD, FRES, FSB
Professor of Zoology, School of Biological Sciences, University of Aberdeen, Aberdeen, United Kingdom

RACHAEL MORRIS-JONES, FRCP, PhD, PCME
Consultant Dermatologist and Honorary Senior Lecturer with a special interest in Infectious Dermatology, Dermatology Department, Kings College Hospital and Kings College London, London, United Kingdom

STEPHEN MORRIS-JONES, MRCP, FRCPath, DTM&H
Department of Clinical Microbiology, Consultant in Infectious Diseases and Medical Microbiology, University College London Hospitals; Honorary Senior Lecturer, University College London, London, United Kingdom

LORRAINE M. NOBLE, PhD, MPhil, DipClinPsychol, CPsychol, CSci, AFBPsS
Senior Lecturer in Clinical Communication, UCL Medical School, University College London, London, United Kingdom

MARIA PAULKE-KORINEK, MD, MSc, PhD
Institute of Specific Prophylaxis and Tropical Medicine, Center for Pathophysiology, Infectiology and Immunology, Medical University of Vienna, Vienna, Austria

ADRIENNE SHOWLER, MD
Resident Physician, Division of Infectious Diseases, Department of Medicine, University of Toronto, Toronto, Ontario, Canada

ANDREW USTIANOWSKI, PhD(Lond), FRCP(Lond), DTM&H
Director, Regional Infectious Diseases Unit, North Manchester General Hospital, Manchester, United Kingdom

L.G. VISSER, MD, PhD
Department of Infectious Diseases, Leiden University Medical Centre, Leiden, Netherlands

URSULA WIEDERMANN, MD, PhD
Professor, Institute of Specific Prophylaxis and Tropical Medicine, Center for
Pathophysiology, Infectiology and Immunology, Medical University of Vienna,
Vienna, Austria

ADRIENNE WILLCOX, RN, PhD, MA(ed), RPE, FHEA, MFTM RCPS (Glasgow)
Nurse Director, A Talent 4 Health Ltd, Woodmancote, Cheltenham, United Kingdom

ALIMUDDIN ZUMLA, MD, MSc, PhD, FRCP(Lond), FRCP(Edin), FRCPath(UK), FSB
Professor of Infectious Diseases and International Health, Division of Infection and
Immunity, University College London Medical School; Consultant Infectious Diseases
Physician, Directorate of Infection, University College London Hospitals NHS Foundation
Trust, London, United Kingdom

Contents

A significant number of travellers sustain travel-related injury or illness, despite receiving pretravel advice. This appears to be due to a combination of inconsistent guidance about risks and recommendations, and partial adherence. This article considers perceptions and attitudes to risk, factors affecting uptake of advice, and features of an effective consultation. A framework is proposed for a pretravel consultation, using a shared decision-making approach. Engaging the traveller as an active participant in maintaining their own health and providing balanced, evidence-based information about risks and benefits is predicted to enhance the effectiveness of the pretravel consultation.

Global uptake of new vaccines shapes the epidemiology of infections, and in turn this changing epidemiology guides vaccine development. Once introduced, surveillance and monitoring of the impact of vaccines on disease and adverse events is vital for further development. This article reviews the use of vaccines as part of routine health care, vaccines that may be required for entry into a destination country, and vaccines that are recommended because of risk during travel. Considerations and advances in the vaccination of travelers are addressed.

This article reviews the normal immune response to vaccines. It describes the effect of different immunosuppressive therapies (glucocorticoids, inhibitors of calcineurin and mTOR, azathioprine, mycophenolate acid, methotrexate, depleting and nondepleting monoclonal antibodies, and tumor necrosis factor antagonists) on critical steps in the cellular and humoral immune responses to vaccines. The impact of age-related involution of thymus and bone marrow on the immune reconstitution in allogeneic hematopoietic cell transplant recipients and human immunodeficiency virus is covered. A practical approach to vaccinating and preparing travelers with severe immunosuppression is proposed.

With industrial development and expanding tourism, many people now have an opportunity to travel to many previously unreachable foreign destinations. Travelers with medical or physical conditions or who are vulnerable because of pregnancy or age (pediatric or elderly traveler), require specialist support and advice before traveling. Immigrants who return to their country of birth to visit relatives and friends should be classified as vulnerable travelers, as they have been shown to carry a disproportionate burden of travel-related morbidity. In this article, we explore the major risks to health and the main preventive strategies appropriate to the most vulnerable travelers.

Blaise Genton and Valérie D'Acremont

A common approach to malaria prevention is to follow the "A, B, C, D" rule: Awareness of risk, Bite avoidance, Compliance with chemoprophylaxis, and prompt Diagnosis in case of fever. The risk of acquiring malaria depends on the length and intensity of exposure; the risk of developing severe disease is primarily determined by the health status of the traveler. These parameters need to be assessed before recommending chemoprophylaxis and/or stand-by emergency treatment. This review discusses the different strategies and drug options available for the prevention of malaria during and post travel.

Sarah J. Moore, Anne Jennifer Mordue (Luntz), and James G. Logan

Protection from the bites of arthropod (insect and acarine) vectors of disease is the first line of defense against disease transmission and should be advised in all cases when traveling abroad. Details are described of the main approaches for the prevention of bites, including topical or skin repellents, impregnated clothing, bed nets, and spatial or aerial repellents and aerosols. The bionomics of the main arthropod vectors of disease are described along with photographic plates and tabulated advice to give the traveler. An in-depth treatment of the different protection methodologies provides an up-to-date overview of the technologies involved.

Rachael Morris-Jones and Stephen Morris-Jones

Travel associated skin disease is extremely common and a frequent cause of the returning traveller seeking medical attention. Widespread cutaneous eruptions usually represent reactive rashes, indicating an underlying systemic infection or allergic reaction. Patients with disseminated or spreading rashes following travel often present with fever and malaise. In contrast, those presenting with localised skin disease such as a blister, nodule, plaque, ulcer etc are usually well in themselves but have sustained a bite/sting/penetrating injury or introduction of infection directly into the skin at the affected site. As a general rule widespread rashes are investigated with blood tests/serology and localised lesions with a skin biopsy for culture and histology.

Herwig Kollaritsch, Maria Paulke-Korinek, and Ursula Wiedermann

Travelers' diarrhea (TD) is the most important health issue among international travelers. In high risk areas, 50–90% of travelers may experience an

etiologies that may lead to jaundice in the returned traveler, visitors of friends and relatives, or new immigrants, and describe the etiology, epidemiology, and pathogenesis of clinical features of each.

An elevated eosinophil count is a common, frequently underrecognized finding in travelers returning from the tropics and elsewhere. Although there are multiple causes of eosinophilia in a traveler, it is often related to an acquired helminth infection. In some cases these infections can be benign and self-limiting, but in others it may lead to severe sequelae for the individual or others. This article outlines the etiology and diagnosis of eosinophilia concentrating on helminth infections.

Improved data collection methods have produced a clearer picture of travel-associated health risks and at-risk travelers. Examination of the causes of mortality and morbidity has led to a change in emphasis on ways of reducing morbidity. There are unanswered questions that relate to the contribution of medical comorbidities on travel-associated illness, how communication can enhance or influence behavior change, and the best strategies to influence the travelers at greatest risk. Enhanced data collection methods and better denominator data are necessary to provide more precise risk information and help inform policy and thereby reduce morbidity in tourists and travelers.

Evaluation of an individual traveler returned from the tropics requires consideration of a greater range of possible diagnoses than would be entertained at home. In trying rapidly to identify the cause of a presenting illness in the traveler, knowledge of their natural history and a carefully taken account of the location of the trip undertaken and potential exposure to exotic infections helps narrow the range of possibilities and thus the amount of laboratory investigation and imaging needed to confirm a diagnosis.

INFECTIOUS DISEASE CLINICS OF NORTH AMERICA

Preface

Travel Medicine

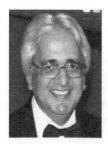 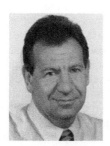 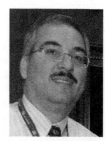

Alimuddin Zumla, MD, MSc, PhD, FRCP(Lond), FRCP(Edin), FRCPath(UK), FSB

Ronald H. Behrens, MB ChB, MD, FRCP(Lond)

Ziad A. Memish, MD, FRCP(Can), FACP, FRCP(Edin), FRCP(Lond), FIDSA

Guest Editors

One of five Americans travel abroad annually, and 38 million visits are to developing and tropical countries. Trauma and accidents are the leading cause of death and injury in travelers. While noncommunicable diseases and climate-related disorders can be important, tropical, infectious, and parasitic diseases now pose an increasing problem for travelers from the United States and Europe to other continents and geographical regions.

The most common cause of ill health in travelers is from diarrhea, as the adage goes, "travel broadens the mind and loosens the bowels." One of the most serious tropical diseases in returning travelers is *Plasmodium falciparum* malaria, which is responsible for an estimated 2 million deaths annually worldwide. Fewer than one in five travelers from the United Kingdom to malaria-endemic regions take prophylactic antimalarial drugs or other mosquito bite preventive measures. Thus, malaria must always be excluded in any ill traveler. Eosinophilia and fever of unknown origin in returning travelers and migrants from the tropics may point toward imported tropical infections or parasitic diseases. Common causes of nonmalarial fever from Africa include rickettsial diseases, filariases, amoebic liver abscess, and Katayama syndrome; from South and South East Asia include enteric fever and arboviral infection; from the Middle East include brucellosis; and from Asia, South America, Mediterranean, and East Africa include visceral and cutaneous leishmaniasis. Human echinococcosis remains highly endemic in regions of South America, Turkey, Mediterranean, Eastern Europe, East Africa, Central Asia, China, and Russia. Sexually transmitted diseases including HIV are endemic globally and pose a great risk to travelers. Rabies continues to cause mortality in certain parts of the world. Because the spectrum of dermatological manifestations seen in travelers while abroad or on return to their home countries is wide, it can be challenging for physicians to recognize and treat such conditions. Of global importance is a wide range of bacterial, viral, and fungal respiratory infections.

In addition to diseases acquired during cross-continental travel, the past two decades have seen a slow resurgence in "tropical" infectious diseases in the West. In Europe giardiasis is considered a travel-related disease but routine surveillance data

Infect Dis Clin N Am 26 (2012) xiii–xvi
http://dx.doi.org/10.1016/j.idc.2012.07.004

id.theclinics.com

from Germany indicate that nearly 50% of infections were acquired during travel within Germany. Within the United States, travelers between the states can be exposed to several "tropical diseases," such as Chagas' disease, viral encephalitides, and leptospirosis.

Thus it is extremely important that physicians globally are aware of the wide spectrum of tropical, infectious, and parasitic diseases their patients may have been exposed to during their travels abroad or within their own countries. It is prudent to inquire about a travel history early on in their consultations, since early diagnosis and treatment of the majority of patients with a potentially fatal infection are required make a rapid and full recovery. With the global emergencies of killer infectious diseases, malaria, tuberculosis, and HIV/AIDS, it has become essential to exclude these early in the consultation. Increased awareness and knowledge among health care providers, family doctors, and hospital emergency departments regarding imported or locally prevalent infectious diseases, early and accurate diagnosis with effective intervention, and treatment measures will reduce morbidity and mortality. In addition to the education of the health care provider, education of the traveler and prescribing preventive measures before travel are of paramount importance. It is also important that those working on the frontlines of medical care globally feel confident in the safe acute management of the health problems travelers present with before specialist help is available.

This special issue of *Infectious Diseases Clinics of North America* on Travel Medicine **consists of 15 articles written by 34** authoritative experts from all around the globe. It gives a comprehensive overview of common travel-associated illnesses and highlights the latest preventive, diagnostic, and treatment measures.

Lorriane Noble, Adrienne Willcox, and Ron Behrens emphasize that pretravel consultation is essential for all travelers since this is intended to educate, motivate, and equip travelers to respond to the health risks posed to themselves by their trips. Despite the ready availability of travel health advice, the number of people who experience travel-related illness or injury each year remains significant, with 8% of travelers from predominantly Western industrialized societies requiring medical intervention during or after their travel.

Joanna Herman and David Hill cover vaccine-preventable diseases and emphasize that prevention is better than cure and that pretravel vaccination is essential for all travelers. Leo Visser describes the problems associated with pretravel vaccination in travelers who are immunosuppressed from any cause and the increased risk they face of acquiring infectious diseases during their travel. Alberto Matteelli, Anna Cristina Carvalho, and Sara Bigoni focus on preventive measures in other vulnerable travelers: those who have health conditions that impose limitations to movement or are associated with a higher susceptibility to health distress or diseases, like pregnant women, children, or the elderly, people with preexisting health problems, and disabled travelers. They classify migrants who return to their country of birth to "Visiting Friends and Relatives" as vulnerable travelers, since they are known to suffer from a disproportionate burden of travel-related morbidities.

Blaise Genton and Valérie D'Acremont emphasize that any traveler to malaria-endemic destinations should be thoroughly informed regarding personal and environmental measures to avoid mosquito bites and that urgent medical advice should be sought as quickly as possible if they develop fever or feel ill.

Travel-associated skin disease is extremely common and a frequent cause of the returning traveler seeking medical attention. In contrast, those presenting with localized skin disease, such as a blister, nodule, plaque, or ulcer, are usually well in themselves but may have sustained a bite or sting that may lead to the introduction of infection. Sarah Moore, Jennifer Mordue (Luntz), and James Logan describe the main approaches for the prevention of bites and stings. They provide an overview of the worldwide distribution of different vectors, the pathogens they carry, and their behavioral activity, in terms of seasonality and time of day. They remind us that tree vector-borne diseases, malaria transmitted by Anopheline mosquitoes, dengue transmitted by Stegomyia (formally Aedes) mosquitoes, and rickettsial infections transmitted by ticks account for half of all systemic febrile illnesses in returned travelers attending travel or tropical-medicine clinics. Rachael and Stephen Morris-Jones in their elegantly illustrated article describe a range of skin abnormalities seen in travelers who seek medical attention on their return from localized infections, penetrating injuries, bites, or stings from insects or an animal. Other skin manifestations may be a marker of an underlying systemic disease acquired while traveling and a diagnosis is best achieved through comprehensive clinical history taking, thorough clinical examination, and focused investigations.

Herwig Kollaritsch, Maria Paulke-Korinek, and Ursula Wiedermann cover travelers' diarrhea, the most important health issue affecting travelers. The risk of acquiring diarrhea is influenced by many factors, such as the destination of the trip, duration of the stay, standard of accommodation, type of travel, age of the traveler, and also by individual risk factors. They describe prevention strategies, including educating travelers about food and water hygiene measures, conditions under which to use prophylactic antibiotics, and vaccination against diarrhea caused by enterotoxigenic *Escherichia coli*.

Sundeep Dhillon highlights that here has been a recent increase in both recreational and adventure travel to extreme environments and environmental hazards, such as weather extremes (hot and cold) and high altitude, frequently pose health problems for travelers. Short-term visitors can adjust to these austere environments provided they have the knowledge and time to acclimatize sufficiently.

Every year millions of people travel to religious, rock, or sporting events from all over the globe, where mass crowding, rapid population movement, and poor hygiene lead to the emergence of a range of infectious diseases, with the potential for spread across the globe. Jaffar Al-Tawfiq and Ziad A. Memish review the risks of infectious diseases and key interventions for their prevention, at mass gatherings.

Rabies is a dreaded and invariably fatal disease and is present in more than 150 countries on all continents. An estimated 55,000 to 70,000 persons die from rabies every year. Christoph Hatz, Esther Kuenzli, and Maia Funk comprehensively cover prevention including vaccination, and detail exposure, prophylaxis, and treatment.

Jaundice and an elevated esosinophil count are common in returning travelers. Liver disease morbidity is common among ill returning travelers, presenting as jaundice. Wilson Chana, Adrienne Showlerc, and Andrea K. Boggildd cover the range of infectious and noninfectious causes of jaundice in travelers.

Andrew Ustianowski and Alimuddin Zumla describe causes of eosinophilia and say that an elevated eosinophil count is a common, frequently underrecognized finding in travelers returning home. Although there are multiple causes of eosinophilia in a traveler, it is often related to an acquired parasite infection.

Examination of the causes of mortality and morbidity has led to a change in emphasis on ways of reducing morbidity. Ronald Behrens and Bernadette Carroll in their article on travel trends and patterns of travel-associated morbidity highlight unanswered questions that relate to the contribution of medical comorbidities on travel-associated illness; how communication can enhance or influence behavior change; and the best strategies to influence the travelers at greatest risk. They provide an overview of the trends in travel and groups of travelers at most risk and examine patterns of morbidity during and after travel.

A traveler with ill health may have a condition that may be noninfective and possibly unrelated to travel; an infectious disease that has a cosmopolitan distribution but may be more common in resource-poor settings; a classical tropical disease which is endemic in a distinct geographical location; or a new or emerging disease not readily identified. Thus evaluation and workup of an individual traveler require the consideration of a wide range of possible diagnoses and urgent laboratory investigations to confirm the diagnosis. Rosemary Daly and Peter Chiodini give a summary outline of laboratory methods for diagnosis of infectious diseases in the returning traveler. They emphasize that in trying to rapidly identify the etiology of the presenting illness in the traveler, knowledge of their natural history and a carefully taken account of the location of the trip undertaken and potential exposure to exotic infections will help narrow the range of possibilities and thus the amount of laboratory investigation and imaging needed to confirm a diagnosis.

Travel Medicine is a young emerging speciality. This Travel Medicine volume of *Infectious Diseases Clinics of North America* comprehensively illustrates the importance of this formal discipline and provides an important addition to the latest literature on the subject. We hope that this volume will serve as a useful guide for physicians, health personnel, travel clinics, and travelers worldwide.

ACKNOWLEDGMENTS

We are very grateful to all the authors for their contributions to this comprehensive volume on Travel Medicine. Our sincere thanks to Stephanie Donley, Clinics Editor, Elsevier Publishing, and their staff for their kind assistance and diligence throughout the development of this special issue. Dr Robert Moellering, Consulting Editor for *Infectious Disease Clinics of North America*, gave his enthusiastic and unflinching support to this project. Adam Zumla provided administrative support to Professor Zumla. We thank our families for their patience during the many long hours spent on this project.

Alimuddin Zumla, MD, MSc, PhD, FRCP(Lond), FRCP(Edin), FRCPath(UK), FSB
Professor of Infectious Diseases and International Health
Department of Infection
Division of Infection and Immunity
University College London Medical School
Directorate of Infection
University College London Hospitals NHS Foundation Trust
London, United Kingdom

Ronald H. Behrens, MB ChB, MD, FRCP(Lond)
Consultant in Travel Medicine, and Director, Travel Clinic
Hospital for Tropical Diseases
Senior Lecturer, London School of Hygiene and Tropical Medicine
Keppel Street
London, United Kingdom

Ziad A. Memish, MD, FRCP(Can), FACP, FRCP(Edin), FRCP(Lond), FIDSA
College of Medicine
Alfaisal University
Deputy Minister for Public Health
Ministry of Health
Riyadh 11176
Kingdom of Saudi Arabia

E-mail addresses:
a.zumla@ucl.ac.uk (A. Zumla)
Ron.Behrens@lshtm.ac.uk (R.H. Behrens)
zmemish@yahoo.com (Z.A. Memish)

Travel Clinic Consultation and Risk Assessment

Lorraine M. Noble, PhD, MPhil, DipClinPsychol, CPsychol, CSci, AFBPsS[a],*,
Adrienne Willcox, RN, PhD, MA(ed), RPE, FHEA, MFTM RCPS (Glasgow)[b],
Ronald H. Behrens, MB ChB, MD, FRCP(London)[c]

KEYWORDS

- Communication • Adherence • Compliance • Concordance • Decision making

KEY POINTS

- Travellers' adherence to preventative strategies is variable, yet little research has considered how to enhance the effectiveness of the pretravel consultation.
- Research in healthcare communication has identified features of an effective consultation which can be applied to travel medicine.
- Responses to pretravel advice are determined by travelers' perceptions of risk, concerns about treatments and preferred risk management strategies.
- A shared decision-making approach encourages professionals and travelers to work in partnership to agree a plan which the traveller is able to follow through.
- In order to reach an informed decision, travelers need balanced, evidence-based information about priority risks which is tailored to their individual circumstances.

TRAVEL CLINIC CONSULTATION AND RISK ASSESSMENT

The pretravel consultation is intended to educate, motivate, and equip travelers to respond to the health risks posed by their trips. Despite the ready availability of travel health advice, the number of people who experience travel-related illness or injury each year remains significant, with 8% of travelers from predominantly Western industrialized societies requiring medical intervention during or after their trip to a preindustrial or developing nation.[1] Evidence continues to accumulate that knowledge of

Disclosures: No funding was received for this work. Lorraine Noble has no financial disclosures or conflicts of interest to disclose. Adrienne Willcox, nurse director of A Talent 4 Health Limited, has received payment and honoraria for educational work from Crucell Ltd, GlaxoSmithKline UK, Novartis Vaccines and Diagnostics Ltd, Pfizer Ltd, and Sanofi Pasteur MSD Ltd. Ron Behrens has received honoraria for acting on advisory boards of NORGINE Pharmaceuticals Ltd and sigma-tau Pharma Limited UK.
[a] UCL Medical School, University College London, Gower Street, London, WC1H 6BT, UK; [b] A Talent 4 Health Ltd, Primrose Bank, Bushcombe Lane, Woodmancote, Cheltenham, GL52 9QQ, UK; [c] Travel Clinic, Hospital for Tropical Diseases, Mortimer Market, London, WC1E 6JB, UK
* Corresponding author.
E-mail address: lorraine.noble@ucl.ac.uk

Infect Dis Clin N Am 26 (2012) 575–593
http://dx.doi.org/10.1016/j.idc.2012.05.007
0891-5520/12/$ – see front matter © 2012 Elsevier Inc. All rights reserved.

travel-related risks and adherence to preventative strategies is variable in travelers who have attended a pretravel consultation.[2,3]

This article focuses on defining the underlying reasons for the difficulties in achieving an optimal response to pretravel advice. This includes a discussion of:

- Expected outcomes of the pretravel consultation
- Conceptions of travel-related risk
- Attitudes toward risk and prevention
- Factors affecting uptake of medical advice

By drawing on evidence and conceptual frameworks from travel medicine and relevant disciplines, a framework for an effective pretravel consultation is proposed. This provides practitioners with the tools to evaluate their own consultations, and those of their trainees, and forms a basis for defining good practice in services that provide pretravel advice.

EXPECTED OUTCOMES OF THE PRETRAVEL CONSULTATION

The structure, organization, and content of the pretravel consultation has been much discussed, particularly the components of risk assessment.[4–7] However, there is at present no nationally or internationally agreed standard for outcomes of the consultation, in the sense of criteria by which an effective pretravel consultation can be measured or judged. Evaluating the effectiveness of a consultation involves examining the process of communication within the consultation and the impact of this on outcomes.[8] Outcomes can be immediate, intermediate, or long term (**Box 1**).

The positive impact of an effective consultation on outcomes is well established and the components of effective communication are well understood.[9–12] Current best practice in health care communication integrates the tasks to be accomplished with the communicative behaviors used to achieve them.[13] However, there is currently no framework for this in travel medicine. The pretravel consultation is complex and densely packed with tasks to be achieved (**Box 2**), which is a lot to accomplish within a single, time-limited consultation, often without the advantage of a preexisting professional-patient relationship.

Moreover, current best practice emphasizes the need for a patient-centered approach and shared decision making,[14–19] in which:

- Patients are involved in decisions as much as they wish
- Information about risk is given in an understandable and unbiased way
- The patient is provided with information about the benefits and risks of the available options, including different treatments and the option of taking no treatment

---

Box 1
Outcomes of a consultation

Immediate

  eg, Understanding and recall of information, satisfaction with the consultation, intention to adhere to recommendations

Intermediate

  eg, Adherence to recommendations

Long term

  eg, Absence of illness, intention to continue healthy behaviors

---

Box 2
Tasks to be achieved in the pretravel consultation

- Establish the traveler's itinerary and other factors that invoke travel-related risks
- Establish relevant medical history and current medication
- Identify and prioritize the travel-related risks relevant to this traveler (and family, if applicable)
- Establish the traveler's previous experience of preventative strategies and identify significant concerns, queries, or potential barriers to adopting an effective preventative regime
- Identify the traveler's need for information and advice
- Discuss the health risks posed by the trip
- Select a preventative regimen that is tailored to the traveler's needs, in line with current evidence and guidance
- Provide information and advice as needed, and check understanding
- Discuss strategies to respond as needed to illness or injury during the trip
- Elicit and address the traveler's concerns and queries
- Negotiate an appropriate and acceptable plan that the traveler feels able to follow through
- Provide advice about follow-up (safety netting)

- Information and advice are tailored to the individual's situation, preferences, and needs
- The professional works in partnership with the patient to achieve a plan that is mutually acceptable

Pretravel advice is within the scope of shared decision making, because it involves making decisions about taking medical treatments (medication and vaccines), which involve both benefits and risks, and a fully informed patient might choose either to have the treatment or not.[15,20]

Although adherence to preventative recommendations has been assessed in travel medicine, little work has examined which features of the pretravel consultation promote or enhance uptake of recommendations. Other mediators of adherence known to be influenced by the health care consultation have also received little attention, such as the traveler's ability to understand and recall information and advice, motivation and intention to follow recommendations, and travelers' confidence in their own ability to follow a recommended course of action (self-efficacy).[21–24]

From this distilled evidence about what constitutes an effective consultation, the following list of outcomes for the pretravel consultation is proposed. By the end of the pretravel consultation, it is expected that travelers will:

- Have been given accurate and relevant knowledge about priority risks to their health and advice on prevention, which is tailored to their individual circumstances, preferences, and needs
- Understand and be able to recall the information and advice
- Be motivated to look after their health and avoid health threats
- Understand the benefits and risks of taking preventative action and not taking preventative action
- Understand how to respond to illness or injuries experienced during the trip
- Have made, in partnership with the health professional, decisions about prevention that accommodate their individual circumstances, preferences, and needs

- Be able to follow the agreed plan, both in terms of prevention and response to illness or injury during the trip, as required

This article considers the extent to which pretravel advice achieves these outcomes and discusses strategies to improve the effectiveness of the consultation.

CONCEPTIONS OF TRAVEL-RELATED RISK

Travel-related risk can be defined as the threat of an adverse event affecting a person's health whilst traveling, which interferes with the trip or necessitates the use of health services. The causes of these events include trauma, acquiring or developing an infection, and illness related to preexisting health conditions (**Box 3**). Social and environmental threats to health, such as road traffic accidents or crime, are valid risks to consider in the pretravel consultation because they can be reduced or avoided by specific interventions. Establishing risk is the basis of the pretravel consultation (**Box 4**).

To make an informed decision, an individual requires information about risks that is understandable, unbiased, tailored to their individual situation, and compares the benefits and risks of potential courses of action. The traveler needs to be in a position to make an informed decision about all the medical interventions being considered,

---

Box 3
Travel-related risks

Journey risks

    eg, Thromboembolism, decompression sickness following recent scuba diving, motion sickness, trips and falls on a cruise

Safety risks

    eg, Unsafe vehicles, fire, carbon monoxide poisoning, assault, rape, theft, sporting or trekking injuries

Environmental risks

    eg, Altitude sickness, sun, heat and cold injuries, air pollution, animal attacks

Food-borne and water-borne risks

    eg, Travelers' diarrhea

Vector-borne risks (including animals)

    eg, Malaria, rabies

Airborne risks

    eg, Influenza

Sexual health and blood-borne viral risks

    eg, Human immunodeficiency virus, hepatitis B and C

Skin health

    eg, Fungal and parasitic infections, wounds

Psychological health

    eg, Fear of flying, culture shock, and reverse culture shock

Data from Field VK, Ford L, Hill DR. Health Information for Overseas Travel. London: National Travel Health Network and Center; 2010. p. 15–57.

> **Box 4**
> **Basic components of a pretravel consultation**
>
> - Establish the probability of the adverse event to the individual/family
>   - Consider epidemiologic evidence and groups at risk
> - Prioritize risks
>   - Common, treatable/avoidable, potentially fatal
> - Select interventions
>   - Based on evidence and effectiveness
>   - Compare the benefits and risks of the adverse event and the interventions
> - Administer the interventions
>   - Discuss the recommendations in the pretravel consultation

particularly those that carry a risk or cost, because adverse reactions to medication and vaccinations can be significant.

Use of the term risk in a consultation implies (1) that there is evidence of a potential hazard (ie, data that could be described in the form of statistics or likelihoods) and (2) that the threat is likely. However, evidence about risks cited in many guidelines comes from a variety of sources, not all of which provide this information. These include:

1. Evidence from randomized controlled trials and controlled trials
2. Epidemiologic studies
3. Observational studies
4. Expert consensus
5. Nonexpert opinion
6. Best guesstimate

In some guidelines, the presence of disease in an area is considered as a risk to travelers, whereas others distinguish between the risk to travelers and the threat to the native population. Inconsistency in determining risk results in variations in guidance. An example is the risk of malaria to tourists to Cambodia (**Table 1**): current evidence shows that the risk to tourists from 13 Western countries is 1 case per 100,000 visits.[32] This compares with a risk of severe neuropsychiatric disturbance resulting from taking mefloquine of 1 case per 10,000 (or 10 cases per 100,000), with risks reported for chloroquine at a similar rate.[25] It is not known how travelers would respond to risks of this likelihood and weigh up the risks and benefits when provided with this information.

Descriptions used to convey the level of threat in international guidelines and in clinical practice include:

Risk everywhere
Risk varies
No known risk
Continuous
Frequent
Infrequent
Rare
High risk
Risk variable
Risk low

Table 1
Statements of malaria risk to travelers to Cambodia from various national and international guidelines and recommendations

Organization	Country	Date	Risk Statement (Abbreviated)
World Health Organization[25]	Global	2011	Malaria risk due predominantly to *Plasmodium falciparum* exists throughout the year in the whole country except in Phnom Penh and Tonle Sap. Negligible risk within the tourist area of Angkor Wat
Advisory Committee on Malaria Prevention[26]	United Kingdom	2007	Risk high in Cambodian western provinces, except no risk in Phnom Penh
Centers for Disease Control[27]	United States	2012	Present throughout the country, except none at the temple complex of Angkor Wat, Phnom Penh, and around Lake Tonle Sap. Moderate risk. *P falciparum* 86%, *Plasmodium vivax* 12%, *Plasmodium malariae* 2%
Deutschen Gesellschaft für Tropenmedizin[28]	Germany	2011	Medium to low risk throughout the country. Minimal risk in the south Mekong region. Malaria free: Phnom Penh, Angkor Wat. *P falciparum* 75%
Expertenkomitee fur Reisemedizin[29]	Switzerland	2011	Low risk (except forested regions during rains). Minimal risk in the south Mekong region. *P falciparum* 86%, *P vivax* 12%, *P malariae* 2%
Société de Medécine des Voyages and la Société Française de Parasitologie[30]	France	2010	*P falciparum* except in Phnom Penh and Tonle Sap; tourist area of Angkor Wat negligible
Società Italiana di Medicina Tropicale[31]	Italy	2003	Risk (except Phnom Penh)

Risk very low
Higher risk
Increased risk
Potential risk
Highest estimated relative risk
Moderate estimated relative risk
Lower estimated relative risk

There is at present no consensus about how these terms relate to the likelihood of an event happening to a traveler. An attempt by the European Commission to standardize descriptors of frequency by attaching percentages to terms such as very common, common, and rare[33] was undermined by evidence that patients held different views about the likelihoods implied by the descriptors, suggesting that such terms should be used with caution.[34] Providing numerical data about the likelihood of the event happening to the traveler is the most transparent approach, and there are established methods for communicating information about risk (**Box 5**).[35–38] However, there is still no consensus within travel medicine about:

- How to discuss risks for which there is no reliable evidence about the likelihood of the adverse event happening to the traveler
- What is an appropriate threshold for deciding whether or not to include a possible adverse event as a risk in a pretravel consultation
- How this threshold might vary according to the severity of the illness or injury.

It is not known whether the emphasis and order of risks presented during the pretravel consultation are congruent with the likelihood and severity of potential health threats (see the article by Behrens and Carroll elsewhere in this issue).

Individuals are less likely to adhere to medical advice when sources contradict each other,[40] but uncertainty in establishing the priority risks to an individual traveler causes variation in advice given. This variation is in addition to the phenomenon of professional noncompliance, in which practitioners deviate from best practice by omitting information or giving inaccurate or irrelevant advice.[41,42] Because travelers often

---

Box 5
Good practice in communicating risk

- Provide unbiased information about the risks and benefits of all reasonable potential options, including doing nothing

- Describe the risk to the individual, not to the population

- Use natural frequencies (eg, 13/100 travelers), rather than percentages (eg, 13%)

- Use common denominators to compare risks (eg, 40/100 compared with 75/100, rather than 2/5 compared with 3/4)

- Present absolute risks (eg, 1/100,000,000 compared with 2/100,000,000), not relative risks (eg, double the risk)

- Use pictorial representation to aid understanding (eg, Cates plot)[39]

- Use verbal descriptors (eg, common, rare) with caution, and clarify the likelihood represented by these descriptors

- Be honest if there is no reliable evidence on which to base an assessment of risk to the individual

- Acknowledge uncertainty about risks, costs, and benefits

seek information from several sources,[43] this inconsistency undermines the credibility of the advice.

Mentioning every conceivable risk is another observed approach, and has been termed the kitchen-sink consultation style[44]:

Quotes from nurse practitioners:

... you may only get a single slot to deal with it, there's very much a case of force feeding somebody [information].

You do see their eyes glaze over sometimes and think, I need to stop now because they're not taking anymore in.

This approach may be the result of defensive practice, or simple optimism that the more information is given, the more will stick. However, overloading a consultation is known to impede understanding, recall, and subsequent adherence to advice,[10,23] and so it does not solve the problem of establishing priorities for an individual traveler.

ATTITUDES TOWARD RISK AND PREVENTION

Guidance phrased in imperative terms (travelers should, must, do, do not, avoid) implies both that it is likely that the adverse event will happen, and that there is a strong association between taking preventative action and staying healthy. However, some travelers remain healthy without taking precautions, whereas others become unwell despite following advice. Most adults have sufficient experience of health care to be aware of this paradox, which results in 'a rational basis for noncompliance'.[45] There are several possible reasons for the apparently inconsistent relationship between taking preventative action and avoiding illness (**Box 6**). The bias caused by overvaluing anecdotal reports in judging the effectiveness of medical advice is not unique to travel medicine, but is particularly relevant in a traveling population with ready access to multiple sources of information, including first-hand accounts from other travelers.

Travelers vary considerably in their tolerance of risk.[21,46] There is an implicit assumption within travel medicine that risks are to be avoided, but, for some travelers, taking risks may be an integral part of having an adventure. For short-term travelers,

---

Box 6

Possible reasons for the inconsistent relationship between taking preventative action, or not, and staying healthy

If the traveler becomes ill, despite taking preventative action:

- The recommended measures did not provide complete protection (eg, because of medication efficacy)

- The traveler partially adhered

- The symptoms or illness had other causes

- Medication side effects were interpreted as illness

- The traveler unintentionally took ineffective measures (eg, counterfeit medication bought during the trip)

If the traveler stays healthy despite not taking preventative action:

- The risk of illness was lower than expected

- The traveler partially adhered

- The traveler took other precautions or naturally engaged in low-risk behavior

the excitement of a holiday mood may be at odds with perceiving a situation as risky and being inclined to follow a preventative routine.

Many studies have shown that travelers arrive at the travel clinic with preexisting knowledge and beliefs about diseases and treatments that, in conjunction with cultural and social norms, have already shaped their perceptions of risk and preferences for engaging in prevention.[47–49] Two conceptual frameworks can be helpful in defining travelers' responses to risks.

The first concerns people's perception of risk and their own ability to respond to it. Research into health beliefs[24] has shown that a person's likelihood of taking action in response to a perceived threat to their health is determined by their perceptions of:

- The severity of the threat
- Their susceptibility to the threat
- The risks, costs, and benefits of taking action
- Their own ability to successfully undertake the required action

Furthermore, a person is more likely to act to avoid a health threat if they intend to take action following their evaluation of the threat, and if there are cues to prompt the behavior nearer the time. There is evidence that travelers' adherence to recommendations is related to their health beliefs and intentions, and that these can be changed by the pretravel consultation.[21,22]

The second conceptual framework concerns preferred responses to risk, and, within this, 2 common approaches can be defined. The first focuses on prevention as a means of minimizing, and ideally eliminating, the risk. An example of this is the precautionary principle, which holds that, if there is a perceived threat of serious harm, preventative action is justified, even in the absence of evidence that harm will ensue.[50] In this approach, the threshold for taking precautions is low, and evidence of a risk is not considered essential.

There is an implicit assumption that a traveler who attends a pretravel consultation intends to take precautions to avoid all the potential risks. However, intention depends on the traveler's perceptions of risk, as discussed earlier. A traveler who believes that a vaccination offers protection against all the diseases that pose a threat to their health may be keen to have a vaccination, but may not have a general intention to follow any other recommendations. Misconceptions about which diseases are preventable by vaccination can therefore overrule advice about antimalarial measures, for example, because the advice may be thought to be irrelevant.[47]

The second approach to responding to risk defines multiple strategies for responding to risk, from identifying a risk to recovery if the adverse event happens (**Box 7**).[51] In this approach, it is assumed that adverse events can happen, despite preventative efforts, hence the need for strategies to minimize harm. There is evidence that some travelers prefer to engage in strategies to minimize harm instead of taking preventative action. For example, in a study of family physicians traveling to south Asia, one of several reasons for nonadherence to chemoprophylaxis was a belief that malaria is easier to treat than prevent.[52] Travelers may show a preference for prevention in response to some risks, but for harm minimization (responding only if required) for other risks. Considering travelers' perceptions, tolerance of risk, and preferred response to risk is therefore fundamental to engaging in a dialogue about travel-related risks.

FACTORS AFFECTING UPTAKE OF MEDICAL ADVICE

Complete adherence to medical recommendations is not the most common response to medical advice.[53] Partial adherence is more common, because people adapt and

---

Box 7
Strategies for responding to risk throughout the life cycle of a crisis

Mitigation

    Identifying risks (eg, risk mapping) and devising strategies to reduce the risk

Preparedness

    Developing the capability to respond to a threat (eg, early warning systems, drills to rehearse responses)

Response

    Activities immediately before, during, or after the crisis to minimize damage or improve recovery

Recovery

    Short-term responses to restore the situation to near normal and long-term strategies to restore life to normal and learn from the event

Data from McLoughlin D. A framework for integrated emergency management. Public Adm Rev 1985;45:165–72.

---

modify regimens according to their health beliefs.[24] Nonadherence can be unintentional (eg, caused by failure of recall) or intentional (eg, caused by beliefs about how much adherence is enough). The more complex the regimen, the less likely people are to adhere,[23] which may because of varying degrees of intentional and unintentional behavior. Even in ideal conditions, expecting full adherence is optimistic. For example, in a study at a Swiss travel clinic, adults traveling to sub-Saharan Africa for less than 3 months who were prescribed mefloquine were given both oral and written information about malaria and prophylaxis, and consented to electronic monitoring of adherence.[54] One-third of travelers (26/81) took all the doses on the expected dates. Variations in adherence included starting the tablets later than 1 week before departure, taking all the tablets but in a random way during the trip, missing doses, stopping the medication during the trip, and stopping the medication on return.

Concerns about side effects are a significant barrier to medication acceptability, particularly regarding antimalarial medication.[55] Explicit discussion in the consultation about medication options and side effects has been shown to change travelers' perceptions of the benefits of taking medication, perceived risks of side effects, and preferences for particular medications.[22,56] There is a known preference to avoid taking medication in the long term, because of fears about toxicity building up over time, which is an issue for longer trips.[48] Concerns about the supposedly synthetic nature of prescribed medication lead some patients to prefer remedies perceived as more natural, including complementary medicines, nutritional supplements, or alternative methods of prevention. A cultural norm to take medication to relieve symptoms, and to stop when symptoms abate, reduces the acceptability of preventative medication in healthy individuals.

Subgroups of travelers are less likely to adhere to preventative strategies, particularly when visiting friends and relatives, on a short business trip, or having a prolonged stay.[47,48] Health beliefs about susceptibility to disease and severity of illness, familial and cultural norms regarding response to health threats, and beliefs about the benefits, risks, and other costs of prevention, account for these patterns of adherence. Exploring the traveler's perspective thus enables the professional to gain an insight into factors that may influence the traveler's behavior. Some practitioners do not themselves follow recommendations, and their beliefs may have a bearing on the advice and sincerity of the message provided to the traveler.[52]

Although response to medical advice is heavily influenced by health beliefs, the climate of the consultation, created by professional-patient communication, also has a major effect on subsequent adherence.[57] Specific features of a consultation have been found to enhance response to medical advice (**Box 8**).[9,10,58–61] An effective working relationship, characterized by trust and rapport, is a key determinant of patient satisfaction and motivation to follow advice.

FRAMEWORK FOR AN EFFECTIVE PRETRAVEL CONSULTATION

The proposed framework is based on the *Calgary-Cambridge Guide to the Medical Interview*, an established, evidence-based structure for the health care consultation that integrates content and process in a series of chronologic tasks.[62] Issues specific to the pretravel consultation are incorporated into the framework (**Table 2**).

In particular, the consultation:

- Explores the traveler's perspective (identifying preexisting knowledge and health beliefs, tolerance of risk, preferred approaches to risk management, and concerns and expectations about preventative strategies)
- Allows for discussion of differing perceptions about priorities and preferred responses to risk
- Incorporates strategies to enhance understanding and recall
- Encourages explicit discussion of potential barriers to adherence

There are 2 key elements to this consultation. The first is the professional's core knowledge base and ability to define the likelihood and severity of risks relevant to the individual traveler, which includes the risks and benefits of all relevant potential courses of action, taking into account the traveler's circumstances, as well as inherent uncertainties. The second is the professional's ability to establish and engage with the

---

Box 8
Communication strategies to enhance adherence to medical recommendations

- Encourage the patient's involvement at the outset and throughout the discussion
- Identify the patient's perspective, knowledge, queries, and concerns
- Provide information that is understandable and well structured:
  - Calibrate the information and language used to the understanding and needs of the individual
  - Clarify any issues, such as patient concerns, queries, or potential barriers raised by either party
  - Chunk information into manageable segments to prevent overload
  - Check understanding and that the patient's needs have been met
- Achieve a shared understanding of the situation, any problems, and possible solutions
- Use positive talk: including empathy, humor as appropriate, encouragement, and support
- Engage in shared decision making, in which patients are involved in decision making as much as they wish
- Consider patients' confidence in their own ability to follow through with the agreed plan and rehearse plans to overcome any barriers

Table 2
Proposed framework for the pretravel consultation

Throughout the Consultation ⇒	Chronologic Tasks	Throughout the Consultation ⇒
Providing structure Explaining the organization of the consultation (eg, providing an overview and signposting topics to be covered) Allocating time according to priorities Varying the amount of information in response to the traveler's need for information, allowing time to digest information and to consider decisions	**Initiating the consultation** Preparing for the consultation The practitioner has evidence-based knowledge of: • Priority travel-related risks, their likelihood and severity • Potential courses of action, risks, and benefits • How this applies to the individual traveler/family • Areas of uncertainty Establishing initial rapport • Travelers feel listened to and that their agenda is identified Establishing the reasons for the consultation • The traveler's expectations, understanding of risks, preferences for preventative action, and attitudes to risk are identified Outcomes of this segment • An agreed problem list • Key decisions to be made **Gathering information** The following information is obtained: Assessing risk • The traveler's itinerary and factors that invoke travel-related risks (cf **Box 3**) • The traveler's relevant medical history and current medication	**Building the relationship** Developing trust, credibility, and rapport Explicitly involving the traveler in selecting priorities and making decisions Identifying and responding to queries and concerns

Exploring the traveler's perspective
- Previous experience of travel-related illness and prevention
- The traveler's relevant knowledge and beliefs
- Further exploration of expectations, preferences, and concerns as needed

Outcomes of this segment
- A priority list of health risks of the trip, tailored to the individual's circumstances
- An understanding of the traveler's perception of risk, motivation to engage in preventative strategies, and preferences for risk management
- An agreed list of topics for which advice will be given

Explanation and planning
Providing information and advice
- Priority risks and recommendations are discussed, tailored to the individual's circumstances, needs, and preferences
- Benefits, risks, and areas of uncertainty are discussed
- Strategies to aid understanding and recall are used, eg, chunking information, checking understanding; strategies for communicating risk (see **Box 5**)

Decision making
- Options are discussed, incorporating the traveler's preferences and addressing queries and concerns
- The traveler is supported in making an informed decision
- Barriers to following the agreed plan are discussed

(continued on next page)

Table 2
(continued)

Throughout the Consultation	Chronologic Tasks	Throughout the Consultation

	Outcomes of this segment
	  • A shared understanding of risks
	  • A mutually agreed plan
	Closing the consultation
	  • Checking that the problem list and any final queries or concerns have been addressed
	  • Forward planning (safety netting)
	Outcomes of this segment
	  • The traveler and the professional are satisfied with the plan
	  • The traveler can understand and recall the information and advice
	  • The traveler intends to follow the plan and feels confident in enacting the plan	

Adapted from Calgary-Cambridge guide to the medical interview – communication process. Available at: http://www.skillscascade.com/handouts/CalgaryCambridgeGuide.pdf. Accessed January 5, 2012; with permission.

traveler's perspective: particularly responding to the traveler's priorities, expectations, preferences, and concerns. These 2 elements in conjunction form the basis of a patient-centered consultation in which informed, shared decision making can take place and the traveler is actively involved in creating a plan that they are able to follow through.

Exploring the traveler's perspective and actively engaging the traveler in negotiating a plan adds to the traditional tasks of a pretravel consultation, which have focused on risk assessment, provision of information, and provision of advice. However, much of the factual information needed by the professional to assess risk can be gathered in advance, by a variety of means, allowing consultation time to be devoted to discussing the implications of the information for the individual. Establishing the traveler's current understanding and need for knowledge and advice reduces time being unnecessarily spent in providing the traveler with information that they already know or do not think they need. Using strategies to manage the amount and pace of information enhances understanding and recall, as well as satisfaction with the consultation. Targeted use of supplementary written information can aid recall of key messages, as well as expanding on lower priority topics (**Box 9**).[63,64] The overriding aim is to promote a partnership between the traveler and the professional; this partnership is known to improve outcomes of care.

FUTURE CHALLENGES

Information management is a particular issue in travel medicine. With so many sources of information available both to travelers and professionals, navigating large quantities of often inconsistent information is required to identify risks that are genuinely relevant to the individual. There is evidence that technology developed for routine tasks, such as online history-taking, is acceptable to patients and improves the use of face-to-face consultation time.[65–67] Clinical decision support technology could be developed to standardize risk assessment by bringing together evidence and guidelines, which could be searched using specific parameters (eg, risks related to the age of the traveler) and could be quickly updated with new evidence.

An additional challenge facing those who provide pretravel advice concerns the travelers who do not seek it. Morbidity and mortality related to travel has consequences beyond the individual traveler, in addition to incurring avoidable health care costs. Engaging with hard-to-reach groups poses difficulties for resource-stretched health care providers, but is the final component of an effective pretravel service. These initiatives often require a different and creative approach; for example,

---

Box 9
Good practice in using supplementary written information

- Consider the individual's ability to read and understand the information (health literacy)
- Select and vet sources to recommend (eg, leaflets or Web sites) that meet the individual's needs
- Explain the purpose of the supplementary information (eg, to aid recall, to provide further detail, to provide advice on topics briefly addressed)
- Point to relevant sections during the consultation to aid recall from episodic memory
- Tailor the information by highlighting areas relevant to the individual
- Encourage follow-up contact if additional questions arise

being promoted by an organization representing the needs of a particular community of travelers.[68] There is a need for evaluated interventions in this area to share good practice.

SUMMARY

A significant number of travelers each year sustain travel-related injury or illness, despite receiving pretravel advice, and this seems to be caused by a combination of inconsistent guidance about risks and recommendations, and partial adherence. A shared decision-making approach to the consultation highlights the role of travelers as active participants in maintaining their own health. This approach encourages health professionals to identify and engage with the traveler's perspective, concerns, and preferences.

A framework for an effective pretravel consultation is described that explicitly recognizes the responsibility shared by the professional and the traveler for identifying the traveler's needs and constructing an acceptable plan. This framework could be used to explore the relationship between process and outcome in the travel clinic setting, and to assess the effectiveness of the pretravel consultation.

Further work is needed to marshal evidence on the likelihood of travel-related risks, and the risks and benefits of potential courses of action, which can be discussed with an individual traveler to inform the process of shared decision making.

ACKNOWLEDGMENTS

The authors thank Dr Jonathan Silverman for permission to adapt the Calgary-Cambridge Guide for the pretravel consultation.

REFERENCES

1. Freedman DO, Weld LH, Kozarsky PE, et al. Spectrum of disease and relation to place of exposure among ill returned travellers. N Engl J Med 2006;354:119–30.
2. Bauer IL. Educational issues and concerns in travel health advice: is all the effort a waste of time? J Travel Med 2005;12:45–52.
3. Hill DR. The burden of illness in international travellers. N Engl J Med 2006;354: 115–7.
4. Hill DR, Ericsson CD, Pearson RD, et al. The practice of travel medicine: guidelines by the Infectious Diseases Society of America. Clin Infect Dis 2006;43: 1499–539.
5. Royal College of Nursing. Competencies: an integrated career and competency framework for nurses in travel health medicine. London: Royal College of Nursing; 2007.
6. Wolfe M, Acosta RW. Structure and organization of the pre-travel consultation and general advice for travelers. In: Keystone JS, Kozarsky PE, Freedman DO, et al, editors. Travel medicine. 2nd edition. Philadelphia: Mosby; 2008. p. 35–45.
7. Field VK, Ford L, Hill DR. Health information for overseas travel. London: National Travel Health Network and Centre; 2010. p. 15–57.
8. Pendleton D. Doctor–patient communication: a review. In: Pendleton D, Hasler J, editors. Doctor–patient communication. London: Academic Press; 1983. p. 5–53.
9. Stewart M. Effective physician-patient communication and health outcomes: a review. CMAJ 1995;152:1423–33.
10. Silverman J, Kurtz S, Draper J. Skills for communicating with patients. 2nd edition. Oxford (United Kingdom): Radcliffe; 2005.

11. Simpson M, Buckman R, Stewart M, et al. Doctor-patient communication: the Toronto consensus statement. BMJ 1991;303:1385–7.
12. Makoul G. Essential elements of communication in medical encounters: the Kalamazoo consensus statement. Acad Med 2001;76:390–3.
13. Kurtz S, Silverman J, Benson J, et al. Marrying content and process in clinical method teaching: enhancing the Calgary-Cambridge guides. Acad Med 1993; 78:802–9.
14. General Medical Council. Good medical practice. London: General Medical Council; 2006.
15. Coulter A, Collins A. Making shared decision-making a reality: no decision about me without me. London: Kings Fund; 2011.
16. Salzburg Global Seminar. Salzburg statement on shared decision-making. BMJ 2011;342:d1745.
17. Fischoff B, Brewer NT, Downs J, editors. Communicating risks and benefits: an evidence-based user's guide. Silver Spring (MD): US Department of Health and Human Services Food and Drug Administration; 2011.
18. Cribb A. Involvement, shared decision-making and medicines. London: Royal Pharmaceutical Society; 2011.
19. European Medicines Agency. Information on benefit-risk of medicines: patients', consumers' and health care professionals' expectations. London: European Medicines Agency; 2009.
20. Coulter A. Involving patients in treatment decisions. NHS Institute for Innovation and Improvement Expert on call webinar. 2010. Available at: http://www.institute.nhs.uk/nhs_alert/expert_on_call/expert_on_call.html. Accessed January 5, 2012.
21. Abraham C, Clift S, Grabowski P. Cognitive predictors of adherence to malaria prophylaxis regimens on return from a malarious region: a prospective study. Soc Sci Med 1999;48:1641–54.
22. Farquharson L, Noble L, Behrens R, et al. Health beliefs and communication in the travel clinic consultation as predictors of adherence to malaria chemoprophylaxis. Br J Health Psychol 2004;9:201–17.
23. Ley P. Communicating with patients: improving communication, satisfaction and compliance. New York: Croom Helm; 1988.
24. Rutter D, Quine L. Social cognition models and changing health behaviours. In: Rutter D, Quine L, editors. Changing health behaviour. Buckingham (United Kingdom): Open University Press; 2002. p. 1–27.
25. World Health Organization. International travel and health. Geneva (Switzerland): WHO; 2011. p. 150, 208.
26. Chiodini P, Hill D, Lalloo D, et al. Guidelines for malaria prevention in travellers from the United Kingdom. London: Health Protection Agency; 2007. p. 48.
27. Centers for Disease Control and Prevention. Infectious diseases related to travel: yellow fever and malaria information, by country. In: CDC Health information for international travel 2012. New York: Oxford University Press; 2012.
28. Deutsche Gesellschaft für Tropenmedizin und Internationale Gesundheit (DTG). Empfehlungen zur Malariavorbeugung [in German]. Available at: http://dtg.org/uploads/media/Malaria_2011.pdf. Accessed January 5, 2012.
29. Bundesamt für Gesundheit Abteilung Übertragbare Krankheiten. Malaria update 2011. Bull BAG 2011;13:280–1 [in German]. Available at: http://www.bag.admin.ch/themen/medizin/00682/00684/01086/index.html?lang=de. Accessed January 5, 2012.
30. Société de Medécine des Voyages and la Société Française de Parasitologie. Recommandations de bonne pratique: protection personelle antivectorielle.

2010 [in French]. Available at: http://www.medecine-voyages.fr/publications/ppavtextecourt.pdf. Accessed January 5, 2012.

31. Bisoffi Z, Napoletano G, Castelli F, et al. Linee guida per la profilassi antimalarica. Giornale Italiano di Medicina Tropicale 2003;8:15–30 [in Italian].

32. Behrens RH, Carroll B, Hellgren U, et al. The incidence of malaria to travellers to south-east Asia: is local malaria transmission a useful risk indicator? Malar J 2010;9:266.

33. European Commission Pharmaceutical Committee. 1998. Guideline on the readability of the label and package leaflet of medicinal products for human use. Brussels (Belgium): European Commission Directorate-General III. p. 22.

34. Berry D, Raynor T, Knapp P, et al. Over the counter medicines and the need for immediate action: a further evaluation of the European Commission recommended wordings for communicating risk. Patient Educ Couns 2004;53:129–34.

35. Edwards A, Elwyn G. Understanding risk and lessons for clinical risk communication about treatment preferences. Qual Health Care 2001;10:i9–13.

36. Edwards A, Elwyn G, Mulley A. Explaining risks: turning numerical data into meaningful pictures. BMJ 2002;324:827–30.

37. Gigerenzer G, Edwards A. Simple tools for understanding risks: from innumeracy to insight. BMJ 2003;327:741–4.

38. Politi MC, Han PK, Col NF. Communicating the uncertainty of harms and benefits of medical interventions. Med Decis Making 2007;27:681–95.

39. Dr Chris Cates' EBM website: Cates plot. Available at: http://www.nntonline.net/visualrx/cates_plot/. Accessed January 5, 2012.

40. Phillips-Howard PA, Blaze M, Hurn M, et al. Malaria prophylaxis: survey of the response of British travelers to prophylactic advice. BMJ 1986;293:932–4.

41. Keystone JS, Dismukes R, Sawyer L, et al. Inadequacies in health recommendations provided for international travelers by North American travel health advisors. J Travel Med 1994;1:72–8.

42. Provost S, Gaulin C, Piquet-Gauthier B, et al. Travel agents and the prevention of health problems among travellers in Quebec. J Travel Med 2002;9:3–9.

43. Leggat PA. Sources of health advice given to travelers. J Travel Med 2000;7:85–8.

44. Willcox A. Nurse-led pre-travel health consultations: evaluating current practice and developing a new model [PhD thesis]. (United Kingdom): University of Warwick; 2010. p. 187.

45. Becker MH. Patient adherence to prescribed therapies. Med Care 1985;23:539–55.

46. Shlim DR. Perspectives: risks travelers face. In: Centers for Disease Control and Prevention, editor. Health information for international travel 2012. New York: Oxford University Press; 2011. p. 20–1.

47. Neave PE, Jones COH, Behrens RH. A review of risk factors for imported malaria in the European African diaspora. J Travel Med 2010;17:346–50.

48. Chen LH, Wilson ME, Schlagenhauf P. Prevention of malaria in long-term travelers. JAMA 2006;296:2234–44.

49. Morgan M, Figueroa-Munoz JI. Barriers to uptake and adherence to malaria prophylaxis by the African community in London, England: focus group study. Ethn Health 2005;10:355–72.

50. Rio Declaration on Environment and Development: Report of the United Nations Conference on Environment and Development. Rio de Janeiro; 1992 (UN Doc./A/Conf.151/26, Vol. I).

51. McLoughlin D. A framework for integrated emergency management. Public Adm Rev 1985;45:165–72.

52. Banerjee D, Stanley PJ. Malaria chemoprophylaxis in UK general practitioners traveling to South Asia. J Travel Med 2001;8:173–5.
53. Osterberg L, Blaschke T. Adherence to medication. N Engl J Med 2005;353: 487–97.
54. Landry P, Iorillo D, Darioli R, et al. Do travelers really take their mefloquine malaria chemoprophylaxis? Estimation of adherence using an electronic pillbox. J Travel Med 2006;13:8–14.
55. Schlagenhauf-Lawlor P, Kain KC. Malaria chemoprophylaxis. In: Keystone JS, Kozarsky PE, Freedman DO, et al, editors. Travel medicine. 2nd edition. Philadelphia: Mosby; 2008. p. 137–57.
56. Senn N, D'Acremont V, Landry P, et al. Malaria chemoprophylaxis: what do the travelers choose, and how does pretravel consultation influence their final decision? Am J Trop Med Hyg 2007;77:1010–4.
57. Kerr J, Weitkunat R, Moretti M, editors. ABC of behavior change: a guide to successful disease prevention and health promotion. London: Elsevier Churchill Livingstone; 2005.
58. Hall JA, Roter DL, Katz NR. Meta-analysis of correlates of provider behavior in medical encounters. Med Care 1988;26:657–75.
59. Haskard-Zolnierek KB, DiMatteo MR. Physician communication and patient adherence to treatment: a meta-analysis. Med Care 2009;47:826–34.
60. Levensky ER, Forcehimes A, O'Donohue WT, et al. Motivational interviewing: an evidence-based approach to counseling helps patients follow treatment recommendations. Am J Nurs 2007;107:50–8.
61. O'Donohue WT, Levensky ER. Promoting treatment adherence: a practical handbook for health care providers. London: Sage Publications; 2006.
62. Calgary-Cambridge Guide to the Medical Interview – Communication Process. Available at: http://www.skillscascade.com/handouts/CalgaryCambridgeGuide. pdf. Accessed January 5, 2012.
63. Noble LM. Written communication. In: Ayers S, Baum A, McManus C, et al, editors. Cambridge handbook of psychology, health and medicine. Cambridge (United Kingdom): Cambridge University Press; 2007. p. 517–21.
64. Carducci A, Calamusa A, de Wet DR, et al. The quality of printed educational resources used in Italian travel clinics. Proceedings of the 11th Conference of the International Society of Travel Medicine, Budapest, Hungary, 24–28 May 2009. Snelville (GA): International Society for Travel Medicine; 2009. p. 76.
65. Pringle M. Using computers to take patient histories. BMJ 1988;297:697–8.
66. Bachman JW. The patient-computer interview: a neglected tool that can aid the clinician. Mayo Clin Proc 2003;78:67–78.
67. Adamson SC, Bachman JW. Pilot study of providing online care in a primary care setting. Mayo Clin Proc 2010;85:704–10.
68. Travelling for Hajj or Umrah? Introducing the Muslim Council of Great Britain meningococcal (ACWY) vaccination package for pilgrims. Available at: http://www.mcb-vac.co.uk/. Accessed January 5, 2012.

Vaccine-Preventable Diseases and Their Prophylaxis

Joanna S. Herman, MBBS, MSc, MRCP, DTMH[a],
David R. Hill, MD, DTMH, FRCP, FFTM (RCPS Glasg), FASTMH[b,c],*

KEYWORDS

- Vaccination • Measles • Polio • Encephalitis • Yellow fever • Hepatitis • Typhoid
- Travel medicine

KEY POINTS

- Vaccination is a key intervention in the prevention of illness in travelers.
- The risk of vaccine-preventable illness in most travelers is low; therefore an individual risk assessment, balancing disease risk with vaccine efficacy and tolerance is key.
- Knowledge of the global epidemiology of vaccine-preventable disease informs an accurate risk assessment.
- Health providers should update routinely recommended vaccines according to national schedules, provide vaccines that may be required for entry to the destination country (e.g. yellow fever vaccine), and administer vaccines based on risk of acquisition during travel.
- In recent years, advances have been made with new vaccine products, understanding of disease risk, and recognition of vaccine adverse events.

The introduction and widespread use of vaccines has had a significant impact on the global incidence of many infectious diseases. Their use has enabled the eradication of some (smallpox), elimination of others in certain regions (eg, poliomyelitis), and dramatic reduction in morbidity and mortality from many (eg, measles, yellow fever [YF], and hepatitis B). Global uptake of new vaccines continues to shape the epidemiology of infections (eg, *Haemophilus influenzae* type b [Hib], *Streptococcus pneumoniae*, and human papillomavirus), and in turn this changing epidemiology guides vaccine development. Once introduced, continued surveillance and monitoring of the impact of the vaccine on both disease and adverse events is vital for further development.

Source of funding: None.
Financial disclosures/declaration of interests: None.
[a] Hospital for Tropical Diseases, Mortimer Market, Capper Street, London WC1E 6JB, UK;
[b] National Travel Health Network and Centre, 250 Euston Road, London NW1 2PG, UK;
[c] Faculty of Infectious and Tropical Diseases, London School of Hygiene and Tropical Medicine, Keppel Street, London WC1E 7HT UK
* Corresponding author. National Travel Health Network and Centre, UCLH NHS Foundation Trust, 250 Euston Road, 5th Floor West, London NW1 2PG, England.
E-mail address: david.hill@quinnipiac.edu

Infect Dis Clin N Am 26 (2012) 595–608
http://dx.doi.org/10.1016/j.idc.2012.05.009
id.theclinics.com

Vaccines may be live-attenuated, inactivated, component, or recombinant. Live (attenuated) vaccines can induce a strong immunologic response similar to that of natural infection, which often results in lifelong immunity. Inactivated vaccines can consist of killed whole organisms (eg, cholera), detoxified exotoxins (eg, tetanus or diphtheria toxoid), soluble capsular antigenic material either alone (eg, pneumococcal) or linked to carrier proteins (eg, Hib), chemically purified components of the organisms (eg, inactivated influenza), or recombinant proteins (eg, hepatitis B). Inactivated vaccines usually require a series of doses for the primary response, with subsequent booster doses to maintain adequate protection. Hepatitis A and B and inactivated polio vaccines have demonstrated long-term immunologic memory.

Vaccination is a key intervention in travel medicine, and is often the reason travelers seek advice before departure; however, vaccine-preventable diseases are uncommon in travelers (usually <1 case per 1000 overseas visits). The decision to vaccinate a traveler involves a risk-benefit assessment based on the risks of disease, the benefits of vaccination, the individual's underlying health, the cost of vaccination, and the risk of adverse events associated with the vaccine.

There are 3 main reasons for vaccinating travelers: vaccination may be recommended as part of routine health care, be required by the destination country, or be recommended because of travel-related risk (**Box 1**).

The pretravel consultation should be used as an opportunity to ensure that the traveler is up to date with routine vaccines according to national guidelines (eg, measles-mumps-rubella [MMR], tetanus). It should then focus on destination-specific vaccines appropriate both for country (eg, YF) and risk from planned activities (eg, rabies, Japanese encephalitis). Many vaccines require more than one dose, and travelers should be aware that receiving incomplete courses of vaccines may lead to incomplete protection. This article reviews the considerations and advances in the vaccination of travelers (see **Box 1, Table 1**).

There are excellent resources to help the provider of travel medicine make decisions as to the appropriate vaccine for the traveler. International resources such as the World Health Organization (WHO) book *International Travel and Health* (www.who.int/ith/en/index.html), and national experts (eg, the US Centers for Disease Control and Prevention [www.who.int/ith/en/index.html] and the UK National Travel Health Network and Center [www.nathnac.org]), should be consulted for up-to-date, evidence-based recommendations.

VACCINES AS PART OF ROUTINE HEALTH CARE
Diphtheria

Diphtheria is now rare in high-income countries. Disease, usually caused by *Corynebacterium diphtheriae,* is transmitted by the respiratory route or by direct contact with infected objects or exudate from skin lesions. Most imported cases in travelers are cutaneous rather than the classic respiratory form with its leathery pharyngeal membrane and systemic intoxication, and are acquired in South Asia. Cutaneous disease presents as a chronic nonhealing ulcer, often contaminated with *Streptococcus* and/or *Staphylococcus*. All travelers should have received a primary course of diphtheria toxoid in childhood with boosting at 10-year intervals if still at risk. Diphtheria vaccine is usually combined with tetanus toxoid.

Influenza

Influenza types A, B, and C are distributed globally. In temperate climates the viruses are seasonal during the winter months, but in the tropics they can circulate year round.

> **Box 1**
> **Vaccines used in international travelers**
>
> *Vaccines administered in the United Kingdom (UK) for age-specific routine health care[a]*
>
> - Diphtheria[b]
> - Tetanus[b]
> - Pertussis[b]
> - Poliomyelitis[b] (also recommended when there is a risk of disease during travel)
> - *Haemophilus influenzae* type b[b]
> - Measles, mumps, and rubella (MMR combination vaccine)
> - Bacillus Calmette-Guérin (BCG)[c]
> - Influenza
> - *Streptococcus pneumoniae*
> - Meningococcal C conjugate
> - Human papillomavirus
>
> *Vaccines that may be required for entry into a destination country*
>
> - Yellow fever (required under International Health Regulations [2005])
> - *Neisseria meningitidis* (serotypes A, C, Y, W 135; required by Saudi Arabia for pilgrims)
>
> *Vaccines that may be recommended because of risk during travel*
>
> - Bacillus Calmette-Guérin (BCG)[c]
> - Hepatitis A
> - Hepatitis B
> - *Salmonella enterica* serotype Typhi
> - Japanese encephalitis
> - Tick-borne encephalitis
> - Rabies
> - Cholera
> - Poliomyelitis
>
> Before administering any vaccine, the manufacturer's complete prescribing information should be consulted.
>
> [a] UK standards for childhood, adolescent, and adult immunization are available from the Department of Health (England) immunization web site (www.immunisation.nhs.uk).
> [b] Usually provided as part of multivalent vaccine products.
> [c] BCG is now administered only to high-risk children in the UK, and for travelers under the age of 16 going to high-risk destinations for at least 3 months (areas with an annual incidence of tuberculosis ≥40 cases/100,000), or health care workers younger than 35 years to same destinations.

Types A and B are responsible for epidemic human disease, with type A producing the most severe illness; type C is found in many animals including pigs and birds. Influenza viruses have the potential for antigenic shift with complete exchange of 1 or more of the 8 influenza genes, potentially leading to a pandemic, for example, pandemic A/H1N1 in 2009 (swine flu), as there is no or limited underlying population immunity. Transmission is most commonly via the respiratory route, but hand to mucous membrane spread also occurs, and virus can survive for hours on fomites.

Table 1
Vaccines for travel: recent advances

Vaccine	Recent Advances	Clinical Relevance
Cholera	Killed whole-cell vaccines provide 67%–84% protection in adults for 2 y	Use in outbreaks being evaluated; consider for aid workers during cholera outbreaks or travelers visiting cholera-endemic areas with limited medical care
Hepatitis A & B	An accelerated schedule (days 0, 7, 21, and 12 mo) achieves seroprotection	Good protection in travelers can be achieved even with impending departure
Influenza	Is the most common vaccine-preventable illness in travelers	Consider vaccine for travelers during risk seasons (see text)
Japanese encephalitis	Inactivated Vero cell vaccine is safe and immunogenic in children; antibodies decline in all recipients by 12 mo. Rare risk in travelers	Carefully select who receives vaccine. Booster is needed 12 mo after primary series for those with ongoing risk
Meningococcal	Conjugate vaccines are more immunogenic in younger age groups	Vaccination for travel to meningitis belt in Africa and for religious pilgrimage to Saudi Arabia
Rabies	Four doses of vaccine after a rabies exposure is now accepted by many countries as adequate protection when combined with RIG	Decreases number of doses of inactivated vaccine
Tick-borne encephalitis	Rare risk in travelers. Accelerated schedule is immunogenic	Balance risk of disease with vaccination
Yellow fever	Rare neurologic and viscerotropic reactions recognized. Higher risk in persons ≥60 yr and with thymus disorders. Breastfeeding infants <30 d old has been associated with YF vaccine virus transmission	Balance risk of disease with vaccine safety. Use new YF vaccination maps to make vaccine recommendations

Abbreviations: RIG, rabies immune globulin; YF, yellow fever.
Adapted from Chen LH, Hill DR, Wilder-Smith A. Vaccination of travelers: how far have we come and where are we going? Expert Rev Vaccines 2011;10(11):1609–20; with permission.

Rapid worldwide dissemination of the virus can occur via air travel. The amount of air traffic can accurately predict the risk of importation into a country, as evidenced by the 2009 pandemic. During seasonal transmission the risk of acquisition during travel can be as high as 1 episode per 100 person-months.[1]

Inactivated and nasally administered live-attenuated vaccines are manufactured annually, based on WHO recommendations regarding the types of A and B viruses that are expected to circulate during the influenza season. All ages can be vaccinated, with the dose and schedule varying according to age. Some countries, such as the United States, recommend annual vaccination of all individuals, including travelers. However, the United Kingdom recommends vaccination only for those considered at increased risk of complications of influenza, such as pregnant women, those aged 65 years and older, children younger than 6 months, and those with chronic underlying disease and immunocompromise (including human immunodeficiency virus [HIV] infection).

Measles

Measles remains endemic in much of the developing world. Although there has been a decline in high-income countries of Europe since it was incorporated into routine childhood vaccination programs more than 20 years ago, in the last several years there has been an increase in cases. Large outbreaks have affected the general population (France, Belgium, Germany, Switzerland, Spain, Romania), or specific groups (eg, the Roma in Italy and Greece, orthodox Jewish communities in Belgium, and traveler communities in the United Kingdom and Norway).[2,3] Such cases have occurred in incompletely and unvaccinated individuals. In northern Europe a contributing factor to low vaccine coverage was the publication in 1998 of an article suggesting a link between MMR vaccine and nonspecific inflammatory conditions of the bowel with resultant childhood disorders such as autism. This association has been discredited and retracted, but not before it had a major impact on vaccine uptake.[4]

The age at which measles is seen has shifted, and it can no longer be regarded as only a disease of childhood. In July 2011 the Health Protection Agency in the United Kingdom reported peak incidence in 10- to 14-year-olds, with the 5- to 9-year and 15- to 19-year groups being the second and third most common age groups affected, respectively.[5] During 2011 in Europe, 79% of cases occurred in those aged 5 years or older. The high mortality seen in the developing world with measles is not seen in industrialized countries, but infection can be severe wherever it occurs.[2]

Measles vaccine is live-attenuated and is usually given with mumps and rubella as MMR. All travelers should check their vaccine status, even for European travel. Persons born before 1957 in the United States and 1970 in the United Kingdom can be assumed to have had natural infection. Summer mass-gathering events popular with teenagers can carry a high risk of transmission, and it is this group that often has low vaccine coverage.

Pertussis

Pertussis or whooping cough, caused by *Bordetella pertussis*, has seen a resurgence in the last decade, as childhood vaccine immunity wanes in adolescents and adults and they develop susceptibility to clinical infection.[6] Such persons can become a source of infection for infants not yet immunized. Travelers should assure that they have received a primary course of pertussis vaccine. If they are going to a country experiencing an outbreak, they can seek adult formulations of pertussis vaccine (usually as tetanus-diphtheria-acellular pertussis vaccine) for a booster.[7]

Polio

Poliomyelitis can develop after infection with poliovirus, a small RNA enterovirus with 3 types (1, 2, and 3). Spread is mainly by the fecal-oral route. Most infections with poliovirus are asymptomatic, with a case/infection ratio of approximately 1:200.

Excellent immunity to disease develops after natural infection. The inactivated Salk vaccine (or IPV) was the first polio vaccine to be licensed in 1955, followed by the live-attenuated oral Sabin vaccine (OPV) in 1961. OPV has been included in the Extended Program on Immunization (EPI) since it was established in 1974. Both OPV and IPV typically contain all 3 poliovirus types. However, during recent efforts at global polio eradication, monovalent and bivalent (1 + 3) OPV has been given.[8] Type 2 poliovirus no longer circulates. OPV is easier and cheaper to administer than IPV, has a rapid action, and produces greater enteric immunity. Rarely, vaccine-associated paralytic poliomyelitis (VAPP) occurs in nonimmune individuals following circulation of vaccine virus in nonimmune populations.

The WHO regions of the Americas, Europe, and the Western Pacific have been declared by the WHO as polio free. In a major public health achievement, India, as one of the 4 remaining countries endemic for polio, was declared polio free in January 2012. With the interruption of wild-type polio transmission in India, there are now 3 polio-endemic countries: Pakistan, Afghanistan, and Nigeria. Having foci of polio in endemic countries can lead to reintroduction and circulation of polio in many countries, as has happened particularly in Africa. Polio can reestablish itself either temporarily or long term, in areas where there is low underlying vaccine coverage. In the last few years this has occurred in Tajikistan, Russia, and China (www.polioeradication.org).

Travelers are at very low risk of infection; however, they should ensure they have received a primary course of vaccine and have been boosted appropriately when traveling to countries at risk.

Tetanus

Clostridium tetani, an anaerobic spore-forming bacillus, has a global distribution. Spores of the bacillus are found in animal feces and are ubiquitous in the environment. Tetanus can develop when spores are introduced through cuts, wounds, punctures, and injection sites, and then germinate. In low-income countries where maternal tetanus vaccine coverage can be low, neonatal tetanus is an important problem. Tetanus vaccine uses a toxoid and is typically given in combination with other antigens such as diphtheria and polio or pertussis. Although most travelers are at very low risk of tetanus, they should ensure that they are up to date with vaccination. A booster dose should be given to those who will not have direct access to medical care in remote areas, and who were vaccinated more than 10 years previously.

VACCINES THAT MAY BE REQUIRED FOR ENTRY INTO A DESTINATION COUNTRY
Yellow Fever

YF is a mosquito-borne viral hemorrhagic fever caused by a flavivirus. There is no specific treatment, and mortality rates can be as high as 50%. YF is endemic in equatorial Africa and in an expanding area of South America.[9] Despite the presence of appropriate *Aedes* spp vectors, it has never been reported in Asia. As a zoonosis in monkeys YF cannot be eradicated, and therefore emphasis is on preventive vaccination and vector control (*Aedes* spp) in urban areas. During the past decade, official reports of YF incidence (50–120 cases a year from South America and 200–1200 cases a year from Africa)[10] probably underestimate the true number of cases, as cases may occur under the level of epidemiologic surveillance. A live-attenuated vaccine has been used for the prevention of YF since 1937, with more than 500 million doses administered.[11] Protective levels of neutralizing antibodies are found in 90% of vaccinees within 10 days and in 99% within 30 days.[12]

YF vaccine is currently the only vaccine that is required under International Health Regulations (IHR) (2005) for entry into YF-endemic countries, and for travel from endemic countries to some *Aedes* spp–infested countries at risk of introduction of the virus. A single dose in healthy individuals gives long-term immunity, but boosting is required under IHR (2005) at 10-year intervals to validate the International Certificate of Vaccination or Prophylaxis for travel purposes. The vaccine must be given at least 10 days before travel.

The risk of YF in travelers is extremely low, and has been estimated to be 0.4 to 4.3 cases per million travelers.[11] However, during epidemic periods it can be higher.[13] Between 1970 and 2010 only 9 cases of YF were reported in unvaccinated travelers from the United States and Europe.[14] The only reported case in a vaccinated traveler comes from a Spaniard who visited West Africa in 1988.

YF vaccine has been considered a well-tolerated vaccine, with mild local and systemic reactions affecting 10% to 30% of vaccine recipients. Anaphylaxis is rare, occurring in 0.8 to 1.8 cases per 100,000 doses. Postvaccination encephalitis has been a recognized risk, particularly for infants vaccinated when younger than 6 months.[11] However, in 2001 a new pattern of serious adverse events was recognized, which have taken two forms: viscerotropic (YEL-AVD) and neurologic (YEL-AND). Neurologic events occur 3 to 28 days (median 14 days) after vaccination, and include fever and headache with meningoencephalitis or central or peripheral signs of demyelination. Nearly all persons recover. The estimated risk is 0.4 to 0.8 cases per 100,000 doses of vaccine.[11,15] By contrast, viscerotropic disease occurs 1 to 8 days (median 3 days) after vaccination, and resembles wild-type infection with fever, multiorgan failure, and a mortality rate exceeding 65%. The estimated risk is 0.3 to 0.4 cases per 100,000 doses of vaccine.[11,15] Risk factors that have been associated with these reactions are age older than 60 years (increasing the risk about 4-fold) and thymus disorders that may have resulted in thymectomy.[16,17]

Vaccination precautions include age older than 60 years, children aged 6 to 9 months, and pregnant and breastfeeding women. There have been recent cases of vaccine virus transmitted to breastfeeding infants, resulting in reversible neurologic disease.[18] Contraindications are children younger than 6 months, egg allergy known to cause anaphylaxis, immunosuppression secondary to HIV (with CD4 <200), long-term steroids, chemotherapy, anti–tumor necrosis factor agents, radiotherapy, receipt of biologically active drugs, or hematological and solid-organ malignancy.

The recognition of the serious adverse events associated with YF vaccine requires that a careful risk assessment is made before administration of the vaccine. Vaccination recommendations have undergone recent reassessment, with new guidelines from WHO that should be consulted before administering YF vaccine.[9] For those who cannot receive vaccine a letter of medical exemption can be issued, which should be taken into account by immigration authorities.

Meningococcal Disease

Meningococcal disease is endemic throughout the world and occurs as sporadic cases, clusters, and large-scale epidemics. In industrialized countries the majority of disease is seen as sporadic cases with occasional outbreaks, but in the meningitis belt of sub-Saharan Africa large epidemics occur.

There are 6 main serotypes: A, B, C, X, Y, and W135. Serotype B is the main public health problem in Europe, Australia, and New Zealand; B and C in the Americas; A and C in Asia; and A in sub-Saharan Africa (although C, X, and W135 have also occurred in Africa).

The meningitis belt, which stretches from Senegal in the west to Ethiopia in the east, has the highest rate of endemic infection globally. Large epidemics occur every 5 to 12 years, predominantly due to serotype A, and the incidence can approach 1% of the population. Epidemics are highly seasonal, occurring during the dry season between December and June, with school-age children at greatest risk. In 2009 there were more than 4000 deaths and 78,000 suspected infections (http://apps.who.int/ghodata/).

A quadrivalent polysaccharide vaccine containing serotypes A, C, Y, and W135 has been available for more than 20 years; conjugated polysaccharide vaccines have been developed in the last 10 years. Conjugate vaccines are more immunogenic in infants and young children, induce a longer duration of protection, and can reduce carriage of the organism. High levels of coverage against meningococcal disease can induce herd immunity. At present there is no widely available vaccine against serotype B.

Most travelers are at low risk, but those who have prolonged close contact with local populations (health care workers, those visiting friends and relatives [VFR travelers], and long-term travelers) should be considered for vaccination. The quadrivalent meningococcal vaccine (A, C, Y, W135) is a requirement for pilgrims traveling to Saudi Arabia for the Hajj and Umrah pilgrimages.

VACCINES THAT MAY BE RECOMMENDED BECAUSE OF RISK DURING TRAVEL
Cholera

In 2010 more than 300,000 cases of cholera and 7500 deaths were reported (http://apps.who.int/ghodata/). This increase was primarily due to the introduction of cholera into Hispaniola in late 2010, where more than 530,000 cases with a case fatality rate of 1.3% have occurred up until April 2012. Historically most cases of cholera have been reported from Africa, but this is likely attributable to gross underreporting in endemic regions of Asia.

Vibrio cholerae is transmitted by the fecal-oral route, and can lead to the sudden onset of profuse watery diarrhea, with the risk of circulatory collapse and death in severe cases. Untreated, more than 50% of severe cases may die, often within hours. The mainstay of treatment is vigorous rehydration (intravenous or oral). In moderate to severe cases antibiotics reduce the volume of diarrhea and duration of excretion of the organism, the latter being important in outbreak settings. Doxycycline, ciprofloxacin, and azithromycin are all effective, although resistance patterns during outbreaks should be determined.

V cholerae relies on an enterotoxin (cholera toxin) to produce diarrhea. The toxin consists of A and B subunits: the B subunit binds to gut epithelial cells and facilitates entry of the A subunit into cells, which induces production of cyclic adenosine monophosphate and resultant electrolyte and water secretion. Current vaccines rely on whole-cell killed V cholerae 01 (classic and El Tor biotypes) with (Dukoral) or without (Shancol) the B subunit, in a 2-dose schedule.[19]

Protection can be expected 1 week after the second dose. There is 60% to 85% protection for 4 to 6 months in all age groups. Protection declines in young children after 6 months, but remains at about 60% after 2 years in older children and adults. Reanalysis of data from the original field trial in Bangladesh indicated that the effectiveness of the whole-cell, cholera toxin B vaccine is enhanced by herd protection that occurs when vaccine coverage is greater than 50%.[20]

Cholera is rare in travelers, and can be a mild illness in healthy persons. The vaccine is recommended for humanitarian aid workers based in refugee settings, and travelers with remote itineraries during cholera outbreaks during which there is limited access to safe water and medical care. An average of 32 clinically compatible cases was reported in the United Kingdom between 2000 and 2009, mostly from South Asia.

Hepatitis A

The risk of hepatitis A infection in travelers has declined over the past 20 years, probably because of improved sanitation at destination countries. The incidence for travel to countries of high or intermediate risk of transmission has declined from 3 to 20 cases per 1000 travelers per month, to 3 to 11 cases per 100,000 persons per month for all travelers and 6 to 28 per 100,000 for those who are presumed to be nonimmune.[21]

South Asia, Africa, and Central America and Mexico are higher-risk areas, but vaccination should also be considered for travel to most other destinations in low-income countries, as vaccination is well tolerated with long-lasting immunity (>20 years) after a primary course. Risk in southern Europe is now minimal, although there have been outbreaks since 2008 in the Czech Republic, Latvia, and Estonia.

VFR travelers are at higher risk of acquiring hepatitis A.[22] Lack of pretravel advice and vaccinations, travel to areas outside usual tourist destinations, longer duration of stay, and prolonged contact with the local population contribute to the higher risk in VFR travelers. Many adult VFR travelers may be immune to hepatitis A, having acquired the infection in childhood when it is often symptomatic. However, their children, if born in a high-income country, will be nonimmune and need vaccination. Hepatitis A vaccine is given either as a single inactivated antigen or combined with hepatitis B or typhoid antigens.

Hepatitis B

Hepatitis B has a global distribution with higher rates in sub-Saharan Africa, parts of South America, South and South East Asia, and China. Approximately 350 million people are estimated to be chronic carriers.

Hepatitis B vaccine uses recombinant surface antigen and is well tolerated. Vaccine can be given alone or in combination with hepatitis A antigens, with both vaccines inducing excellent immunity. Ninety-nine percent of recipients of a combined hepatitis A and B vaccine seroconverted 1 month after a zero, 1-month, and 6-month schedule.[23] An accelerated schedule (zero, 7 days, 21 days, and 12 months) is approved; more than 60% seroconverted to hepatitis B at 1 month.

Because of the potential to develop acute fulminant hepatitis, or chronic liver disease and hepatocellular carcinoma with long-term infection, vaccination should be offered to those considered at risk, and in particular those traveling to countries with a prevalence of more than 2% of hepatitis B surface antigen.[24] Risk factors include occupation, prolonged travel, medical and dental treatment, and travel with chronic medical problems or during pregnancy that may require medical intervention while abroad. VFR travelers and young children who may be in close contact with the local population also should be encouraged to receive vaccine. Advice on behavioral risk reduction should be given at the same time. Most countries routinely vaccinate their children against hepatitis B.

Japanese Encephalitis

Japanese encephalitis (JE) is the most important cause of epidemic encephalitis worldwide, with approximately 35,000 to 50,000 cases annually.[25] The flavivirus is transmitted by dusk-biting *Culex* spp mosquitoes that breed in paddy fields, with pigs and birds as amplifying hosts. JE is endemic in much of South and South East Asia, the Western Pacific, and China, with a tendency to summer epidemics in temperate regions. Most infections are subclinical, but if disease develops there is a 20% to 30% fatality rate, and up to 50% of cases have long-term neurologic sequelae.

JE is rare in travelers, with only 55 cases reported in unvaccinated travelers between 1973 and 2008, and an estimated incidence of less than 1 case per million travelers.[26] The risk varies according to destination, duration and season of travel, and activities.

An inactivated Vero cell–derived vaccine (Ixiaro) was licensed in 2009. Immunogenicity is comparable with that of the now discontinued mouse brain vaccine (JE-VAX) following

2 doses given 28 days apart. However, the duration of protection is limited, and those who remain at risk should be boosted at 12 to 15 months.[27] Only 40% of vaccinees will seroconvert after a single dose. There are other JE vaccines (including live-attenuated vaccines) available in Asia. Vaccination is recommended for long-term travelers to endemic areas and for short-term travelers who have an appropriate level of exposure in rural transmission areas.

Rabies

Rabies is a zoonotic disease caused by an RNA lyssavirus, which infects humans and other mammals. It is endemic worldwide, but has the highest incidence in humans in Asia and Africa where 95% of deaths occur. Globally it is estimated that more than 55,000 people die of rabies every year. Transmission can occur following contact with the saliva from an infected wild or domestic animal, most often via a bite, but occasionally from a scratch or saliva contact with an open wound. Once symptoms of the disease develop, rabies is nearly always fatal. Dogs are the source of 99% of human rabies deaths and of rabies exposures in travelers.

Rabies prevention involves both preexposure and postexposure vaccination. Several tissue-culture vaccines are available: human diploid cell, chick embryonated egg vaccine, and Vero cell vaccine. Preexposure, 3 doses are given on days 0, 7, and 21 or 28. In healthy persons, long-term immunity ($\geq$10 years) is likely. For travelers, a single primary course is usually sufficient, and boosting is usually not necessary.[28]

Vaccination is recommended for both adults and children traveling to areas where medical care is not readily accessible, those traveling for long periods through rabies-endemic countries, those involved in risk activities (eg, running, cycling), and those who have occupational risk (veterinarians, laboratory workers handling the virus). Young children may be at higher risk because of their tendency to approach animals.

All travelers, whether or not they have received preexposure vaccine, should be advised that thorough wound cleansing (copious water and use of soap) is necessary following an exposure. For those who have received preexposure vaccine, 2 doses (days 0 and 3) of vaccine are needed. If preexposure vaccine has not been given, the traveler will need to have postexposure vaccine (5 doses on days 0, 3, 7, 14, and 28) and rabies immune globulin. Some countries no longer recommend the fifth postexposure dose.[28,29] Human and equine rabies immune globulin are biologics in short supply, often obtained only after travel to a referral center. Vaccines are safe in those with immunosuppression, but their antibody response may be suboptimal.

Tick-Borne Encephalitis

Tick-borne encephalitis (TBE) is the most common arbovirus transmitted by ticks in Europe; approximately 10,000 cases are reported each year across Europe and Russia. TBE also occurs in China, but data are limited. Over the past decade the geographic distribution and reported incidence of disease have increased.[30,31] About a third of persons infected develop clinical symptoms after 4 to 28 days; two-thirds will recall a tick bite. Case fatality rates vary from 1% in the European subtype to 20% in the Far-Eastern subtype, but neurologic deficits are frequent in those that recover.

TBE is a rare disease in travelers, with an estimated risk of 1 case per 10,000 person-months during TBE transmission season in those unvaccinated.[32] Exposure is usually during travel or work in rural forested areas of Central Europe during the months of March to November. Consumption of unpasteurized dairy products can also transmit TBE. No antiviral treatment is available.

Prevention of TBE includes protective clothing, insect repellents applied to both skin and clothes, and vaccination (currently only available in Europe and Canada). TBE vaccines are inactivated, and require 3 doses over 12 months, with a booster at 3 years. Vaccination is recommended for persons who are living in TBE-endemic areas, those at occupational risk (eg, farmers, loggers, hunters), and those traveling to rural endemic areas below 1400 m during late spring and summer.

Typhoid

Enteric fever (typhoid and paratyphoid fevers) remains a public health problem in many developing countries, but has largely disappeared from high-income countries, where it is almost always seen in returning travelers. The WHO estimates that there are 21 million cases each year including 200,000 deaths.[33] Infection with Salmonella Typhi or S Paratyphi A, B, or C can result in enteric fever. Whereas infection with S Paratyphi B and C may be milder, S Typhi and S Paratyphi A can produce severe disease with indistinguishable clinical syndromes.[34] The case fatality rate can be as high as 30% in endemic countries without adequate treatment, but rates are much lower in travelers.[35]

In endemic regions S Typhi is regarded as the most frequent cause of disease, but in travelers in recent years S Paratyphi has been seen with about equal frequency, possibly because current typhoid vaccines do not protect against S Paratyphi.[36] The highest risk of enteric fever is in travelers to South Asia. Data from both the United States and United Kingdom indicate that more than 65% of imported enteric fever is from India, Pakistan, and Bangladesh,[36,37] with risk of infection calculated to be as high as 37 cases per 100,000 visits by VFR travelers to Bangladesh, compared with to less than 1 case per 100,000 visits for travel to other developing countries.

Increasing prevalence of multidrug-resistant strains of S Typhi and S Paratyphi complicates effective therapy.[33] Resistance to chloramphenicol, ampicillin, or co-trimoxazole (trimethoprim-sulfamethoxazole) has been widespread since the 1990s, and there has been increasing resistance to ciprofloxacin because of its frequent use. At present most strains remain sensitive to ceftriaxone, cefixime, and azithromycin.

The killed whole-cell typhoid vaccine was abandoned because of a high rate of unpleasant adverse events. There are currently two vaccines available: an oral live-attenuated Ty21a strain (Vivotif) and a parenteral inactivated capsular polysaccharide vaccine containing the virulence (Vi) antigen either singly or combined with hepatitis A antigen. Vi antigen enhances infectivity of S Typhi and contributes to protection of the pathogen against host defenses. The oral vaccine lacks the Vi antigen, but contains immunogenic cell wall polysaccharides that induce a secretory immunoglobulin A and cell-mediated immune response against intracellular bacilli. Neither vaccine is protective against S Paratyphi.

Primary vaccination with Ty21a consists of 3 or 4 (depending on the country where immunized) enteric-coated capsules taken on days 1, 3 and 5 (and 7). There is rapid seroconversion after a single dose of the Vi antigen vaccine, but it should be repeated at 3-yearly intervals if at continued risk (polysaccharide vaccines have no boosting effect). Both vaccines are well tolerated.

Efficacy of both vaccines is suboptimal, with rates of 55% to 75%[38] reported in endemic populations. Vaccine-induced immunity can be overcome by a high inoculum. Thus, it must be emphasized to travelers that the vaccine offers only moderate protection against typhoid and no protection against paratyphoid, and therefore food hygiene measures remain important.

Vaccination should be targeted at travelers to the Indian subcontinent, particularly VFR travelers. Extensive rural travel in other developing regions merits vaccine consideration.

Tuberculosis

It is uncommon to acquire tuberculosis (TB) during travel.[39,40] Those at greatest risk are VFR travelers, health care workers, and those who are resident in endemic regions. The estimated incidence in long-term travelers to highly endemic regions is 3.5 infections per 1000 person-months of travel, and of active disease 0.6 per 1000 person-months of travel.[39] In Peace Corps volunteers the incidence rate for infection ranged from 0 to 5 cases per 1000 person-months.[40] To assess incidence rates of infection, observational studies have looked at tuberculin skin test (TST) conversions.[41] However, these studies have limitations because most lack a control group, making bias an issue.

Risk is determined by the amount (frequency and duration) of exposure to a source case, and individual factors that determine the probability of an individual becoming infected if exposed. Tubercle bacilli are rapidly dispersed outdoors and become nonviable in sunlight. By contrast, if indoors in a room with no ventilation, a high density of bacilli remain viable and suspended as droplet nuclei in the air for prolonged periods of time, with a subsequent greater risk of infection.

Transmission of *Mycobacterium tuberculosis* (MTB) during flights has been examined. The ventilation system on modern aircraft prevents random distribution of MTB, both by the airflow pattern and filters that trap the bacilli. The WHO has published guidelines for management of those with possible exposure on aircraft, and recommends tracing of passengers who sat in the same row or 2 rows adjacent to smear-positive cases for at least 8 hours (and further criteria if multidrug-resistant or extremely drug–resistant MTB).[42] In contrast to WHO guidelines, others have suggested a low risk of transmission during air travel, questioning the utility of screening.[41]

Bacillus Calmette-Guérin (BCG) vaccination is part of most countries' routine immunization schedule. BCG provides protection against disseminated disease and TB meningitis in infants and young children, but this protection wanes with age and is significantly lower 10 to 15 years after vaccination.[43] Current United Kingdom recommendations for BCG vaccination for travel are to immunize children younger than 16 years who are traveling to a country with an annual incidence of TB of at least 40 cases per 100,000 population, and staying for at least 3 months. Health care workers up to the age of 35 years visiting high-incidence countries can also be immunized.

If BCG vaccine is not given, persons can be screened with TST or an interferon-γ release assay before and after travel. The best practice for travel-medicine practitioners is to ensure that travelers are aware of the risk of TB, and to educate them to seek early medical advice should they develop any of the cardinal symptoms (fever, cough, weight loss), so that prompt investigation and treatment can be instigated.

SUMMARY

Vaccines are usually highly effective in protecting travelers against many infectious diseases. Each traveler needs to be considered individually, with vaccination based on a careful risk-benefit assessment. Several important new vaccines are in development including those for dengue, meningococcal disease group B, and malaria, as well as a killed YF vaccine. Physicians involved in travel medicine should ensure they are up to date with latest vaccine developments, to afford their travelers the best protection.[44]

REFERENCES

1. Mütsch M, Tavernini M, Marx A, et al. Influenza virus infection in travelers to tropical and subtropical countries. Clin Infect Dis 2005;40(9):1282–7.

2. Muscat M, Bang H, Wohlfahrt J, et al. Measles in Europe: an epidemiological assessment. Lancet 2009;373(9661):383–9.
3. Mankertz A, Mihneva Z, Gold H, et al. Spread of measles virus d4-Hamburg, Europe, 2008-2011. Emerg Infect Dis 2011;17(8):1396–401.
4. Deer B. How the case against the MMR vaccine was fixed. BMJ 2011;342:c5347.
5. Health Protection Agency. Measles cases in Europe update to end-July 2011. Health Protection Report. Available at: http://www.hpa.org.uk/hpr/archives/2011/news3411.htm#msls07. Accessed June 29, 2012.
6. Guiso N, Wirsing von Konig CH, Forsyth K, et al. The global pertussis initiative: report from a round table meeting to discuss the epidemiology and detection of pertussis, Paris, France, 11-12 January 2010. Vaccine 2010;29(6):1115–21.
7. Centers for Disease Control and Prevention. Updated recommendations for use of tetanus toxoid, reduced diphtheria toxoid and acellular pertussis (tdap) vaccine from the Advisory Committee on Immunization Practices, 2010. MMWR Morb Mortal Wkly Rep 2011;60(1):13–5.
8. Sutter RW, John TJ, Jain H, et al. Immunogenicity of bivalent types 1 and 3 oral poliovirus vaccine: a randomised, double-blind, controlled trial. Lancet 2010;376(9753):1682–8.
9. Jentes ES, Poumerol G, Gershman MD, et al. The revised global yellow fever risk map and recommendations for vaccination, 2010: consensus of the informal WHO working group on geographic risk for yellow fever. Lancet Infect Dis 2011;11(8):622–32.
10. World Health Organization. Yellow fever in the WHO African and American regions, 2010. Wkly Epidemiol Rec 2011;86(34):370–6.
11. Staples JE, Gershman M, Fischer M. Yellow fever vaccine: recommendations of the Advisory Committee on Immunization Practices (ACIP). MMWR Recomm Rep 2010;59(RR-7):1–27.
12. Monath TP, Nichols R, Archambault WT, et al. Comparative safety and immunogenicity of two yellow fever 17D vaccines (Arilvax and YF-VAX) in a phase III multicenter, double-blind clinical trial. Am J Trop Med Hyg 2002;66(5):533–41.
13. Monath TP. Review of the risks and benefits of yellow fever vaccination including some new analyses. Expert Rev Vaccines 2012;11(4):427–48.
14. Barnett ED. Yellow fever: epidemiology and prevention. Clin Infect Dis 2007;44(6):850–6.
15. Lindsey NP, Schroeder BA, Miller ER, et al. Adverse event reports following yellow fever vaccination. Vaccine 2008;26(48):6077–82.
16. Barwick Eidex R, Yellow Fever Vaccine Safety Working Group. History of thymoma and yellow fever vaccination [letter]. Lancet 2004;364(9438):936.
17. Khromava AY, Barwick Eidex R, Weld LH, et al. Yellow fever vaccine: an updated assessment of advanced age as a risk factor for serious adverse events. Vaccine 2005;23(25):3256–63.
18. Kuhn S, Twele-Montecinos L, MacDonald J, et al. Case report: probable transmission of vaccine strain of yellow fever virus to an infant via breast milk. CMAJ 2011;183(4):E243–5.
19. Shin S, Desai SN, Sah BK, et al. Oral vaccines against cholera. Clin Infect Dis 2011;52(11):1343–9.
20. Ali M, Emch M, von Seidlein L, et al. Herd immunity conferred by killed oral cholera vaccines in Bangladesh: a reanalysis. Lancet 2005;366(9479):44–9.
21. Mütsch M, Spicher VM, Gut C, et al. Hepatitis A virus infections in travelers, 1988-2004. Clin Infect Dis 2006;42(4):490–7.
22. Bui YG, Trepanier S, Milord F, et al. Cases of malaria, hepatitis A, and typhoid fever among VFRs, Quebec (Canada). J Travel Med 2011;18(6):373–8.

23. Thoelen S, Van Damme P, Leentvaar-Kuypers A, et al. The first combined vaccine against hepatitis A and B: an overview. Vaccine 1999;17(13–14):1657–62.
24. Centers for Disease Control and Prevention. CDC health information for international travel 2012. Atlanta (GA): US Department of Health and Human Services, Public Health Service; 2012.
25. Fischer M, Lindsey N, Staples JE, et al. Japanese encephalitis vaccines: recommendations of the Advisory Committee on Immunization Practices (ACIP). MMWR Recomm Rep 2010;59(RR-1):1–27.
26. Hills SL, Griggs AC, Fischer M. Japanese encephalitis in travelers from non-endemic countries, 1973-2008. Am J Trop Med Hyg 2010;82(5):930–6.
27. Eder S, Dubischar-Kastner K, Firbas C, et al. Long term immunity following a booster dose of the inactivated Japanese encephalitis vaccine Ixiaro®. Vaccine 2011;29(14):2607–12.
28. World Health Organization. Rabies vaccines: WHO position paper. Wkly Epidemiol Rec 2010;85(32):309–20.
29. Robertson K, Recuenco S, Niezgoda M, et al. Seroconversion following incomplete human rabies postexposure prophylaxis. Vaccine 2010;28(39):6523–6.
30. Centers for Disease Control and Prevention. Tick-borne encephalitis among U.S. travelers to Europe and Asia—2000-2009. MMWR Morb Mortal Wkly Rep 2010; 59(11):335–8.
31. World Health Organization. Vaccines against tick-borne encephalitis: WHO position paper. Wkly Epidemiol Rec 2011;86(24):241–56.
32. Rendi-Wagner P. Risk and prevention of tick-borne encephalitis in travelers. J Travel Med 2004;11(5):307–12.
33. Crump JA, Mintz ED. Global trends in typhoid and paratyphoid fever. Clin Infect Dis 2010;50(2):241–6.
34. Bhan MK, Bahl R, Bhatnagar S. Typhoid and paratyphoid fever. Lancet 2005; 366(9487):749–62.
35. Connor BA, Schwartz E. Typhoid and paratyphoid fever in travellers. Lancet Infect Dis 2005;5(10):623–8.
36. Final report: pilot of enhanced enteric fever surveillance in England, Wales, and Northern Ireland. Health Protection Agency. Available at: http://www.hpa.org.uk/webw/HPAweb&HPAwebStandard/HPAweb_C/1206575041900?p=1158945066450. Accessed June 29, 2012.
37. Lynch MF, Blanton EM, Bulens S, et al. Typhoid fever in the United States, 1999-2006. JAMA 2009;302(8):859–65.
38. World Health Organization. Typhoid vaccines: WHO position paper. Wkly Epidemiol Rec 2008;83(6):49–59.
39. Cobelens FGJ, van Deutekom H, Draayer-Jansen IWE, et al. Risk of infection with *Mycobacterium tuberculosis* in travellers to areas of high tuberculosis endemicity. Lancet 2000;356:461–5.
40. Jung P, Banks RH. Tuberculosis risk in us Peace Corps volunteers, 1996 to 2005. J Travel Med 2008;15(2):87–94.
41. Abubakar I. Tuberculosis and air travel: a systematic review and analysis of policy. Lancet Infect Dis 2010;10(3):176–83.
42. World Health Organization. Tuberculosis and air travel. Guidelines for prevention. 3rd edition. Geneva (Switzerland): World Health Organization; 2008.
43. Smith PG, Fine PE. BCG vaccination. In: Davies PD, editor. Clinical tuberculosis. London: Chapman & Hall Medical; 1998. p. 417–31.
44. Chen LH, Hill DR, Wilder-Smith A. Vaccination of travelers: How far have we come and where are we going? Expert Rev Vaccines 2011;10(11):1609–20.

The Immunosuppressed Traveler

L.G. Visser, MD, PhD*

KEYWORDS

- Immunocompromised • Immunosuppressive agents • Travel health information
- Vaccines • Tumor necrosis factor antagonist • Immune reconstitution
- Hematopoietic cell transplantation • HIV

KEY POINTS

- Clonal proliferation of T- and B-cells is a central event in mounting an effective immune response against pathogens and vaccines.
- Most immunosuppressive drugs reduce the number of effector T- and/or B-cells by blocking this clonal expansion.
- Age-related changes of the thymus may explain why immune reconstitution after high dose chemotherapy, allogeneic haematopoietic cell transplantation, or during combined anti-retroviral therapy for HIV may remain incomplete.
- These considerations can be used to propose a practical approach to travellers with severe immunosuppression.

INTRODUCTION: IMMUNOSUPPRESSION REFERS TO LOSS IN QUALITY OR QUANTITY OF CELLULAR AND/OR HUMORAL IMMUNE COMPONENTS

The human immune system is affected by age, disease, and medication. If a condition results in loss in numbers or functional defects of cellular and/or humoral immune components, the term immunosuppression or immunocompromised is used. Primary immunodeficiencies such as X-linked agammaglobulinemia, are inherited. When loss in quality or quantity results from disease or its therapy, the immunodeficiency is classified as secondary. This article focuses on travelers with secondary immunodeficiencies, including prolonged administration of high-dose corticosteroids, treatment with immunosuppressive drugs such as alkylating agents and antimetabolites, as well as treatments with therapeutic monoclonal antibodies and treatments consequent to hematopoietic malignancies, human immunodeficiency virus (HIV) infection, and treatment with irradiation (**Fig. 1**).[1]

Determination of the degree of immunosuppression may be a challenge, especially because the effects of new therapeutic modalities, such as monoclonal antibodies and

Conflicts of interest: L.G. Visser has served on speakers' bureaus for Abbott, Crucell and Sanofi.
Department of Infectious Diseases, Leiden University Medical Centre, C5P-41, Albinusdreef 2, 2333 ZA Leiden, Netherlands
* Corresponding author.
E-mail address: l.g.visser@lumc.nl

Infect Dis Clin N Am 26 (2012) 609–624
http://dx.doi.org/10.1016/j.idc.2012.06.003
0891-5520/12/$ – see front matter © 2012 Elsevier Inc. All rights reserved.

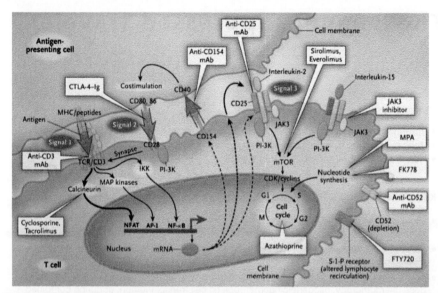

Fig. 1. Activity of immunosuppressive drugs in the T-cell. Each of the steps involved in the activation and proliferation of T-cells can be the target of an immunosuppressive drug: 1) destruction of reacting T-cells through binding of monoclonal IgG1 antibodies (mAb) to CD52; 2) interference with the co-stimulatory signals; 3) blocking the intracellular signal of the antigen-recognising T-cell receptor (TCR) by cyclosporine and tacrolimus; 4) inhibition of DNA synthesis and cell proliferation by molecular-target- of-rapamycin (mTOR) inhibitors sirolimus and everolimus, mycophenolic acid (MPA), azathioprine, cyclophosphamide and metothrexate; and 5) modulation of the effector T-response. CDK, cyclin-dependent kinase; IKK, inhibitor of nuclear factor-kB kinase; MAP, mitogen-activated protein; MHC, major histocompatibility complex; MPA, mycophenolic acid. (*From* Halloran PF. Immunosuppressive drugs for kidney transplantation. N Engl J Med 2004;351:2715–29; with permission.)

tumor necrosis factor (TNF) inhibitors, on the effectiveness and safety of vaccines has not been fully characterized. However, it is relevant as the incidence or severity of some vaccine-preventable diseases must be balanced, with the lowered efficacy of the vaccines or even harm they may cause as can occur with live, attenuated vaccines. This article reviews the normal immune response to vaccines and explores the effect of different immunosuppressive treatments on critical steps in the cellular and humoral immune responses to vaccines. Practical approaches to dealing with travelers with severe immunosuppression are suggested.

THE NORMAL IMMUNE RESPONSE: CLONAL PROLIFERATION IS A CENTRAL EVENT IN MOUNTING AN EFFECTIVE IMMUNE RESPONSE

Only a few naive T and B cells are able to recognize a given antigen. This number is too small for a useful response against a vaccine or pathogen. In order to mount an effective immune response, it is crucial these few T- and B-cells clone and multiply in numbers.

During a primary immune response, when the immune system is exposed to antigens or pathogens for the first time, naive CD4$^+$ T cells in lymph nodes or spleen recognize peptide antigens on the surface of dendritic cells and are activated through the binding of these antigens to their T-cell receptors. This activation, together with costimulatory signals delivered by the antigen-presenting dendritic cell, result in the activation of 3 signal transduction pathways results in the T cell: (1) the calcium-calcineurin-nuclear factor of activated T cells (NFATT) pathway, (2) the RAS-mitogen–activated protein (MAP) kinase-activating protein (AP)-1 pathway, and (3) the nuclear factor-κB (NF-κB) pathway.[2,3] The most important result of this activation is the production of the cytokine interleukin (IL)-2 by the activated T cells. Binding of IL-2 to its CD25 receptor on the surface of the activated T cell is necessary for its survival and leads to cell division, and gives rise to a clone of thousands of T cells that all bear the same antigen receptor.[4(p346)] After 4 to 5 days of growth, the activated CD4+ T cells differentiate into helper and regulatory effector and memory T cells.

Activation of naive CD8+ T cells requires costimulatory signals from dendritic cells and help from CD4+ effector T cells that recognize related antigens presented on the surface of the same dendritic cells.[4(p383)] This stimulates CD8+ T cells to produce IL-2, which drives their own proliferation and differentiation into cytotoxic effector and memory cells.

Naive B cells that have bound antigen to their surface immunoglobulin receptors require costimulatory signals from CD4+ helper T cells that respond to the same antigen for these B cells to survive, proliferate, and differentiate in antibody-producing plasma cells and memory B cells. One month after immunization, memory B cells are present at their maximum levels.[4(pp388–97)] Through their highly repetitive structure, bacterial polysaccharides can induce mature B cells to proliferate and produce antibodies without the help of T cells (so-called T-cell-independent antigens), although costimulatory signals from dendritic cells may be necessary for their survival and differentiation.

In contrast with a primary immune response, a secondary immune response, consequent to a new exposure to the same antigen or pathogen, starts with the proliferation of memory T and B cells on recognition of the antigen. Because memory cells to a given antigen are a 100-fold to 1000-fold more prevalent than at the primary exposure, and because memory cells are more sensitized to activation by antigen than naive cells, a more rapid and vigorous response ensues.

Taken together, a clonal expansion of either naive or memory T and B cells following appropriate stimulatory signals of antigen-presenting cells is essential to acquire sufficient numbers of effector and memory T and B cells for an effective immune response.

THE WAY IMMUNOSUPPRESSIVE DRUGS WORK: REDUCING NUMBERS

Each of the steps discussed earlier can be the target of an immunosuppressive drug (**Fig. 1**): (1) destruction of reacting T and/or B cells, (2) interference with the costimulatory signals, (3) blocking the intracellular signal of the antigen-recognizing T-cell receptor, (4) inhibition of DNA synthesis and cell proliferation, and (5) modulation of the effector T-cell or B-cell response. The net result of all but the last step is that the clonal expansion is blocked.

As a result, the primary immune response to new (vaccine) antigens (or neoantigens) is likely to be severely hampered, with a resultant poor antibody response following vaccination. In general, the secondary immune response by memory T and B cells to revaccination with vaccine antigens that have been seen before (recall antigens) is better conserved. There are more T and B memory cells present that are able to react to the antigen and these cells are able to respond to lower levels of antigen. However, because the clonal expansion of memory cells are inhibited, the resulting antibody levels are lower and duration of protection may be shortened compared with the normal host response.

As a general rule, revaccination of a traveler on immunosuppressive therapy with inactivated vaccines usually results in protective antibodies, albeit producing lower titers of antibodies. In case of primary immunization, additional doses may be necessary to achieve protective antibody titers. For this reason, measuring antibody levels after vaccination is advised.

Live, attenuated vaccines, such as yellow fever vaccine, need to replicate to induce a protective immune response resulting in the clearance of the vaccine strain virus without disease. Inhibition of the clonal expansion of T and B cells may lead to delayed and less effective clearance of the replicating virus, increasing the risk of severe vaccine-associated disease and adverse events. Therefore, the administration of live, attenuated vaccines while immunosuppressed is always contraindicated.

Glucocorticoids

The biologic function of glucocorticoids is to limit and resolve inflammatory responses to avoid tissue damage.[5] During inflammation, increased cortisol levels dampen local and systemic inflammatory reactions, facilitating resolution of the inflammatory response.[6] Glucocorticoid receptors belong to a large family of 48 nuclear receptors. After binding of glucocorticoid to its nuclear receptor, the complex moves from the cytosol to the nucleus and promotes or prevents gene expression at the level of RNA synthesis from the DNA template (transcription).[7] The glucocorticoid's nuclear receptor is expressed in virtually all cells, and has different isoforms with distinct functions in different cell types.[5] In addition, it has been proposed that glucocorticoids may modulate around 1% of the genome.[6] As a consequence, the metabolic and immunologic effects of glucocorticoid therapy are complex and diverse.

Glucocorticoids limit leukocyte trafficking to the site of inflammation[6] and release of proinflammatory eicosanoids such as prostaglandins and leukotrienes.[8] In macrophages, the glucocorticoid-receptor complex interferes with the transcriptional activation of the RAS-MAP kinase–activator protein 1 (AP-1) and the NF-κB pathway, thereby suppressing a broad range of responses of these cells to inflammation-inducing stimuli (proinflammatory signals).[7]

In naive T cells, glucocorticoids inhibit activation of transcriptions factors such as AP-1, NF-κB, and nuclear factor of activated T cell (NFAT),[6] making these cells less responsive to activating signals and more prone to programmed cell death (apoptosis).[8]

Glucocorticoids are widely used to suppress rejection of organ transplants and to treat immune-mediated inflammatory or allergic diseases. Although the responsiveness to treatment with glucocorticoids may vary between individuals and over time, it is generally assumed that a daily dose of prednisone of less than 10 mg does not result in significant immune suppression. Most guidelines consider live, attenuated vaccines to be contraindicated if the cumulative dose of oral or parenteral prednisone is greater than 280 mg.

The antiinflammatory potency differs between different glucocorticoid analogs (**Table 1**). In addition, the systemic immune-suppressive activity of glucocorticoid analogs may be less than prednisone through the alterations in their bioavailability. An oral controlled release formulation of budesonide, for example, is used in the treatment of inflammatory bowel disease and its antiinflammatory activity is 15 times more

Table 1
Antiinflammatory potency of different glucocorticoid analogs

Glucocorticoid	Relative Antiinflammatory Activity
Hydrocortisone	0.25
Prednisone	1
Methylprednisone	1.25
Dexamethasone	5.12

potent than that of prednisone. However, budesonide is rapidly metabolized by cytochrome P-450 enzymes in the liver after oral administration.[9] As a result, the systemic bioavailability (approximately 10%–15%) and ensuing systemic side effects, such as suppression of pituitary-adrenal function, are reduced.[10]

Because of the interindividual differences in responsiveness to glucocorticoids, it is difficult to estimate the biologic half-life of these drugs. In general, it is better to defer live, attenuated virus vaccination for at least 1 month after discontinuation of systemically absorbed glucocorticoid therapy (≥280 mg). The numbers of CD4+ and CD8+ T cells in blood should be determined to exclude lymphopenia caused by long-standing T-cell apoptosis.

Inhibitors of Intracellular Signal Transduction from the Antigen-Recognizing T-cell Receptor (Cyclosporin A, Tacrolimus, Sirolimus, Everolimus)

Cyclosporin and tacrolimus block the clonal expansion of activated T cells by interfering with the transmission of signals from the antigen–T-cell receptor complex to the nucleus. Both drugs inhibit the intracellular enzyme calcineurin in a dose-dependent way, although tacrolimus is more potent than cyclosporin. Activated calcineurin allows transcription factors to migrate from the cytoplasm to the nucleus, where they induce the transcription of several cytokine genes. Inhibition of calcineurin leads to reduced production of cytokines such as IL-2 which is required for survival and clonal proliferation of the activated T-cell, and reduced expression of CD40 ligand on the cell membrane of the T-cell which is required for T-cell help to B-cells. As a consequence, the clonal expansion of B cells is inhibited, the numbers of helper effector T cells reduced, and CD40 ligand and cytokine production from these T cells is then inhibited. B-cell proliferation to T-cell–independent antigens is reduced.

Cyclosporin and tacrolimus are extensively used in organ transplantation but also in the treatment of graft-versus-host disease, atopic eczema, and so forth.

The elimination half-life of cyclosporin and tacrolimus is between 8.4 and 27 hours[11] and 8.5 hours,[12] respectively, meaning that the immunosuppressive effect can last up to 7 days for cyclosporin and 3 days for tacrolimus following cessation of treatment.

Sirolimus (also known as rapamycin) and its derivative everolimus inhibit the intracellular enzyme mammalian target of rapamycin (mTOR). This serine/threonine kinase is widely expressed among many cell types, and its complex biology is not completely elucidated. Immune cells use intracellular signaling through mTOR to modulate their response to the environment.[13,14]

Inhibition of mTOR by sirolimus or everolimus has numerous, and sometimes opposite, effects on differentiation, maturation, and function of antigen-presenting dendritic cells (DC) and macrophages. Sirolimus and everolimus inhibit DC differentiation and maturation in vitro, reduce antigen uptake by pinocytosis and endocytosis, increase migration of activated DC to lymph nodes, impede maturation of DC and their ability to stimulate effector T cell responses, stimulate IL-12 production of macrophages in response to bacterial antigens (LPS), but impair interferon (IFN)-α and IFN-β production by plasmacytoid DC in response to viral vaccines.

In CD4+ T cells, inhibition of mTOR prevents the signal of the IL-2 cytokine receptor from activating cell proliferation. Instead, the activated T cells die through programmed cell death (apoptosis),[4(p660)] whereas the proliferation of regulatory T cells (T_reg) remains unaffected, promoting tolerance.[13]

Patients treated with sirolimus are better able to control viremia with cytomegalovirus than patients treated with calcineurin inhibitors. Sirolimus is thought to promote the metabolic switch from glycolysis to fatty acid oxidation, thereby enhancing differentiation to CD8+ memory T cells.[14]

In addition, the clonal expansion of B cells is inhibited by preventing the signal from the IL-4 cytokine receptor from activating the B-cell proliferation.[4(p660),13]

A principal toxic effect of sirolimus not related to immunosuppression is impaired wound healing.

The metabolism and elimination of sirolimus and everolimus is strongly influenced by variability in enterocyte P-glycoprotein and CYP3A4 activity. Comedication affecting these P-glycoprotein levels or CYP3A4 activity alters the pharmacokinetics of these drugs. The terminal half-life of sirolimus and everolimus are 62 ± 12 hours and 18 to 35 hours, respectively, with immunosuppression lasting up to 18 and 9 days after stopping treatment.[15,16]

Drugs that Destroy Dividing Cells (Azathioprine, Mycophenolate, Methotrexate, Cyclophosphamide)

Azathioprine, mycophenolic acid (MPA), methotrexate (MTX), and cyclophosphamide interfere with DNA synthesis and are cytotoxic to rapidly dividing cells, such as activated T or B cells.

Because this cytotoxic effect is not selective, continuously dividing tissues such as bone marrow, gut epithelium, and skin can be affected, limiting the dose that can be safely given.

The prodrug azathioprine (AZA) undergoes extensive metabolic transformations and is converted into metabolically active 6-thioguanine nucleotides (6-TGN) and 6-methyl-mercaptopurine ribonucleotides (6-MMRP).[17] 6-TGN is phosphorylated into 6-thioguanosine-5'-triphosphate (6-TGTP) and can be incorporated into DNA and RNA causing strand breakage and inhibition of DNA repair and replication processes. 6-MMRP inhibits purine synthesis. This cytotoxic effect leads to the inhibition of clonal expansion of activated T or B cells. In addition, 6-TGTP specifically binds to small guanosine triphosphatases instead of endogenous guanosine triphosphate, leading to apoptosis of activated T cells receiving costimulatory signals from dendritic cells via CD28. The immunosuppressive effect of AZA at clinically relevant doses (2.5 mg/kg) is predominantly by apoptosis. The incorporation of 6-TGN into DNA may induce mutagenic oxidative damage to DNA in the skin of patients treated with azathioprine when exposed to ultraviolet A from sunlight and increase the risk of squamous cell skin carcinoma.[18]

The biologic availability of AZA is variable, ranging from 16% to 72%.[17] The half-life of 6-TGN ranges from 3 to 13 days, meaning that the immunosuppressive effect can last up to 2 months following cessation of treatment.

MPA is a potent inhibitor of the type II isoform of inosine monophosphate dehydrogenase (IMPDH). This type II isoform of IMPDH is mostly found in activated T and B cells. MPA inhibits guanosine synthesis and ultimately DNA synthesis and proliferation of T and B cells. In addition, MPA induces apoptosis of activated T cells and B cells, and decreases immunoglobulin production by B cells.[19] MPA also decreases the recruitment of lymphocytes and monocytes into inflammatory tissues and the capacity in vitro of dendritic cells to efficiently present antigens to T cells. As a result, immuno-suppressive treatment regimens containing MPA severely disrupt both primary and secondary immune responses, implying that vaccination does not result in a protective antibody response.[20]

MPA was found to be highly active against yellow fever (median effective concentration [EC_{50}] 0.08 ± 0.05 µg/mL) and dengue virus in vitro.[19,21]

The mean elimination half-life of MPA ranges from 9 to 17 hours, with an immunosuppressive effect lasting for at least 5 days.[22]

MTX is a folate antagonist commonly used in low doses (0.3–0.6 mg/kg or 7–15 mg per week) in the treatment of rheumatoid arthritis and other chronic immune-mediated inflammatory diseases.[23,24]

In the cell, MTX is converted to polyglutamated forms that inhibit cell proliferation by inhibiting dihydrofolate reductase, resulting in the suppression of purine and thymidine synthesis. Polyglutamated MTX is also a competitive inhibitor of other folate-dependent enzymes leading to the cellular release of adenosine, which has a wide range of antiinflammatory effects.[23,25] In addition, polyglutamated MTX selectively induces apoptosis of activated naive as well as memory T cells and clonal deletion of activated naive T cells, possibly triggered by altered DNA strands produced in the absence of thymidine.[24] The immunosuppressive activity of MTX is more prolonged than the plasma half-life might suggest. Polyglutamated MTX metabolites accumulate in the tissues, explaining the prolonged inhibitory effects on the immune response. The half-life of the biologic activity of inducing apoptosis after removing the drug was around 3 days.[24] Because of the intracellular accumulation, the immunosuppressive activity may last up to 4 weeks after stopping MTX.

The absorption in the proximal jejunum and the renal tubular secretion and reabsorption of MTX are variable between patients.[23] Together with the accumulation of polyglutamated metabolites of MTX, it is therefore impossible to determine a lowest dose, below which live, attenuated vaccines, such as yellow fever vaccine, can be safely administered.

There have been no published reports of lethal complications following inadvertent administration of yellow fever vaccine during MTX treatment.[26] This may be partly explained by the observation that MTX can inhibit the replication of 17D yellow fever virus at therapeutic serum concentrations (EC_{50} 0.07 µg/mL).[21]

Antibodies that Deplete Lymphocytes or Interfere with Cell Function

In contrast with inhibitors of signal transduction and cytotoxic drugs, monoclonal antibodies have the potential to interfere with the immune response in a precise way, which has prompted an ongoing search for new humanized immunosuppressive monoclonal antibodies that trigger the removal of specific T or B cells (depleting antibodies) or block the function of their target antigen without killing the cells that carry it (nondepleting antibodies). In the last decade, more than 10 immunosuppressive monoclonal antibody products have been approved by the US Food and Drug Administration, and many more are in development.

Monoclonal antibodies are produced by immortalized cell clones derived from a fusion of a myeloma cell line with a single B cell, and are characterized by identical antibody structure and the affinity and specificity of the antigen-binding site.[27] Through several modifications, rodent monoclonal antibodies have been humanized to varying degrees to prevent rapid immune-mediated clearance: (1) chimeric antibodies that have a constant region derived from human immunoglobulin (Ig) G and a variable region derived from parental rodent IgG; (2) in complementarity-determining region (CDR)–grafted antibodies, only the CDR that contains the antigen-binding site within variable region is of rodent origin; and (3) antibodies that have been fully humanized. Fully humanized monoclonal IgG antibodies have the longest half-life, approaching that of human IgG (25 days). The half-life of nondepleting antibodies is important because it can predict the duration of the immunosuppressive effect.

Alemtuzumab and rituximab are examples of depleting monoclonal antibodies. The humanized monoclonal IgG1 antibody alemtuzumab is directed against CD52 expressed by most T and B lymphocytes. Alemtuzumab leads to a massive depletion of the lymphocyte population from which complete recovery can take several years, if ever, in older patients. In one study, B-cell numbers returned to normal between 3 and 6 months, whereas the number of T cells was only around 200×10^6 cells per liter after 9 months and remained subnormal for the duration of the study (36 months).[28] Alemtuzumab is used in the treatment of chronic lymphocytic leukemia and is being investigated in several immune-mediated inflammatory disorders such as multiple sclerosis.

The chimeric IgG$_1$ anti-CD20 monoclonal antibody rituximab eliminates more than 95% of CD20$^+$ B-cell precursors, from pre–B-cell stage to pre–plasma-cell stage, for a period of 6 to 9 months.[29] During this period, antibody responses to vaccines are severely hampered because many antibody-producing plasma cells are short-lived and require replacement from CD20$^+$ precursors, and because antigen-presenting B cells are lacking to activate CD4$^+$ helper T cells. Also, the number of memory B cells in the bone marrow of patients treated with rituximab is reduced.[30] B cells that return from the bone marrow to the peripheral blood after depletion have a predominantly immature (CD27$^-$IgD$^-$) or naive (CD27$^-$IgD$^+$) phenotype rather than memory B-cell (CD27$^+$) phenotype.[31,32] The delayed development of new memory cells seems to persist for several years after rituximab treatment.[33]

Timing of vaccination is therefore critical in patients treated with rituximab. Primary immunizations with new vaccines should preferably be given before treatment because long-lived plasma cells are not affected by rituximab. After treatment, it may take more than a year to mount an effective primary response. Secondary immune responses to revaccination with recall antigens need to be postponed for 6 months or longer after rituximab.[34,35] Primary immunizations with live, attenuated vaccines such as yellow fever vaccine need to be postponed for at least 12 months after the last dose of rituximab.

Antibodies that Modulate the Immune Response

Treatment with TNF antagonists has improved the lives of many patients with rheumatoid arthritis or other immune-mediated inflammatory diseases. TNF-α and TNF-β (or lymphotoxin [LT]-α) belong to a large family of 19 cytokines that regulate apoptosis and differentiation or proliferation of T and B cells.[36,37] TNF-α is a homotrimer and is synthesized by macrophages, natural killer (NK), T cells, and B cells in membrane-associated TNF (mTNF) and soluble TNF (sTNF) forms. LT-α is mainly produced in a membrane-bound form by NK, T cells, and B cells.[4(p383)] TNF plays a key role in the local containment of bacterial and mycobacterial infections in the human host.

There are 2 classes of TNF antagonists: soluble TNF receptors and TNF monoclonal antibodies. These classes differ in structure, function, and pharmacokinetics. The soluble TNF receptor, etanercept, consists of 2 extracellular domains of human TNF receptor-2 fused to the Fc fragment of human IgG1. Etanercept binds only 1 TNF molecule per molecule of etanercept, and has a lower affinity for mTNF than for sTNF. Etanercept readily dissociates from both mTNF and sTNF after binding and has a short half-life (4 days).[38] These characteristics may explain the reduced effect on the inhibition of T-cell activation and IFN-γ production as well as the lower risk of reactivation of latent tuberculosis in comparison with the TNF monoclonal antibodies.[39]

There are currently 4 approved TNF monoclonal antibodies: infliximab, adalimumab, golimumab, and certolizumab pegol. Infliximab is a chimeric monoclonal antibody composed of a murine antigen–binding variable region and a human IgG1 constant region. Adalimumab and golimumab are humanized monoclonal antibodies with both human variable and constant regions. Certolizumab pegol consists of human antigen-binding fragments bound to polyethylene glycol. The TNF monoclonal antibodies infliximab, adalimumab, and golimumab have longer half-lives (9.5 days, 14.7–19.3 days, and 11 days, respectively), and may simultaneously bind several TNF molecules, and bind mTNF at a higher level.[40]

During TNF antagonist treatment, the secondary immune response to inactivated vaccines and the antibody response to polysaccharide vaccines are effective, although titers may be lower in comparison with healthy controls.[41] Secondary immunization with yellow fever is unremarkable, probably because vaccinees are still protected by circulating antibodies from a previous vaccination.[42] Primary vaccination with yellow fever and other live, attenuated vaccines should be avoided at all costs. If yellow fever vaccination is required for future travel, it should be given 3 to 4 weeks before the start of therapy with TNF antagonists.

AGE-RELATED INVOLUTION OF THYMUS AND BONE MARROW RESULTS IN INCOMPLETE IMMUNE RECONSTITUTION

From the first year of life, there is a gradual decrease of the thymic epithelial space where naive CD4$^+$ helper, CD8$^+$ cytotoxic, and CD4$^+$CD25^{++} regulatory T cells are formed. At the age of 70 years, the thymic epithelial space has shrunk to 10% of the original thymic volume. It is estimated that, by the age of 105 years, the thymus will have ceased generating naive T cells.[43]

During this process of thymopoiesis (proliferation, maturation, and selection of T cells) a vast repertoire of different T-cell receptors are created through recombinant rearrangement of the T-cell receptor gene segments. The net result of the gradual age-related thymic involution is a decreasing output of naive T cells into the peripheral circulation and an increasing restriction of the peripheral T-cell receptor repertoire, limiting the range of antigens to CD4$^+$ and CD8$^+$ T cells that are available for mounting a response to a foreign antigen. Similar changes occur in the bone marrow, where the accumulation of fat results in a decreased production of naive B cells.[44] As a result, the peripheral lymphocyte pool at an older age is primarily shaped by previously encountered antigens, based on the extant memory cells. In time, these memory cells reach their replicative limit, leaving older individuals vulnerable even to infections that they have previously successfully dealt with in the past.

These changes may help to explain the reduced efficacy of the immune system in old age, with increased susceptibility to infectious diseases, and reduced response to vaccination.

For example, 4 weeks after the first dose (primary immunization) with hepatitis A vaccine (HAV), seroconversion rates (anti-HAV$\geq$20 IU/mL) and geometric mean titers of anti-HAV antibodies were lower after the age of 40 years.[45] Subjects aged more than 60 years had a seroconversion rate of 60% after the first dose.

Similar findings were reported for yellow fever vaccine in elderly travelers aged between 60 and 81 years.[46] Viremia was more common in the elderly (86%) and persisted longer than in younger volunteers (aged 18–28 years). Ten days after vaccination, seroprotection was attained by 50% of the elderly participants compared with 77% of the young. At day 14, all vaccinees were protected, but the geometric mean titer of neutralizing antibodies was lower in the elderly.

The impaired ability of the aged immune system to rapidly clear yellow fever vaccine virus may offer an explanation for the increased risk of yellow fever vaccine–associated visceral disease in the elderly.

These age-related changes may explain why immune reconstitution may be incomplete after high-dose chemotherapy, allogeneic hematopoietic cell transplantation, or T-cell or B-cell–depleting monoclonal antibody treatment, and during combined antiretroviral therapy for HIV.[47]

Allogeneic Hematopoietic Cell Transplantation

During the preconditioning of recipients of allogeneic hematopoietic cell transplants with cytotoxic drugs, depleting monoclonal antibodies, and total body irradiation, most of the host immune response are destroyed as both malignant and normal hematopoietic cells are destroyed. Rebuilding of the adaptive T-cell and B-cell immunity after transplantation takes months to years, and while this occurs, there is an increased susceptibility to certain bacterial, viral, and fungal infections, and a reduced responsiveness to vaccines.

After transplantation, an initial increase in T cells consequent to a homeostatic proliferation of transferred donor T cells and surviving host T cells occurs. The relative contribution of both T-cell sources depends on the dosage of donor T cells in the graft and intensity of preconditioning of the recipient. Although host-derived and donor-derived memory T cells contribute to the adaptive immunity early after transplantation, the immunoprotection is incomplete because the recipient's T-cell receptor repertoire is at most patchy, limited by the initial T cell source for expansion. After 3 to 6 months, the numbers of these cells progressively decreases from replicative exhaustion or activation-induced cell death.[47,48]

For a functionally complete immune reconstitution, it is essential that the peripheral T-cell compartment is replenished by naive T cells generated from the thymus.

The efficiency of generating naive T cells is compromised in older age, poor recovery from thymic injury following preconditioning therapy, and graft-versus-host disease (GVHD). In children and young adults (aged 2–19 years), normal numbers of naive T cell are produced within 1 year after transplantation; in older adults (aged 20–59 years), this occurs after 2 to 3 years.[48] Until then, they should be considered severely immunosuppressed. Full recovery from thymic injury caused by chemotherapy or total body irradiation may eventually occur in young persons. In GVHD, mature donor T cells cause thymic epithelial cell injury that reduces thymic output of naive T cells. In younger persons, thymopoiesis can recover within a year, but, in older patients, such recovery may not occur.[48]

In the first months to years after transplantation, antibodies are produced by surviving host plasma cells that have some resistance to the preconditioning treatment. Naive B cells start to appear 2 months after transplantation, and originate from donor cells.[49] The B-cell compartment does not become completely reconstituted until 1 to 2 years after transplantation, or longer when GVHD occurs.

Recipients of hematopoietic cell transplants are routinely revaccinated 6 months to 1 year after transplantation as antibodies to vaccine-preventable diseases gradually decline in the years following transplantation.[50] These patients should be considered as never vaccinated and receive a complete and full-dose series of childhood vaccines. Secondary T-cell responses to vaccines received (by the donor) before transplantation can be detected at 1 to 6 months after transplantation. Secondary B-cell responses (antibody production) to protein vaccines (eg, tetanus toxoid) received before transplantation can be found at 6 to 12 months after transplant. Primary T-cell and antibody responses to new vaccines, as well as B-cell responses to polysaccharide vaccines, only develop 1 or more years later after transplantation. As outlined earlier, the optimal timing may differ depending on age, preconditioning, and GVHD. For practical reasons, current guidelines recommend routine immunizations at 6 to 12 months after transplantation.[50]

There are limited data on when vaccination with inactivated travel-related vaccines can be expected to induce an immune response after hematopoietic cell transplantation. As discussed earlier, this response depends on time after transplantation, age, preconditioning, active GVHD, and current immunosuppressive therapy. The antibody response to vaccination should be tested 1 month or later after the last dose.

Although case reports have been published on uneventful yellow fever vaccination in 2 hematopoietic cell transplant recipients,[51,52] and yellow fever vaccination is considered optional in certain conditions,[50] extreme caution is advised, especially in the older adult in whom the recommended 2 years after transplantation may be insufficient for full immune reconstitution.

Immune Reconstitution Under Antiretroviral Therapy for HIV

Successful antiretroviral therapy (ART) of HIV effectively suppresses viral replication to less than the detection limits and is associated with a large decrease in AIDS-defining conditions.[53] Most of the initial increase in numbers of CD4$^+$ T cells (20–30 cells/μL per month) during the first 1 to 6 months of ART is a result of release of memory and effector T cells from lymph nodes and spleen where they were trapped in response to viral replication and immune activation.[54] CD4$^+$ numbers increase further over the next 2 years (5–10 cells/μL per month) as the production of homeostatic proliferation of mature CD4$^+$ cells, from naive CD4$^+$ T cells by the thymus and with an increased life span of both these cells. After 2 years, CD4$^+$ numbers increase more slowly (2–5 cells/μL per month) for the next 7 years. When the production of naive CD4$^+$ T cells is limited, the T-cell receptor repertoire remains truncated, even when the numbers of CD4$^+$ T cells have normalized.

Suboptimal to poor antibody responses to primary immunization with inactivated or polysaccharide vaccines are expected in patients with (persistent) low CD4$^+$ T cell numbers (less than 400 cells/μL), high plasma HIV RNA levels, active disease, or old age at time of vaccination, and a nadir CD4$^+$ T cell of less than 200 cell/μL before the start of ART.[55] In these circumstances, serologic testing 4 to 8 weeks after vaccinations is advisable. Because of lower antibody titers following vaccination, the duration of protection may be shorter in HIV-infected people. As an example, following hepatitis A vaccination, a retrospective study of HIV-infected adults with, respectively, 11% and 21% less than 1000 and greater than or equal to 1000 HIV RNA copies/mL did not have protective antibodies against hepatitis A ($\geq$10 mIU/mL) 6 to 10 years later.[56]

Primary vaccination with yellow fever vaccine has been shown to be immunogenic and safe in most HIV-infected patients in 2 retrospective cohort studies.[57,58] Suppressed HIV RNA levels (<50 copies/mL) and higher numbers of CD4$^+$ T cells were associated with a better immunologic response. Duration of protection was less than 10 years in 23% of the vaccinees in one of the studies.[57] Yellow fever vaccination should be delayed in patients who have a CD4$^+$ T cell count less than 350 cells/μL and who are not receiving ART. Yellow fever vaccination should be avoided in patients who have a CD4$^+$ T cell count less than 200 cells/μL.

A PRACTICAL APPROACH TO TRAVELERS WITH SEVERE IMMUNOSUPPRESSION
How Can this Information be Applied in Daily Travel Medicine Practice?

Step 1. Determine the effect of the underlying condition and/or its immunosuppressive treatment on the likely immune response of the traveler
The theoretic outline given earlier can be used to determine whether and how the immunosuppressive treatment affects critical steps in the cellular and humoral immune response to pathogens and vaccines. If possible, restore the gastric acid barrier. Many patients on immunosuppressive treatment receive proton pump inhibitors. Antacids double the risk of traveler's diarrhea.[59] Consult the treating physician if treatment with antacids can be stopped safely.

Step 2. Is yellow fever vaccination required because of risk of infection?
Many travelers who have received yellow fever vaccination in the past and who are now on immunosuppressive treatment still have protective antibodies levels, even if

vaccination was more than 10 years previously. Revaccination with yellow fever vaccine can almost always be avoided by determining whether the traveler still has protective neutralizing antibody levels from a previous vaccination. For the United States, information about serologic testing can be obtained through the state health department or the Centers for Disease Control and Prevention's Division of Vector-Borne Diseases on 970-221-6400.

Primary immunization with yellow fever vaccine and other live, attenuated vaccines should be avoided in severely immunosuppressed travelers. Some travelers are willing to temporarily stop their immunosuppressive treatment to be able to receive primary immunization with yellow fever vaccine. **Table 2** shows the minimal time until immune reconstitution. As indicated earlier, thymic injury (eg, irradiation) and old age may compromise full recovery.

Immunosuppressive therapy should be restarted, preferably 4 weeks after vaccination. The decision to stop immunosuppressive therapy should therefore not be taken lightly, because it may take 3 to 4 months before immunosuppression is resumed. In the meanwhile, exacerbation of the immune-mediated inflammatory disease may occur.

Step 3. Check antibodies titers

The immune response to primary immunization is likely to be poor in immunosuppressed travelers and additional doses may be required before protective antibody titers are reached. For this reason, it is advised to measure antibody titers 4 to 8 weeks after vaccination. Travelers born before 1950 or in a country highly endemic for hepatitis A should be checked for anti–hepatitis A antibodies because they may have acquired hepatitis A infection during childhood and, if so, do not require hepatitis A vaccination.

Revaccination with inactivated vaccines of a traveler on immunosuppressive therapy will result in protective antibodies in most cases, albeit at lower levels and for a shorter period of time. Revaccination may be required at shorter intervals. Therefore, it is useful to determine antibody titers before the next journey to decide whether revaccination is required.

Table 2
Minimal duration of immunosuppressive activity[a]

Drug	Duration
Prednisone	1 mo[b]
Cyclosporin	7 d
Tacrolimus	3 d
Sirolimus	18 d
Everolimus	9 d
Azathioprine	2 mo
Mycophenolic acid	5 d
Methotrexate	1 mo
Alemtuzumab	>1 y
Rituximab	1 y
Etanercept	1 mo
Infliximab, adalimumab, golimumab, certolizumab	3 mo

[a] Old age and thymic injury may prolong time until full immune reconstitution.
[b] Numbers of CD4+ and CD8+ T cells in blood should be determined to exclude lymphopenia caused by long-standing T-cell apoptosis.

Step 4. Give travel health information
In addition to general travel health information, special attention should be given to skin care (sun protection and treatment of infected insect bites), hand hygiene (alcoholic rubs), early antibiotic treatment of traveler's diarrhea, transportation of medicines, and travel health and evacuation insurance.[60,61]

SUMMARY

Clonal proliferation of T and B cells is a central event in mounting an effective immune response against pathogens and vaccines. Most immunosuppressive drugs reduce the number of effector T and/or B cells by blocking this clonal expansion. Aging and injury to the thymus lead to a decreased output of naive T cells to the peripheral circulation. These age-related changes explain why immune reconstitution after high-dose chemotherapy, allogeneic hematopoietic cell transplantation, or during combined antiretroviral therapy for HIV may remain incomplete. These considerations should be used to formulate a pragmatic and logical vaccination program for travelers with severe immunosuppression.

REFERENCES

1. Recommendations of the Advisory Committee on Immunization Practices (ACIP). General recommendations on immunization. MMWR 2011;60(RR02):1–64.
2. Halloran PF. Immunosuppressive drugs for kidney transplantation. N Engl J Med 2004;351:2715–29.
3. Ingelfinger JR, Schwartz RS. Immunosuppression — the promise of specificity. N Engl J Med 2005;353:836–8.
4. Murphy K, Travers P, Walport M. Janeway's immunobiology. 7th edition. New York: Garland Sciences; 2008. p. 346.
5. Rhen T, Cidlowski JA. Antiinflammatory action of glucocorticoids — new mechanisms for old drugs. N Engl J Med 2005;353:1711–23.
6. Perretti M, D'Acquisto F. Annexin A1 and glucocorticoids as effectors of the resolution of inflammation. Nat Rev Immunol 2009;9:62–70.
7. Glass CK, Saijo K. Nuclear receptor transrepression pathways that regulate inflammation in macrophages and T cells. Nat Rev Immunol 2010;10:365–76.
8. Serhan CN, Chiang N, Van Dyke TE. Resolving inflammation: dual anti-inflammatory and pro-resolution lipid mediators. Nat Rev Immunol 2008;8:349–61.
9. Edsbäcker S, Andersson T. Pharmacokinetics of budesonide (Entocort EC) capsules for Crohn's disease. Clin Pharmacokinet 2004;43:803–21.
10. Rutgeerts P, Löfberg R, Malchow H, et al. A comparison of budesonide with prednisolone for active Crohn's disease. N Engl J Med 1994;331:842–5.
11. Dunn CJ, Wagstaff AJ, Perry CM, et al. Cyclosporin: an updated review of the pharmacokinetic properties, clinical efficacy and tolerability of a microemulsion-based formulation (Neoral®)1 in organ transplantation. Drugs 2001;61: 1957–2016.
12. Hooks MA. Tacrolimus, a new immunosuppressant–a review of the literature. Ann Pharmacother 1994;28:501–11.
13. Thomson AW, Turnquist HR, Raimondi G. Immunoregulatory functions of mTOR inhibition. Nat Rev Immunol 2009;9:324–37.
14. Ferrer IR, Araki K, Ford ML. Paradoxical aspects of rapamycin immunobiology in transplantation. Am J Transplant 2011;11:654–9.
15. Mahalati K, Kahan BD. Clinical pharmacokinetics of sirolimus. Clin Pharmacokinet 2001;40:573–85.

16. Kirchner GI, Meier-Wiedenbach I, Manns MP. Clinical pharmacokinetics of everolimus. Clin Pharmacokinet 2004;43:83–95.

17. de Boer NK, van Bodegraven AA, Jharap B, et al. Drug insight: pharmacology and toxicity of thiopurine therapy in patients with IBD. Nat Clin Pract Gastroenterol Hepatol 2007;4:686–94.

18. Anstey A, Lear JT. Azathioprine; clinical pharmacology and current indications in autoimmune disorders. BioDrugs 1998;9:33–47.

19. Ritter ML, Pirofski L. Mycophenolate mofetil: effects on cellular immune subsets, infectious complications, and antimicrobial activity. Transpl Infect Dis 2009;11: 290–7.

20. Struijk GH, Minnee RC, Koch SD, et al. Maintenance immunosuppressive therapy with everolimus preserves humoral immune responses. Kidney Int 2010;78:934–40.

21. Neyts J, Meerbach A, McKenna P, et al. Use of the yellow fever virus vaccine strain 17D for the study of strategies for the treatment of yellow fever virus infections. Antiviral Res 1996;30:125–32.

22. Staatz CE, Tett SE. Clinical pharmacokinetics and pharmacodynamics of mycophenolate in solid organ transplant recipients. Clin Pharmacokinet 2007;46:13–58.

23. Grim J, Chládek J, Martínková J. Pharmacokinetics and pharmacodynamics of methotrexate in non-neoplastic diseases. Clin Pharmacokinet 2003;42:139–51.

24. Genestier L, Paillot R, Fournel S, et al. Immunosuppressive properties of methotrexate: apoptosis and clonal deletion of activated peripheral T cells. J Clin Invest 1998;102(2):322–8.

25. Chan ES, Cronstein BN. Methotrexate–how does it really work? Nat Rev Rheumatol 2010;6:175–8.

26. da Mota LM, Oliveira AC, Lima RA, et al. Vaccination against yellow fever among patients on immunosuppressors with diagnoses of rheumatic diseases. Rev Soc Bras Med Trop 2009;42:23–7.

27. Nelson AL, Dhimolea E, Reichert JM. Development trends for human monoclonal antibody therapeutics. Nat Rev Drug Discov 2010;9:767–74.

28. CAMMS223 Trial Investigators, Coles AJ, Compston DA, Selmaj KW, et al. Alemtuzumab vs. interferon beta-1a in early multiple sclerosis. N Engl J Med 2008;359: 1786–801.

29. Edwards JC, Cambridge G. B-cell targeting in rheumatoid arthritis and other autoimmune diseases. Nat Rev Immunol 2006;6:394–403.

30. Rehnberg M, Amu S, Tarkowski A, et al. Short- and long-term effects of anti-CD20 treatment on B cell ontogeny in bone marrow of patients with rheumatoid arthritis. Arthritis Res Ther 2009;11:R123.

31. Leandro MJ, Cambridge G, Ehrenstein MR, et al. Reconstitution of peripheral blood B cells after depletion with rituximab in patients with rheumatoid arthritis. Arthritis Rheum 2006;54:613–20.

32. St.Clair EW. Good and bad memories following rituximab therapy. Arthritis Rheum 2010;62:1–5.

33. Muhammad K, Roll P, Einsele H, et al. Delayed acquisition of somatic hypermutations in repopulated IGD+CD27+ memory B cell receptors after rituximab treatment. Arthritis Rheum 2009;60:2284–93.

34. van Assen S, Holvast A, Benne CA, et al. Humoral responses after influenza vaccination are severely reduced in patients with rheumatoid arthritis treated with rituximab. Arthritis Rheum 2010;62:75–81.

35. Pescovitz MD, Torgerson TR, Ochs HD, et al, Type 1 Diabetes TrialNet Study Group. Effect of rituximab on human in vivo antibody immune responses. J Allergy Clin Immunol 2011;128:1295–302.

36. Aggarwal BB. Signalling pathways of the TNF superfamily: a double-edged sword. Nat Rev Immunol 2003;3:745–56.
37. Croft M. The role of TNF superfamily members in T-cell function and diseases. Nat Rev Immunol 2009;9:271–85.
38. Lobo ED, Hansen RJ, Balthasar JP. Antibody pharmacokinetics and pharmaco-dynamics. J Pharm Sci 2004;93:2645–68.
39. Wallis RS. Tumour necrosis factor antagonists: structure, function, and tubercu-losis risks. Lancet Infect Dis 2008;8:601–11.
40. Rigby WF. Drug insight: different mechanisms of action of tumour necrosis factor antagonists - passive-aggressive behaviour? Nat Clin Pract Rheumatol 2007;3: 227–33.
41. Visser LG. TNF-α antagonists and immunization. Curr Infect Dis Rep 2011;13: 243–7.
42. Scheinberg M, Guedes-Barbosa LS, Mangueira C, et al. Yellow fever revaccina-tion during infliximab therapy. Arthritis Care Res 2010;62:896–8.
43. Lynch HE, Goldberg GL, Chidgey A, et al. Thymic involution and immune recon-stitution. Trends Immunol 2009;30:366–73.
44. Siegrist CA, Aspinall R. B-cell responses to vaccination at the extremes of age. Nat Rev Immunol 2009;9:185–94.
45. Genton B, D'Acremont V, Furrer HJ, et al. Hepatitis A vaccines and the elderly. Travel Med Infect Dis 2006;4:303–12.
46. Roukens AH, Soonawala D, Joosten SA, et al. Elderly subjects have a delayed antibody response and prolonged viraemia following yellow fever vaccination: a prospective controlled cohort study. PLoS One 2011;6(12):e27753.
47. Williams KM, Hakim FT, Gress RE. T cell immune reconstitution following lympho-depletion. Semin Immunol 2007;19:318–30.
48. Krenger W, Blazar BR, Holländer GA. Thymic T-cell development in allogeneic stem cell transplantation. Blood 2011;117:6768–76.
49. Bosch M, Khan FM, Storek J. Immune reconstitution after hematopoietic cell transplantation. Curr Opin Hematol 2012;19:324–35.
50. Ljungman P, Cordonnier C, Einsele H, et al, Center for International Blood and Marrow Transplant Research, National Marrow Donor Program, European Blood and Marrow Transplant Group, American Society of Blood and Marrow Transplan-tation, Canadian Blood and Marrow Transplant Group, Infectious Disease Society of America, Society for Healthcare Epidemiology of America, Association of Medical Microbiology and Infectious Diseases Canada, Centers for Disease Control and Prevention. Vaccination of hematopoietic cell transplant recipients. Bone Marrow Transplant 2009;44:521–6.
51. Gowda R, Cartwright K, Bremner JA, et al. Yellow fever vaccine: a successful vacci-nation of an immunocompromised patient. Eur J Haematol 2004;72:299–301.
52. Yax JA, Farnon EC, Cary Engleberg N. Successful immunization of an allogeneic bone marrow transplant recipient with live, attenuated yellow Fever vaccine. J Travel Med 2009;16:365–7.
53. Thompson MA, Aberg JA, Cahn P, et al, International AIDS Society-USA. Antire-troviral treatment of adult HIV infection: 2010 recommendations of the Interna-tional AIDS Society-USA panel. JAMA 2010;304:321–33.
54. Corbeau P, Reynes J. Immune reconstitution under antiretroviral therapy: the new challenge in HIV-1 infection. Blood 2011;117:5582–90.
55. Geretti AM, Brook G, Cameron C, et al, BHIVA Immunization Writing Committee. British HIV Association guidelines for immunization of HIV-infected adults 2008. HIV Med 2008;9:795–848.

56. Crum-Cianflone NF, Wilkins K, Lee AW, et al, Infectious Disease Clinical Research Program HIV Working Group. Long-term durability of immune responses after hepatitis A vaccination among HIV-infected adults. J Infect Dis 2011;203: 1815–23.

57. Veit O, Niedrig M, Chapuis-Taillard C, et al, Swiss HIV Cohort Study. Immunogenicity and safety of yellow fever vaccination for 102 HIV-infected patients. Clin Infect Dis 2009;48:659–66.

58. Pacanowski J, Lacombe K, Campa P, et al. Plasma HIV-RNA is the key determinant of long-term antibody persistence after yellow fever immunization in a cohort of 364 HIV-infected patients. J Acquir Immune Defic Syndr 2012;59:360–7.

59. Soonawala D, Vlot JA, Visser LG. Inconvenience due to travelers' diarrhea: a prospective follow-up study. BMC Infect Dis 2011;11:322.

60. Jong EC, Freedman DO. Chapter 8. Immunocompromised travelers. In: Brunette GW, editor. The yellow book. CDC health information for international travel 2012. Oxford University Press; 2012.

61. Kotton CN, Ryan ET, Fishman JA. Prevention of infection in adult travelers after solid organ transplantation. Am J Transplant 2005;5(1):8–14.

Visiting Relatives and Friends (VFR), Pregnant, and Other Vulnerable Travelers

Alberto Matteelli, MD*, Anna Cristina C. Carvalho, MD, PhD,
Sara Bigoni, MD

KEYWORDS

- Traveler • VFR • Pregnancy • Pediatric • Elderly • Vulnerable

KEY POINTS

- Visiting relatives and friends travelers have a disproportionate burden of travel-related morbidity and are less prone to adopt preventive measures.
- The travel associated risks for the pregnant traveler vary across the trimester of pregnancy and depend on the preexisting medical conditions and obstetric problems.
- Very young children and the older traveler have a weaker immune system, which increases the risk of infectious diseases and severe forms of malaria during travel: the need for appropriate pre-travel immunization and chemoprophylaxis is increased.
- In general, live vaccines should be avoided during pregnancy.
- Food and water precautions during travel are particularly recommended to vulnerable travelers like children, pregnant women and elderly.

INTRODUCTION

With industrial development and expanding tourism, many people now have an opportunity to travel to many previously unreachable foreign destinations. Travelers with medical or physical conditions or who are vulnerable because of pregnancy or age (pediatric or elderly traveler), require specialist support and advice before traveling. Qualified travel agencies and accredited travel medicine clinics should provide the necessary information to help travelers with disabilities or health problems plan their trip. Web-based advice providing information on travel health may provide inappropriate or irrelevant advice. Internet sources should be consulted where the body is internationally recognized or if a health professional recommends it.

The authors have nothing to disclose.
Institute of Infectious and Tropical Diseases, Spedali Civili Hospital, University of Brescia, 1 Piazzale Spedali Civili, Brescia 25100, Italy
* Corresponding author.
E-mail address: matteelli@med.unibs.it

Infect Dis Clin N Am 26 (2012) 625–635
http://dx.doi.org/10.1016/j.idc.2012.07.003

id.theclinics.com

Immigrants who return to their country of birth to visit relatives and friends should be classified as vulnerable travelers, as they have been shown to carry a disproportionate burden of travel-related morbidity.

In this article, we explore the major risks to health and the main preventive strategies appropriate to the most vulnerable travelers.

VISITING RELATIVES AND FRIENDS TRAVELERS
Definition

The definition of VFR, as a group of travelers commonly referred to as "visiting friends and relatives," is continuously changing, as the trend and character of travel changes.

The "classic" VFR is defined as a traveler who is of a different ethnicity in relation to the host country population but similar to that of the destination population, and whose intended purpose of travel is to visit friends or relatives, where there is a risk for tropical infectious diseases (eg, malaria).

However, following extensive immigration and increasing global mobility, second-generation or third-generation immigrants challenge this definition. Several scenarios highlight the problems of VFR definition in the current era. In the literature, authors have used different terms for VFRs, for example, the foreign-born traveler ("immigrant" VFR) from the child or non–foreign-born spouse of an immigrant traveler ("traveler VFR"), although they may well travel to the same destination visiting friends or relatives. Recently, a new definition of VFR was proposed based on 2 fundamental criteria, with the exclusion of race, ethnicity, or administrative/legal status (eg, immigrant) and where a gradient of risk (both infectious and noninfectious) exists between where he or she currently lives and where he or she travels to visit. This definition underlines the importance of hazards that are not infectious diseases (eg, road accidents, injuries, crime, pollution etc) together with classical infectious hazards (eg, malaria, waterborne infections).[1,2]

A debate on the definition of VFR continues, confirming the importance of this group of travelers in the discipline of travel medicine.[3]

Travel-Associated Risk

There are several health determinants that are attributed to the higher risk of both travel-related infectious and noninfectious diseases among VFR. These are best categorized under broad groupings, including the socioeconomic status of travelers (eg, level of schooling, legal status, financial barriers to pretravel health care), preexisting health conditions (eg, immunodeficiency, age), behaviors (eg, for sexually transmitted diseases, last-minute travel plans, and longer trips), and the environment (eg, pollution or the possibility of having access to safe food, clean water, and sanitary conditions at the destination).[1,2]

Malaria

In 2010, 71% of malaria cases imported into the United States among civilians was among VFRs, who also constituted 53% of all severe malaria cases.[4] Similar data came from Europe: data from GeoSentinel[5] show that VFRs who traveled to sub-Saharan Africa had more than 8 times the odds of receiving a diagnosis of malaria than other tourist travelers. In the same study, *falciparum* malaria accounted for 86.8% of illness in the immigrant VFR group, 63.3% in the traveler VFR group, and 44.0% in the tourist traveler group.

Increased incidence of malaria may relate to both travelers and their journey. VFRs may travel to and stay in remote rural areas for long periods and have closer contact with local populations because they are familiar with the destination through historical links and have a lower perception of risk of malaria. VFRs seek pretravel advice less frequently than other groups of travelers, and are less compliant with antimosquito measures and malaria chemoprophylaxis. Many VFRs presume they are immune against malaria; however, in most VFRs, especially those who emigrated to endemic countries a decade or more previously, immunity will have waned and is no longer protective. The lack of perceived malaria risk is the predominant reason for low uptake of chemoprophylaxis. On average, 10% to 31% of VFR travelers from Canada used chemoprophylaxis, and the high cost was one important contributing factor to the low uptake.[6]

This evidence suggests a need for social and culturally targeted messages through the media to enhance access to medical travel advice and, where possible, reimburse chemoprophylaxis medication to reduce the economic disincentive in using the drugs against malaria. These should be done in collaboration with health workers in travel medicine, anthropologists, health education professionals, and health authorities.[3]

Hepatitis A

In 2009, a Swedish study[7] described that 52% of the travel-associated cases of hepatitis A occurred in VFR travelers from East Africa; most occurring in children (age <14 years). A Dutch Schiphol Airport Survey[8,9] conducted between 2002 and 2009 assessing knowledge, attitudes, and practices of travelers regarding hepatitis A, concluded that VFRs sought travel health advice less frequently than non-VFR travelers. VFRs also traveled more frequently to high-risk and intermediate-risk destinations, and VFRs who traveled to both high-risk and low-risk to intermediate-risk destinations had lower levels of disease awareness and knowledge and planned to undertake more risk activities than non-VFR travelers.

Adult VFR travelers born in developed countries, and all child VFR travelers without a history of hepatitis A or vaccination, should be considered for vaccination.[8]

Tuberculosis

Travel to an area where tuberculosis is endemic constitutes a risk for acquiring tuberculosis infection.[10] The risk is determined by exposure to an infective case, the duration of the exposure, and individual factors (immunosuppression, immunity), and so is linked to travel characteristics (destination, duration of travel, crowded conditions, living principally indoors or outdoors, and so forth). VRF travelers will be at similar exposure to risk as other tourists whose travel itinerary is similar.

Preventive Strategies: Pretravel Health Counseling for VFRs

Pretravel counseling of VFRs may present several barriers, depending on the travelers themselves (eg, absence of awareness of travel-related health risks) and on the travel health services (eg, expensive, far away, not easily accessible). Where possible, clinics should incorporate culturally sensitive educational materials, provide translators, and provide handouts in relevant languages to the population they serve.

Travel immunization recommendations and requirements for VFRs are the same as other tourists. However, since VFRs often travel to visit tropical rural areas, private homes, and overcrowded settings, they have as a consequence an increased risk for infectious diseases and are more likely to require the majority of the available vaccines.[10,11]

Assessment of routine vaccinations (measles, tetanus, and so forth), particularly for children, is important. Polio vaccination should always be boosted in combination with tetanus and diphtheria, in all adult travelers, regardless of travel destination and duration. For hepatitis A, immunity should not be assumed. Adult VFR travelers, especially if young, may be nonimmune if they do not have a history of immunization. Yellow fever vaccination has to be verified in VFR travelers and administered as recommended by World Health Organization (WHO) guidance.

VFR travelers to endemic areas should be made aware of malaria risk, especially the threat to children. Preventive measures, prophylactic medications, and barrier methods (eg, bed nets) should be recommended, as they apply to all tourists. Travelers should buy antimalarial drugs before departure, as counterfeit drugs are widely sold in many developing countries. Chemoprophylaxis drugs should be sufficient to cover the whole period of travel and adjustments of total prescribed tablets for a prolongation of the visit may be required and should be discussed.[13]

Health advisors need to educate the travelers on personal hygiene behavior: frequent handwashing, as well as avoiding high-risk foods, including dairy products, undercooked foods, fresh meat, and fish and untreated water. Particular advice to young children and parents on the avoidance of petting local dogs should be strongly made, as the prevalence of rabies is significant in many countries.[12]

The Pediatric VFR

Children of immigrants who settled in the European Union or the United States commonly accompany their parents back to their native countries.[14–16] They constitute a population at great risk because they lack immunity to many infectious agents and will be in close contact and proximity with the local population and exposed to a more hazardous environment.

THE PREGNANT TRAVELER

The 21st century is being characterized by an increasing global mobility involving many groups of the population, including pregnant women. When a pregnant woman decides to travel, there are many aspects of risk and health she should consider. Most importantly, she should seek pretravel advice well before (4–6 weeks) departure and ideally before purchasing her tickets, allowing her to change travel plans without financial consequences.

General Risks

There are no formal evidence-based recommendations on actual threats and contraindications to travel during pregnancy. Some important risk factors that may be considered as relative contraindications to traveling, which may differ across the stage of pregnancy, are preexisting medical conditions (eg, diabetes, heart disease) or obstetric problems (eg, history of ectopic pregnancy, history of miscarriage, multiple gestations in present pregnancy, incompetent cervix).[12,17] The American Academy of Obstetrics and Gynecology[18] suggests the safest period for traveling is in the second trimester of pregnancy, where the risks of an adverse events are similar to or smaller than those described for the third trimester.

Airlines and some travel companies place restrictions on travel during pregnancy and these need to be confirmed before a reservation. Most airlines allow a pregnant women to fly up to the 36th week of gestation, but documentation should be carried to support the stage of pregnancy. Air travel during pregnancy, however, has other associated risks. Normal complications of pregnancy, including spontaneous fetal loss (spontaneous abortion or intrauterine fetal demise), are increased,[19] as is a risk of venous thromboembolism, especially during flights longer than 8 hours.[20,21]

There are a number of precautions that pregnant travelers should take in avoiding infectious and communicable diseases. The most frequent disease acquired during travel is traveler's diarrhea. Dehydration and electrolyte imbalance are dangerous for the mother and for the fetus and thereby liberal rehydration with an electrolyte solution should be advised.[22] Azithromycin would be the most appropriate antibiotic therapy should this be needed, but this decision should be made by a health professional. Hepatitis E infection has a more severe clinical course during pregnancy and has been associated with fulminant hepatic failure and death in a proportion of pregnant women. There is currently no vaccine available for hepatitis E.[23]

Malaria with *Plasmodium falciparum* during pregnancy carries substantial morbidity to mother and baby. Pregnant women are more likely (by a factor of 3) to develop severe malaria, with complications including hypoglycemia, miscarriage, stillbirth, and premature labor.[24–26] Women travelers should be advised against visiting malarious areas when pregnant. Chemoprophylaxis should always be used if pregnant women travel, but none of the current regimens have a licensed indication for use during pregnancy.[27] Chloroquine is considered safe during pregnancy, although its use is limited to chloroquine-sensitive areas.[27] Mefloquine is considered safe after the 16th week of pregnancy, but the Centers for Disease Control and Prevention and WHO suggest it can be used also during the first trimester if the pregnant woman is going to travel in a high-risk area. Doxycycline is in some countries contraindicated during pregnancy. There is some evidence from Sweden that it is safe for use in the early stages of pregnancy, as its effects on the development of the epiphyseal plates and staining of teeth occur in the later stages of pregnancy. The safety of atovaquone-proguanil combination during pregnancy is unknown, but its component drugs have been used through pregnancy without any toxicity or teratogenicity.[27,28]

Immunization in Pregnancy

A number of infections that occur during travel can be prevented by the administration of safe and effective vaccines.[29] However, none of the widely used travel vaccines are licensed for use during pregnancy and their use should be based on a risk-and-benefit assessment. Hepatitis A and B, influenza, tetanus-diphtheria, polio, and typhoid vaccines are generally considered safe during pregnancy and are recommended. Japanese encephalitis, meningococcal meningitis, pneumococcal, and yellow fever vaccines should be used when benefits outweigh the risks. The risk is that of an effect on the fetus or pregnancy that is unknown. Yellow fever vaccination is only recommended after the sixth month of pregnancy and in case of imminent epidemic or if the pregnant woman is travelling to areas of high risk of infection.[30,31] There is evidence of passage of live virus through breast milk for breastfeeding infants, so it should not be administered to such travelers. The live attenuated Japanese encephalitis vaccine should be avoided in pregnancy unless the likely risk is considered substantial.[12,17,32,33]

PEDIATRIC TRAVELERS
Introduction

Traveling can be an exciting experience for children, full of fun and discoveries. International pediatric travelers are estimated to be 1.9 million each year.[34] The very young traveler (younger than 1 year) may be prone to acquire infectious diseases because of his immature immune system. Unsupervised play around pools and on the beach can lead to a child drowning, which is one of the most frequent causes of death in young travelers.

Weighing the risks and benefits of traveling with children is essential before departure. Children with underlying chronic diseases should be properly evaluated to determine the risks associated with traveling abroad and what measures are required for a safe journey. A medical kit with appropriate content should be prepared. Travel health insurance is especially important for pediatric travelers and all existing illnesses should be declared so they are covered by the policy.

Chemoprophylaxis for malaria is recommended for all ages from infants onward. Children visiting friends and relatives in sub-Saharan countries have the highest risk of acquiring malaria.[35] Complications with severe malaria are frequent in children. Initial symptoms of malaria are often difficult to differentiate from other febrile diseases of childhood. Chemoprophylaxis for children is adjusted by their body weight. An important factor in selecting a regimen is the ease of administration in infants and young children. No current drug regimens are formulated as a syrup or dispersible powder; they are all tablets. Mefloquine is a practical regimen, as it is administered weekly and the crushed tablet can be hidden in syrup or solid food. Atovaquone-proguanil is made as a pediatric dose, but is a sugar-coated tablet that needs to be taken daily, which in very young infants can lead to difficulties in administration. Doxycycline should not be given to children younger than 8 years.[36] Personal protective measures based on insect repellents should be combined with chemoprophylaxis. DEET is the most effective repellent and is considered safe when used in concentrations of 30% or less on exposed skin (avoid mucosal contact) in children older than 2 months.[34,37–39]

Food and water hygiene should be maintained during travel to reduce enteric infections, which are an important cause of traveler's diarrhea. Children should receive disinfected water, which should be either sterilized by using a filtration system or halogen treatment, or sealed bottled water. When a child develops diarrhea, adequate treatment with oral rehydration solutions should be provided. For young infants, at least 100 mL should be given for each loose stool and a regular volume given throughout the day to ensure a good urine output. Antimotility drugs, in particular diphenoxylate, are not recommended for children with diarrhea. Data on empiric use of antibiotics are lacking but when used in cases of moderate to severe diarrhea, azithromycin is the antibiotic most appropriate for use in children (once a day for 3 days), as fluoroquinolones are not recommended because of the potential risk of cartilage damage.[34]

Mode of Transport

The choice of the mode of transport is another aspect to consider when traveling with children. A healthy baby can travel by air 48 hours after birth, but should ideally wait until at least 1 week of life. The partial pressure of oxygen at cruising altitude is the equivalent of breathing 15% oxygen at sea level. Oxygen desaturation may be clinically relevant in children with respiratory insufficiency or cardiovascular diseases or who are premature; in such cases, a medical evaluation is recommended before traveling.[19,40] A frequent problem associated with air travel is earache, related to changes in cabin air pressure during takeoff and landing, which often leads to crying. Feeding the infant or letting the infant suck on a pacifier to stimulate swallowing may reduce the eardrum pressure.

Car accidents are the main cause of death among travelers, and a leading cause of traumatic injuries in children. Infants and young children should always be placed in a car seat. Parents should be advised to bring along a car seat, as they are often not provided in many developing countries. All car passengers should wear seat belts when traveling.[34,41,42]

THE OLDER TRAVELER

In recent years, an increasing number of older individuals are traveling, and with an aging population this trend will increase. WHO estimates that the world's population aged 60 and older will double from about 11% to 22% between 2000 and 2050; by 2050 there will be 2 billion in this age group.[43,44] Longer life expectancy allows opportunity for the retired population to spend more time traveling and taking more adventuresome journeys.

General Recommendations

In general, older travelers (>65 years of age) should always seek a pretravel consultation and a risk assessment for their planned journey and itinerary. The older traveler may have a number of preexisting morbidities, including cardiovascular disorders, diabetes mellitus, chronic respiratory diseases, and renal insufficiency, and frequently are using several medications in managing their medical condition. Travelers who require regular monitoring of their medication, such as anticoagulation or blood glucose, need to be fully prepared for this process to be undertaken during their journey or be trained to test themselves with glucose-monitoring equipment. Web sites of medical associations for diverse chronic diseases are available and can offer additional information regarding traveling with specific health conditions.[45]

Travel insurance is critical for all travelers, but is particularly important for older travelers with chronic health conditions. In developing countries, the public medical infrastructure may be limited and inadequate and the private health care expensive. Many older travelers have high premiums on their travel insurance and have their existing morbidities excluded for their travel policy. They should be strongly advised to have their existing medical problems insured and be prepared to pay for private hospital insurance cover, as statistically, their health problems are more likely to be related to their existing medical problem than a newly acquired health problem.

Cruises are particularly popular among older travelers and senior citizens. Passengers older than 65 years have the most emergency visits to health clinics on cruise ships, of which respiratory tract infection, injuries, motion sickness, and gastrointestinal illness are the most frequent diagnoses.[46] The leading cause of death among older travelers is cardiovascular events and other preexisting medical complications.[47]

Specific preventive measures

The recommendations for vaccination in the elderly traveler in general follow that for younger travelers. Older travelers have reduced quality of cell-mediated immunity.[48–52] This increases their susceptibility to some infectious diseases. As the routine immunization of children was established in the late 1940s, travelers born before that may not have received routine childhood vaccination, such as diphtheria, tetanus, and poliomyelitis. They should receive a full primary course. Influenza vaccination and pneumococcal polysaccharide vaccine should be routinely provided to anyone older than 65.[53]

In older individuals, the seroconversion following vaccination is lower. Serious adverse events and death in vaccinees aged 65 years or older[54–56] after yellow fever vaccination are well established. Older travelers and their physicians need to decide on the risks and benefits of yellow fever vaccination when traveling with a low risk of exposure.

Elderly travelers face a more serious and life-threatening risk of malaria if they are infected. Mühlberger and colleagues,[57] described that patients older than 60 with falciparum malaria had a risk of death and cerebral complication increased, respectively, by a factor of 5.74 and 3.29 times higher than younger patients. Antimalarial prophylaxis agents are well tolerated by the elderly. Atovaquone-proguanil is considered safe for elderly patients, although clinical studies involving this age group are still limited. Drug interaction between proguanil and warfarin can increase the anticoagulant effect of warfarin; however, adverse events related to this potential interaction have not been described.[36]

Post-Travel Consultation

If returned travelers are symptomatic, they should attend for a post-travel review and investigation.[58-60]

In a recent prospective study involving 89,521 ill travelers recorded in the Geosentinel Surveillance Network database, international travelers older than 60 years were more likely to be male, to be resident in North America and Canada, and to travel for tourism. Acute diarrhea, respiratory disease, and dermatologic complaints were the syndromes most frequently reported among elderly travelers. The proportionate morbidity of age-associated conditions was significantly higher among older travelers: there was a linear positive relationship between age and the proportion of death, heart disease, and lower respiratory tract infections.[61,62]

REFERENCES

1. Barnett ED, MacPherson DW, Stauffer WM, et al. The visiting friends or relatives traveler in the 21st century: time for a new definition. J Travel Med 2010;17: 163–70.
2. Behrens RH, Stauffer WM, Barnett ED, et al. Travel case scenarios as a demonstration of risk assessment of VFR travelers: introduction to criteria and evidence-based definition and framework. J Travel Med 2010;7(3):153–62.
3. Angell SY, Cetron MS. Health disparities among travelers visiting friends and relatives abroad. Ann Intern Med 2005;142(1):67–73.
4. Mali S, Kachur SP, Arguin PM, Division of Parasitic Diseases and Malaria, Center for Global Health; Centers for Disease Control and Prevention (CDC). Malaria surveillance—United States, 2010. MMWR Surveill Summ 2012;61(2):1–17.
5. Leder K, Tong S, Weld L, et al, Geosentinel Surveillance Network. Illness in travelers visiting friends and relatives: a review of the GeoSentinel Surveillance Network. Clin Infect Dis 2006;43:1185–93.
6. Dos Santos CC, Anvar A, Keystone JS, et al. Survey of use of malaria prevention measures by Canadians visiting India. Can Med Assoc J 1999;160:195–200.
7. Askling HH, Rombo L, Andersson Y, et al. Hepatitis A risk in travelers. J Travel Med 2009;16(4):233–8.
8. Angell SY, Behrens RH. Risk assessment and disease prevention in travelers visiting friends and relatives. Infect Dis Clin North Am 2005;19(1):49–65.
9. Evan Genderen PJ, van Thiel PP, Mulder PG, et al, Dutch Schiphol Airport Study Group. Trends in knowledge, attitudes, and practices of travel risk groups toward prevention of hepatitis A: results from the Dutch Schiphol airport survey 2002 to 2009. J Travel Med 2012;19(1):35–43.
10. Rieder HL. Risk of travel-associated tuberculosis. Clin Infect Dis 2001;33(8): 1393–6.
11. Gautret P, Wilder-Smith A. Vaccination against tetanus, diphtheria, pertussis and poliomyelitis in adult travelers. Travel Med Infect Dis 2010;8(3):155–60.
12. Keystone JS. CDC Health Information for International Travel. Yellow Book. Chapter 8. Advising Travelers with Specific Needs—Immigrants Returning Home to Visit Friends & Relatives (VFRs). New York: Oxford University Press; 2012. Available at: http://wwwnc.cdc.gov/travel/yellowbook/2012/chapter-8-advising-travelers-with-specific-needs/immigrants-returning-home-to-visit-friends-and-relatives-vfrs.htm. Accessed June 25, 2012.

13. Pavli A, Maltezou HC. Malaria and travelers visiting friends and relatives. Travel Med Infect Dis 2010;8(3):161–8.
14. Valerio L, Roure S, Sabrià M, et al. Epidemiologic and biogeographic analysis of 542 VFR traveling children in Catalonia (Spain). A rising new population with specific needs. J Travel Med 2011;18:304–9.
15. Arnáez J, Roa MA, Albert L, et al. Imported malaria in children: a comparative study between recent immigrants and immigrant travelers (VFRs). J Travel Med 2010;17(4):221–7.
16. Hagmann S, Benavides V, Neugebauer R, et al. Travel health care for immigrant children visiting friends and relatives abroad: retrospective analysis of a hospital-based travel health service in a US urban underserved area. J Travel Med 2009; 16(6):407–12.
17. World Health Organization. International Travel and Health 2012. Travelers with pre-existing medical conditions and special needs. Available at: http://www. who.int/ith/precautions/medical_conditions/en/. Accessed June 25, 2012.
18. American College of Obstetricians and Gynecologists. Air travel during pregnancy. ACOG committee opinion No. 443. Obstet Gynecol 2009;114:954–5.
19. Withers A, Wilson AC, Hall GL. Air travel and the risks of hypoxia in children. Paediatr Respir Rev 2011;12:271–6.
20. Hezelgrave NL, Whitty CJ, Shennan AH, et al. Advising on travel during pregnancy. BMJ 2011;342:d2605.
21. Geerts WH, Bergqvist D, Pineo GF, et al. Prevention of venous thromboembolism: American College of Chest Physicians Evidence-Based Clinical Practice Guidelines. Chest 2008;133:381S–453S.
22. Agnew CL, Ross MG, Fujino Y, et al. Maternal/fetal dehydration: prolonged effects and responses to oral rehydration. Am J Physiol 1993;264:197–203.
23. Navaneethan U, Al Mohajer M, Shata MT. Hepatitis E and pregnancy: understanding the pathogenesis. Liver Int 2008;28(9):1190–9.
24. McGready R, Ashley EA, Nosten F. Malaria and the pregnant traveler. Travel Med Infect Dis 2004;2:127–42.
25. Royal College of Obstetricians and Gynaecologists. The diagnosis and treatment of malaria in pregnancy. Greentop Guideline No 54B. 2010. Available at: http://www. rcog.org.uk/files/rcog-corp/GTG54bDiagnosisTreatmentMalariaPregnancy0810.pdf. Accessed July 25, 2012.
26. Desai M, Kuile FO, Nosten F, et al. Epidemiology and burden of malaria in pregnancy. Lancet Infect Dis 2007;7(2):93–104.
27. Schlagenhauf P, Petersen E. Malaria chemoprophylaxis: strategies for risk groups. Clin Microbiol Rev 2008;21(3):466–72.
28. Lalloo DG, Hill DR. Preventing malaria in travelers. BMJ 2008;336(7657): 1362–6.
29. Boggild AK, Castelli F, Gautret P, et al, Geosentinel Surveillance Network. Vaccine preventable diseases in returned international travelers: results from the GeoSentinel Surveillance Network. Vaccine 2010;28(46):7389–95.
30. Staples JE, Gershman M, Fischer M, Centers for Disease Control and Prevention (CDC). Yellow fever vaccine: recommendations of the Advisory Committee on Immunization Practices (ACIP). MMWR Recomm Rep 2010;59(RR-7):1–27.
31. Canadian Immunization Guide. 7th edition. 2006. Available at: http://www.phac-aspc.gc.ca/im/is-cv/index-eng.php. Accessed July 25, 2012.
32. Rose SR. Pregnancy and travel. Emerg Med Clin North Am 1997;15(1):93–111.
33. Suh KN, Mileno MD. Challenging scenarios in a travel clinic: advising the complex traveler. Infect Dis Clin North Am 2005;19:15–47.

34. Weinberg N, Weinberg M, Maloney S. CDC health information for international travel. Yellow book. Chapter 7: international travel with infants and children. New York: Oxford University Press; 2012. Available at: http://wwwnc.cdc.gov/travel/yellowbook/2012/chapter-7-international-travel-infants-children/traveling-safely-with-infants-and-children.htm. Accessed June 25, 2012.

35. Schlagenhauf P, Adamcova M, Regep L, et al. Use of mefloquine in children—a review of dosage, pharmacokinetics and tolerability data. Malar J 2011;10:292.

36. Arguin PM, Mali S. Malaria. In: CDC health information for international travel. Yellow book. Chapter 3 – Infectious diseases related to travel. New York: Oxford University Press; 2012. Available at: http://wwwnc.cdc.gov/travel/yellowbook/2012/chapter-3-infectious-diseases-related-to-travel/malaria.htm#1939. Accessed June 25, 2012.

37. Maloney SA, Weinberg M. Prevention of infectious diseases among international pediatric travelers: considerations for clinicians. Semin Pediatr Infect Dis 2004;15:137–49.

38. Shlim DR. Self-diagnosis and treatment of travelers' diarrhea. In: Keystone JS, Kozarsky PE, Freedman DO, et al, editors. Travel medicine. 1st edition. Philadelphia: Elsevier Ltd; 2004. p. 201–4.

39. Mackell S. Traveler's diarrhea in the pediatric population: etiology and impact. Clin Infect Dis 2005;41:S547–52.

40. Bossley C, Balfour-Lynn IM. Is this baby fit to fly? Hypoxia in aeroplanes. Early Hum Dev 2007;83:755–9.

41. Summer AP, Fischer PR. Pediatric, neonatal and adolescent travelers. In: Keystone JS, Kozarsky PE, Freedman DO, et al, editors. Travel Medicine. 2nd edition. Philadelphia: Elsevier Limited; 2008. p. 223–33.

42. Lo Bue P. Tuberculosis. In: CDC health information for international travel (Yellow book) 2012. Chapter 3: infectious diseases related to travel – tuberculosis. Available at: http://wwwnc.cdc.gov/travel/yellowbook/2012/chapter-3-infectious-diseases-related-to-travel/tuberculosis.htm. Accessed June 25, 2012.

43. World Health Organization. 10 facts on ageing and life course. Available at: http://www.who.int/features/factfiles/ageing/en/index.html. Accessed June 25, 2012.

44. Driessen SO, Cobelens FG, Ligthelm RJ. Travel-related morbidity in travelers with insulin-dependent diabetes mellitus. J Travel Med 1999;6(1):12–5.

45. Yanni E, Cantor A. CDC Health Information for International Travel. Yellow Book. Chapter 8: Travelers with disabilities - advising travelers with specific needs. New York: Oxford University Press; 2012. Available at: http://wwwnc.cdc.gov/travel/yellowbook/2012/chapter-8-advising-travelers-with-specific-needs/travelers-with-disabilities.htm. Accessed June 25, 2012.

46. World Health Organization. International travel and health – travel by sea. 2012. Available at: http://www.who.int/ith/mode_of_travel/sea_travel/en/index.html. Accessed June 25, 2012.

47. Suh KN. The elderly traveler. In: Keystone JS, Kozarsky PE, Freedman DO, et al, editors. Travel medicine. 2nd edition. Philadelphia: Elsevier Limited; 2008.

48. Bourée P. Immunity and immunization in elderly. Pathol Biol 2003;51:581–5.

49. Centers for Disease Control and Prevention (CDC). Emergency preparedness and response. Heat stress in the elderly. Available at: http://www.bt.cdc.gov/disasters/extremeheat/elderlyheat.asp. Accessed June 25, 2012.

50. Franceschi C, Monti D, Sansoni P, et al. The immunology of exceptional individuals: the lesion of centenarians. Immunol Today 1995;16:12–6.

51. Paganelli R, Scala E, Quintil, et al. Humoral immunity in aging. Aging 1994;6:143–50.

52. Ben-Yehuda A, Weksler ME. Immune senescence: mechanisms and clinical implications. Cancer Invest 1992;10:525–31.
53. World Health Organization (WHO). Vaccine-preventable diseases and vaccines. In: International travel and health. 2012. Available at: http://www.who.int/ith/chapters/ith2012en_chap6.pdf. Accessed June 25, 2012.
54. Martin M, Weld LH, Tsai TF, et al, GeoSentinel Yellow Fever Working Group. Advanced age a risk factor for illness temporally associated with yellow fever vaccination. Emerg Infect Dis 2001;7(6):945–51.
55. Struchiner CJ, Luz PM, Dourado I, et al. Risk of fatal adverse events associated with 17DD yellow fever vaccine. Epidemiol Infect 2004;132(5):939–46.
56. Centers for Disease Control and Prevention (CDC). Yellow fever vaccine. Recommendations of the Advisory Committee on Immunization Practices (ACIP). MMWR Recomm Rep 2010;59(RR-7). Available at: http://www.cdc.gov/mmwr/pdf/rr/rr5907.pdf. Accessed June 25, 2012.
57. Muhlberger N, Jelinek T, Behrens RH, et al. Age as a risk factor for severe manifestations and fatal outcome of falciparum malaria in European patients: observations from TropNetEurop and SIMPID Surveillance Data. Clin Infect Dis 2003;36(8):990–5.
58. World Health Organization. International travel and health. Medical examination after travel. Available at: http://www.who.int/ith/precautions/medical_examination/en/index.html. Accessed June 25, 2012.
59. Steffen R, Kane MA, Shapiro CN, et al. Epidemiology and prevention of hepatitis A in travelers. JAMA 1994;272:885–9.
60. Taylor DN, Pollard RA, Blake PA. Typhoid in the United States and the risk to the international traveler. J Infect Dis 1983;148:599–602.
61. Gautret P, Guadart J, Leder K, et al. Travel-associated illness in older adults (> 60 y). J Travel Med 2012;19:169–77.
62. National Prevention Information Network (NPIN). The elderly. Available at: http://www.cdcnpin.org/scripts/population/elderly.asp. Accessed June 25, 2012.

Malaria Prevention in Travelers

Blaise Genton, MD, PhD, DTMH[a,b,*],
Valérie D'Acremont, MD, PhD, DTMH[c,d]

KEYWORDS

- Malaria • Chemoprophylaxis • Travel • Prevention • Stand-by emergency treatment

KEY POINTS

- The risk of acquiring malaria depends on the length and intensity of exposure; the risk of developing severe disease is primarily determined by the health status of the traveler.
- Malaria prevention relies on **A**wareness of risk, **B**ite avoidance, **C**ompliance with chemoprophylaxis, and prompt **D**iagnosis in case of fever.
- Mefloquine, atovaquone/proguanil (A/P) and doxycycline are >90% effective to prevent malaria; the incidence of adverse events is highest for mefloquine followed by doxycycline and A/P.
- Misconceptions such as malaria being a trivial illness, repellents being unsafe in children, or mefloquine leading to suicide need to be discussed to improve adherence of travelers to preventive measures.
- The most important message is to advise the traveler to seek medical care in case of fever during or after travel.

A case history

A couple with two children aged 2 and 4 years are planning a safari to the Serengeti Park in the United Republic of Tanzania, followed by a one-week stay on the west coast of Zanzibar. The 37-year old husband is not willing to take chemoprophylaxis as he has lived in Senegal in the past and has never developed malaria. His 36-year old wife does not use contraceptive measures as the couple plans to conceive another child. How would you advise this family for their forthcoming trip?

Conflicting interests: Blaise Genton has received research and travel grants from Novartis Pharma to study the safety and efficacy of artemether/lumefantrine for the treatment of malaria in non-immune travelers, and the impact of the introduction of artemether/lumefantrine as first-line treatment on child mortality and malaria transmission in Tanzania.

[a] Infectious Diseases, Department of Medicine, Travel Clinic Department of Ambulatory Care and Community Medicine, University Hospital, Bugnon Street, 1011 Lausanne, Switzerland;
[b] Swiss Tropical & Public Health Institute, University of Basel, Socinstrasse, 4002 Basel, Switzerland;
[c] Travel Clinic Department of Ambulatory Care and Community Medicine, University Hospital, Bugnon Street, 1011 Lausanne, Switzerland; [d] Global Malaria Program, World Health Organization, Appia, 1202 Geneva, Switzerland
* Corresponding author. CHUV/Policlinique Médicale Universitaire, Rue du Bugnon 44, CH-1011 Lausanne, Switzerland.
E-mail address: Blaise.genton@unibas.ch

Infect Dis Clin N Am 26 (2012) 637–654
http://dx.doi.org/10.1016/j.idc.2012.05.003
0891-5520/12/$ – see front matter © 2012 Elsevier Inc. All rights reserved.

APPROACH TO PREVENTING MALARIA

A common approach would be to apply the "A, B, C, D" rule for malaria prevention: **A**wareness of risk, **B**ite avoidance, **C**ompliance with chemoprophylaxis, and prompt **D**iagnosis in case of fever.

WHAT IS THE RISK?

The risk of acquiring malaria depends on the exposure period and the intensity of malaria; the risk of developing severe disease is primarily determined by the traveller's health status.

Exposure Assessment

The risk of acquiring malaria depends on the intensity of malaria transmission. Malaria occurs in most of sub-Saharan Africa, in large areas of Asia, in parts of South East Asia, in Oceania, in Haiti and in Central and Southern America, as well as in limited areas of Mexico, the Dominican Republic, North Africa and the Middle East (**Fig. 1**). The risk is quite disparate, even within a country. It is greater in rural areas and often fluctuates with the seasons, showing peaks during the rainy season. The transmission of malaria decreases with increasing altitude, and usually does not occur in highland areas (above 2,000 meters).[1]

In order to estimate the absolute risk of acquiring malaria during travel to a specific destination, an accurate numerator, i.e. the number of travelers to each destination who become ill with malaria, and denominator, i.e. the total number of travelers visiting each destination, are required. Without access to this type of data it is very difficult to calculate a precise risk in many regions . Added to which, information on chemoprophylaxis use and adherence to medication is often not usually available, and thus no differentiation is made between attack rates among chemoprophylaxis users and non-users. In the 80's, the incidence of malaria in European travelers using no chemoprophylaxis was 15.2/1'000 travelers per month in East Africa, and 24.2/1'000 travelers per month in West Africa.[2] When information on chemoprophylaxis use was not factored in, the incidence rates of malaria were only 1.7/1'000 travelers in East Africa, 3.8/1'000 travelers in West Africa, 41/1'000 in Oceania, and 0.01–0.1 in Latin America, the Far East and the Middle East.[3]

More recent analyses of traveler's databases have confirmed that the highest risk of acquiring malaria is in Africa and Oceania, with an intermediate risk in Southern Asia and the lowest risk is in Central America, South East Asia and South America.[4,5]

During the last decade, malaria has declined considerably,[6,7] thanks to the large scale implementation of effective control measures such as insecticide-impregnated bed-nets, indoor residual spraying and the use of very effective drugs [artemisinine-based combinations (ACTs)]. The reduction of malaria transmission worldwide is also reflected by the very low risk of imported malaria in Europe from India or Latin America, e.g. 1/1'000–3'000 per year of exposure.[8,9] Long term travelers, back-packers, and travelers visiting friends and relatives (VFR) are at higher risk of acquiring malaria.

In addition to transmission intensity, the level of parasite resistance to chemoprophylactic agents is an important factor in the risk assessment. Resistance to chloroquine is widespread outside Central America, the Middle East and China. Resistance to mefloquine is limited to South East Asia, particularly Thailand and Cambodia.

When assessing exposure, the travel itinerary should be detailed to determine the risk of acquiring malaria. The main factors to consider include:

- Level of transmission in the areas to be visited
- Duration of exposure

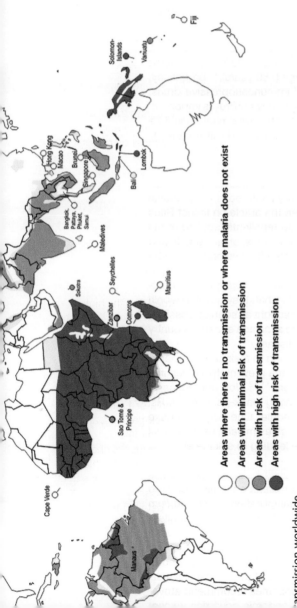

Areas where there is no transmission or where malaria does not exist

Areas with minimal risk of transmission

Areas with risk of transmission

Areas with high risk of transmission

...ansmission worldwide.

d to rural versus urban areas
on
of travel (back-pack vs package holiday).

sment

of the traveler's should be considered in assessing the risk of developing
aria. Risk factors for severe disease include: age (>60 years),[10] pregnancy,
ficiencies (e.g. HIV, asplenia), and the use of immunosuppressive drugs.
ng these factors when choosing an appropriate antimalarial drug is important.
of reliable diagnostic services and safe and effective treatment should be
d, so as to provide appropriate advice on self-diagnosis and self-treatment.

PREVENTION PER SE
and Non Drug Interventions

s to malaria-endemic destinations need to be fully informed about personal
nmental measures to avoid mosquito bites (see the article on Insect Bites
in this issue). These measures include mosquito repellents (applied to the
se of clothes that provide full coverage, window screens, or air-conditioned
rnight. Insecticide-impregnated bed nets are very effective and should be
ded, especially for long-term travelers.
ost malaria deaths in travelers are due to delays in the diagnosis and treat-
avelers should be encouraged to think of malaria when they develop febrile
during or after travel. Medical advice should be sought as soon as possible,
veler should be reminded to mention their visit to a malaria endemic country
propriate tests are undertaken to exclude the disease.
s should be reminded of the importance of adhering to their chemoprophy-
en. Evidence shows that non adherence to malaria preventative measures
n, and ranges between 30% to 55% of travelers.[11,12] Non adherence to
emoprophylaxis is particularly a problem among back-packers, VFRs,
travelers and those using a daily dosing schedule. One way to reduce
ence problems is to discuss misconceptions such as malaria being a trivial
ellents being unsafe in children, or mefloquine leading to suicide etc.[13]

phylaxis

ard recommendation for any traveler visiting a malaria endemic area is to
ar antimalarial drugs to prevent growth and multiplication of *Plasmodium*
Chemoprophylaxis does not prevent infection, but avoids clinical manifes-
d protects against the development of severe disease. There are several
ohylactic agents that are active against *Plasmodium falciparum* and non
species. However, all but primaquine, do not prevent relapses a phenom-
ciated with *P. vivax* and *P. ovale* infection. Because of the almost universal
of *Plasmodium falciparum* to chloroquine, all countries recommend atova-
quanil, mefloquine, or doxycycline for malaria-endemic countries, except

Table 1
Drugs used for prophylaxis

Drug	Dose	Schedule	Indication	Contra-Indications
Atovaquone-proguanil Adult tablet contains 250 mg atovaquone and 100 mg proguanil Pediatric tablet 62.5 mg–25 mg	>40 kg 1 tablet 31–40 kg 3 Pediatric tablets 21–30 kg 2 Pediatric tablets 11–20 kg 1 Pediatric tablet 9–10 kg[a] 3/4 Pediatric tablet 5–8 kg[a] 1/2 Pediatric tablet	Begin 1–2 d before travel to malarious areas. Take daily while in the malarious area and for 7 d after leaving the area	All areas	Contraindicated in individuals with severe renal impairment (creatinine clearance <30 mL/min) Not recommended for prophylaxis in children weighing <5 kg, pregnant women, and women breastfeeding infants weighing <5 kg
Mefloquine 228 mg base (250 mg salt)	>45 kg 1 tablet 25–44.9 kg 3/4 tablet[b] 16–24.9 kg 1/2 tablet[c] 10–15.9 kg 1/4 tablet <9.9 kg[d] 5 mg per kg[e]	Begin ≥1–2 wk before travel to malarious areas. Take weekly on the same day of the week in the malarious area and for 4 wk after leaving the area	Areas with mefloquine sensitive-strains of *Plasmodium*	Contraindicated in people allergic to mefloquine or related compounds (quinine, quinidine) and in people with any present or past history of psychiatric disorders, or seizures Not recommended for persons with cardiac conduction abnormalities
Doxycycline	100 mg Children ≥8 y of age: 2 mg/kg up to adult dose of 100 mg/d	Begin 1–2 d before travel to malarious areas. Take daily while in the malarious area and for 4 wk after leaving the area	All areas	Contraindicated in children <8 y of age and pregnant women
Primaquine	30 mg base (52.6 mg salt) Children 0.5 mg/kg base (0.8 mg/kg salt) up to adult dose	Begin 1–2 d before travel to malarious areas. Take daily while in the malarious area and for 7 d after leaving the area For terminal prophylaxis, take the same dose daily for 14 d after departure from malaria area	All areas especially with high prevalence of P. vivax Prolonged exposure to P. vivax and/or P. ovale	Contraindicated in people with G6PD deficiency, pregnant and lactating women, unless the infant being breastfed has a documented normal G6PD level

Abbreviation: G6PD, glucose-6-phosphate dehydrogenase.
a Off label less than 11 kg bodyweight.
b Reduction of the dose in women after 7th dose to 1/2 tablet.
c Reduction of the dose in women after 7th dose to 1/4 tablet.
d Off label less than 5 kg.
e Preparation through pharmacist.

the drug regimen chosen is appropriate for that individual's particular health and risk factors. Travelers should be reminded that any drug taken for chemoprophylaxis must be used in conjunction with personal protective measures to prevent mosquito bites, and all anti-malarial drugs have the potential to cause adverse reactions. If there is a concern about tolerance, malaria prophylaxis may be initiated several weeks before departure to ensure any adverse effects are detected and the regimen altered before departure. Because of the problem of counterfeit medication in many countries, travelers should be advised to purchase anti-malarial medication prior to departure.

Details (dosage per body weight, schedule, indications and contra-indications) of the main drugs used for prophylaxis are given in **Table 1**.

Chloroquine or Hydroxychloroquine

Chloroquine is a synthetic 4-aminoquinoline. Its use is limited to areas with chloroquine-sensitive parasites. Apart from its bitter taste, chloroquine is well tolerated. Retinal toxic effects may occur with long-term daily doses (>100 g total dose). Chloroquine is contraindicated in individuals with psoriasis or a history of epilepsy.

Mefloquine

Mefloquine is a quinoline methanol. It is one of the first line drugs for the prevention of malaria for travelers to chloroquine-resistant areas. The most frequently reported minor side effects are: nausea, strange vivid dreams, dizziness, mood changes, insomnia, headaches, and diarrhea. Approximately 1% to 5% of mefloquine users may have to discontinue prophylaxis because of adverse reactions. Tens of millions of travelers have used mefloquine as prophylaxis. Severe reactions have been reported from 1 in 6'000–13'000 users. Women tend to experience more neuropsychological reactions than men.[14] Severe reactions have often been observed particularly in individuals who have contraindications to using the drug. Absolute contraindications include a past history of psychiatric disorders. Most of the adverse reactions are only mild and self limiting. Splitting the dose into ½ a tablet taken twice per week has shown to reduce the frequency and intensity of adverse events.[15] Twenty-two reports of deaths, including five suicides, in association with the use of mefloquine have been reported; however, information on the denominator (number of mefloquine users) is lacking, but is approximately 35–40 million,[16] and no association with mefloquine has been confirmed.

Since a protective therapeutic drug level is attained after three weekly doses, some physicians propose taking "loading doses", of two doses per week in the week prior to departure, or to start earlier (more than 2 weeks). This schedule is reported to produce an increase in side-effects.

Atovaquone/Proguanil

Atovaquone/proguanil is a fixed drug combination of atovaquone and proguanil in a single tablet. It is effective as a causal (acting at the liver stage) as well as suppressive (acting at the blood stage) prophylactic drug. Thanks to these properties, atovaquone/proguanil can be stopped one week after leaving the malarial endemic area. Atovaquone/proguanil is effective everywhere, including areas with multi-drug resistant parasites, even though several documented cases of atovaquone/proguanil resistance have been reported from parasites acquired in sub-Saharan Africa.[17,18] Atrovaquone/proguanil prophylaxis has proved to be safe and well tolerated.[19] The most frequent adverse events are gastrointestinal, such as nausea, vomiting, abdominal pain or diarrhea. Serious adverse events such as fulminant hepatitis and extensive rash have been reported. Headaches and oral ulceration are not uncommon.

Doxycycline

Doxycycline is an antibiotic that inhibits parasite protein synthesis. Doxycycline is effective against chloroquine and mefloquine resistant strains of parasites. It can cause gastrointestinal adverse reactions, and rarely esophageal ulceration, unlikely to occur if the drug is taken with food and fluids. An extensive report on doxycycline as a chemoprophylactic and treatment agent against malaria has recently been published by a panel associated with CDC.[20] Despite reports of skin sensitivity in 7% to 21% of people using doxycycline for prophylaxis (100 mg/day), a blinded study reports that doxycycline has similar rates of cutaneous adverse events as other antimalarials.[14] The phenomenon of photosensitivity may be a dose dependent reaction, with 21% of users taking 150 mg/day reporting a rash, against 32% of users taking 200 mg/day dose reporting a skin problem. The problem of women developing vaginal candidiasis has no published supporting evidence. The potential of an interaction in women using the the oral contraceptive is frequently cited in the literature.[21] The rate of contraception failure in women treated with antibiotics was between 1.2% and 1.6%, a similar rate as in those without treatment. There is at present, no clear evidence to confirm this interaction. The authors of the CDC report thus do not recommend taking special contraceptive measures.

Primaquine

Primaquine is an 8-aminoquinoline which is active against developing liver stages (causal prophylaxis), liver hypnozoites, asexual forms and gametocytes. Several studies have shown efficacy of primaquine for malaria prevention in non- and semi-immune subjects.There is limited data of its use in travelers. The protective efficacy against both *P. falciparum* and *vivax* infections, when given at a dose of 0.5 mg/kg/day (30 mg for an adult) is around 85% to 93%.[22] With its causal effect , primaquine can be discontinued within a week after departure from malaria-endemic areas. Primaquine is not considered a first line chemoprophylactic but as an alternative in individuals who are not glucose-6-phosphate dehydrogenase (G-6-PD) deficient and cannot use a first line agent. Commonly reported adverse events include nausea and abdominal pains, which can be reduced through taking it with food. Methemoglobinemia and oxidant induced hemolytic anemia can occur in individuals with G-6-PD deficiency, especially among those of Mediterranean, African and Asian origin. Because of the haemolytic potential, limited safety data and it only being available on an unlicensed basis, primaquine is not much used.

How to Choose a Chemoprophylactic Agent?

The main criteria for choosing appropriate chemoprophylactic agents should be the following: level of parasite drug resistance (chloroquine and mefloquine resistance) in the destination, the presence of contraindications, and importantly travelers' preferences based on the nature of adverse drug reactions, schedule, and cost. Appropriate chemoprophylactic agents for parasite resistant areas are summarised in **Table 1**. The choice lies between atovaquone/proguanil, doxycycline and mefloquine. There is no difference in terms of protective efficacy between the three regimens, which ranges between 92% and 95%. Contraindications for each of these drugs are summarized in **Table 1**. The safety and tolerability are based on limited data and one study that has assessed the rate and nature of adverse events in a blinded fashion. Four drug regimens were compared in a double-blind manner: atovaquone/proguanil, doxycycline, mefloquine, and chloroquine/proguanil.[14] The latter combination is still being recommended by WHO for areas endemic for *P. vivax* and falciparum with emerging chloroquine-resistant parasites.[23] Most European and North American countries do not recommend this combination as it has a low protective efficacy. In the above study, chloroquine/proguanil had the highest proportion of mild to moderate adverse events (45%), followed by mefloquine (42%), doxycycline (33%) and atovaquone proguanil (32%). Details of the proportion of travelers with significant adverse events with each drug regimen, for known adverse event categories, are illustrated in **Fig. 2**.

A recent Cochrane review published in 2010 has described the efficacy, safety and tolerability of atovaquone/proguanil, doxycycline and mefloquine.[24] Using eight randomized or quasi-randomized studies (4,240 participants) the rate of adverse events with atovaquone/proguanil or doxycycline was equivalent. Atovaquone/proguanil had generally fewer adverse events than mefloquine [relative risk (RR): 0.72, 95% confidence intervals (CI) 0.60 to 0.85], less gastrointestinal (RR 0.54) and less neuropsychiatric events (RR 0.86). Doxycycline had fewer neuropsychiatric adverse events than mefloquine (RR 0.84).

The incidence of adverse events with mefloquine was slightly higher. The rate of adverse events is one of a number of factors to take into account when advising on chemoprophylaxis. A number of issues need to be explored with the traveler. The nature of adverse events, regimen schedule, duration of intake and cost are all likely to affect choice and adherence. Patients may have personal reasons for choosing one drug rather than the other, including for example a positive or negative past experience with a specific drug. At the Lausanne University Hospital's Travel Clinic, the different options discussed with clients are shown in **Table 2**. This table has been tested in a formal study to better understand the travelers' preferences and the determinant(s) of their choice. Travelers visiting malaria-endemic areas who had access to this table, but no additional information were asked what their first choice of chemoprophylactic was. 44% of the clients chose mefloquine (Mephaquine 24%, Lariam 20%), 21% Malarone, and 19% doxycycline. After the consultation (consisting of a discussion and consideration of potential contraindications), 50% of the clients

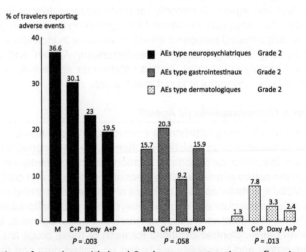

Fig. 2. Proportion of travelers with level 2 adverse events using mefloquine, chloroquine/proguanil, doxycycline, or atovaquone/proguanil. (*Data from* Schlagenhauf P, Tschopp A, Johnson R, et al. Tolerability of malaria chemoprophylaxis in non-immune travellers to sub-Saharan Africa: multicentre, randomised, double blind, four arm study. BMJ 2003;327(7423):1078.)

Table 2
Summary of efficacy, tolerance, dosage, schedule and price for drugs used as malaria chemoprophylaxis (chart used as a basis for discussion between the traveler and health care provider in the travel clinic, University of Lausanne)

Drug	Efficacy	Adverse-Events (AE)			Regimen	Price in Switzerland and Swiss francs (CHF)			
Name of Antimalarial Tablet	Level of Protection (%)	% Total of Travelers with AE	% of Travelers Who Needed to Consult a Doctor for AE	Main Serious AE	Duration Number of Tablets that Must be Taken	For a 7-d Trip	For a 14-d Trip	For a 21-d Trip	For a 28-d Trip
Lariam® Mephaquine® (generic)	90	88	11	Anxiety, bad dreams, depression, dizziness, headache	Long 1 each week (1 wk before and 4 wk after)	42 34	42 34	84 68	84 68
Malarone®	90	81	7	Nausea, diarrhoea, mouth ulcers	Short 1 tablet each day (2 d before and 7 d after)	125	125	187	187
Supracycline® (doxycycline)	90	83	6	Vaginal thrush, sunburn	Long 1 each day (2 d before, and 4 wk after)	36	46	54	54

Data from Schlagenhauf P, Tschopp A, Johnson R, et al. Tolerability of malaria chemoprophylaxis in non-immune travellers to sub-Saharan Africa: multicentre, randomised, double blind, four arm study. BMJ 2003;327(7423):1078.

Table 3
Considerations when discussing drugs for malaria chemoprophylaxis

Drug	Reasons to Prefer Usage of This Drug	Reasons to Avoid Usage of This Drug
Atovaquone/ proguanil	Good for last-minute travelers because the drug is started 1–2 d before travel Some people prefer to take medicine daily Good choice for short trips because the medicine needs to be taken for only 7 d after traveling rather than 4 wk Well tolerated—side effects uncommon Pediatric tablets are available and may be more convenient	Cannot be used by women who are pregnant or breastfeeding a child that weighs <5 kg Cannot be taken by people with severe renal impairment Is more expensive than other options (especially for long trips) Some people (including children) would rather take medicine weekly
Mefloquine	Some people would rather take medicine weekly Good choice for long trips because it is taken only weekly Can be used during pregnancy Can be given to the whole family Is relatively inexpensive	Cannot be used in areas with mefloquine resistance Cannot be used in patients with past or present psychiatric conditions Cannot be used in patients with seizure disorder Not recommended for people with cardiac conduction abnormalities Not a good choice for last-minute travelers because protective drug concentration is only reached after 2 wk or more Some people would rather take a medication weekly For short trips, some people would rather not take medication for 4 wk after travel

Doxycycline	Some people prefer to take a daily medicine	Cannot be used by pregnant women and children aged <8 y
	Good for last-minute travelers because the drug is started 1–2 d before travel	Some people would rather take a medicine weekly
	Tends to be the least expensive antimalarial	For short trips, some people would rather not take medication for 4 wk after travel
	People who are already taking doxycycline long-term to prevent acne do not have to take an additional medicine	People may want to avoid the increased risk of sun sensitivity
	Doxycycline can also prevent some bacterial infections (such as rickettsial infections and leptospirosis), so it may be preferred by people planning to hike, camp, and swim in fresh water	Some people are concerned about the potential of getting an upset stomach from doxycycline
Primaquine	It is the most effective medicine for preventing P. vivax, so it is a good choice for travel to places with high P. vivax endemicity	Cannot be used in patients with glucose-6-phosphate dehydrogenase (G6PD) deficiency
	Good choice for short trips because the medicine needs to be taken for only 7 d after traveling rather than 4 wk	Cannot be used in patients who have not been tested for G6PD deficiency
	Good for last-minute travelers because the drug is started 1–2 d before travel	Cannot be used by pregnant women
	Some people prefer to take medicine daily	Cannot be used by women who are breastfeeding, unless the infant has also been tested for G6PD deficiency
		Some people (including children) would rather take medicine weekly
		Some people are concerned about the potential of getting an upset stomach from primaquine

Adapted from Centers for Disease Control. Infectious diseases related to travel: malaria. Yellow book. Available at: http://wwwnc.cdc.gov/travel/yellowbook/2012/article-3-infectious-diseases-related-to-travel/malaria.htm. Accessed December 22, 2011.

selected mefloquine (37% Mephaquine and 14% Lariam), 24% opted for Malarone, and 19% doxycycline.[25]

Besides distinct patterns of parasite prevalence and medical contraindications, there are other reasons to consider the use or avoidance of a particular drug and these are listed in **Table 3**.

STAND-BY EMERGENCY TREATMENT

Malaria can be successfully treated early in the course of the disease. Travelers should therefore be advised to seek medical assistance as soon as they develop symptoms. With the global decline of malaria and the growing number of countries approaching near malaria elimination, the potential risk of serious drug reactions with chemoprophylaxis use is becoming an important part of a risk benefit calculation, A number of European countries (e.g. Switzerland, Germany and Austria) recommend the use of stand-by emergency treatments (SBET) with atovaquone/proguanil, artemether/lumefantrine and probably, in the near future, dihydroartemisinine/piperaquine during travel to countries where the risk of acquiring malaria is lower than the risk of serious adverse drug reactions from widespread use of chemoprophylaxis. Most of the standby drug combinations are well tolerated and very efficacious in non immune travelers, although only artemether/lumefantrine has been studied in large populations of immune and non-immune malaria patients.[26] All these drug combinations can be given to children >5 kg. Travelers prescribed SBET for use when they develop a fever need to be counselled to (1) seek immediate medical advice and where this is not possible within 24 hours, self treat but seek care as soon as possible afterwards and (2) that at least 6 days should have elapsed between arrival in the malaria area and self-treating. The dosage and regimens of the different combinations for SBET are detailed in **Table 4**. Although SBET has several advantages over chemoprophylaxis, including fewer adverse drug reactions, lower cost, no adherence problem, evidence shows that only a few travelers actually use their standby treatment (1.4%).[27]

There was hope that availability of reliable and cheap rapid diagnostic tests for malaria (mRDT) could be used to better identify travelers with actual malaria. Unfortunately, studies of travelers with malaria have shown that mRDT are not used with accuracy as sick individuals have difficulty following the procedures and interpreting their results.[28]

SBET is an option for travelers who visit low endemic areas, but also for travelers who do not want to take chemoprophylaxis, or choose a suboptimal drug regimen, or require a poorly effective drug regimen because of medical reasons. Long-term residents who live in remote areas may also decide to use the the mRDT and SBET combination, with or without chemoprophylaxis. The advantages and disadvantages of chemoprophylaxis and stand-by emergency treatment are summarized in **Table 5**.

MALARIA PREVENTION FOR PARTICULAR GROUPS
Very Short-Term Travelers (<7 Days) or Frequent Travelers

The risk may be lower for travelers staying in city centres in a malaria-endemic area for <1 week, and for those who make repeated short-term trips to urban settings than it is for other travelers. Chemoprophylaxis with atovaquone/proguanil is a good option for such travelers as the total duration of medication is much shorter than other regimens.

Long-Term Travelers (>6 Months)

Long-term travelers are at a higher risk of malaria than short-term travelers with more prolonged exposure. Observational studies have shown that this group of

Table 4
Drugs used for stand-by emergency treatment of malaria

Drug	Dosing	Schedule	Contra-Indications	Advantages
Atovaquone-proguanil (AP) (250 mg/100 mg)	>40 kg 4 tablets 31–40 kg 3 tablets 21–30 kg 2 tablets 11–20 kg 1 tablet 9–10 kg[a] 3/4 tablet 5–8 kg[a] 1/2 tablet	Daily dose to be taken orally for 3 consecutive days To be taken with fatty food	Contra-indicated in individuals with severe renal impairment (creatinine clearance <30 mL/min) Not recommended in children weighing <5 kg, pregnant women, women breastfeeding infants weighing <5 kg, and those on AP prophylaxis	One daily dose Good for expatriates because of long shelf-life (3 y) Possible to switch for chemoprophylaxis with same agent
Artemether-lumefantrine (20 mg/120 mg)	>35 kg 4 tablets 25–35 kg 3 tablets 15–25 kg 2 tablets 5–15 kg 1 tablet	3-d treatment schedule with a total of 6 oral doses. The patient should receive the initial dose, followed by the second dose 8 h later, then 1 dose twice per day for the following 2 d. To be taken with fatty food	Not recommended in children weighing <5 kg, pregnant women, women breastfeeding infants weighing <5 kg, and those on mefloquine prophylaxis	Excellent safety and efficacy profile demonstrated in the largest sample size of non-immune patients with malaria Almost no resistance described
Dihydroartemisinin-piperaquine Adult tablet 40 mg/320 mg Pediatric tablet 20 mg/160 mg (Not yet available)	>75 kg 4 tablets 36–75 kg 3 tablets 24–35 kg 2 tablets 13–23 kg 1 tablet 7–12 kg 1 Pediatric tablet 5–6 kg 1/2 Pediatric tablet	Daily dose to be taken orally for 3 consecutive days	Not recommended in pregnant women, women breastfeeding infants weighing <5 kg, and children weighing <5 kg	One daily dose Almost no resistance described

Abbreviation: AP, atovaquone-proguanil.
[a] Off label under 11 kg bodyweight.

Table 5	
Advantages and disadvantages of chemoprophylaxis versus standby emergency treatment (SBET)	
Advantages	**Disadvantages**
Chemoprophylaxis	
Opportunity to test tolerability of the drug before departure and to change to an alternative if necessary	Usually more expensive than SBET
Higher safety of chemoprophylaxis for travelers with co-morbidities	Travelers read the the leaflet and stop the medication due to fear of adverse drug reactions
Possible interactions with current medication can be assessed before departure	Full adherence is only observed in about one third of the travelers
Appropriate to prevent mild and severe episode of malaria in areas with high level of transmission	In areas with low malaria risk, the risk of serious adverse events largely exceeds the risk of severe malaria
SBET	
Rare adherence problems if appropriate (written) information	Increased incidence rate of adverse drug reactions when taken as treatment. Mefloquine is not advised for this indication
Usually cheaper than prophylaxis	Need to take atovaquone/proguanil and artemether/lumefantrine with fatty food because of their lipophilic property
Medication always available on site on time	Severe drug reactions can occur without close medical supervision
0.5%–1.4% of all travelers to whom SBET medication has been prescribed will finally use it	SBET use in febrile travelers ($\sim$10% of all travelers) has been 5%–17%, but Plasmodial infection could be confirmed retrospectively in only 11%–17% of SBET-users only
At present, no malaria deaths reported linked to the use of SBET (surveillance data from Germany, Switzerland and Austria)	—

Adapted from Kollaritsch HH, Nödl H. Malaria. Österreichische Ärztezeitung 2010;12:37–51.

people under-use personal preventive measures and are poorly adherent to chemo-prophylaxis. Several strategies can be recommended (i) chemoprophylaxis for an initial period and then review after a local assessment of the malaria risk, the avail-ability of reliable diagnostic tests, and medical facilities. If the risk is considered very low and there is good medical support, the use of chemoprophylaxis can be stopped, (ii) SBET, and/or seasonal chemoprophylaxis taken during peak seasons. Extensive discussion needs to take place, including a clear description of the high risk areas, and an explanation that long-term use of chemoprophylactic drugs do not lead to toxicity or ill health, Confusion arising from discordant recommendations given by friends or expatriates living in the destination country (dispelling myths about immunity) may impact on adherence and needs to be discussed during the pre-travel consultation.[29] Details on the duration for the safe use of chemoprophy-lactic drugs are included in **Table 6**. An emphasis should be placed on measures to avoid mosquito bites, through the use of insecticide-impregnated bed nets, frequent

Table 6
Safety of chemoprophylactic drugs for long-term use

Antimalarial Agent	Advice on Long-Term Use
Chloroquine	Safe for long-term use No limit but caution if use >5 y (need for ophthalmic examination every 6–12 mo thereafter)[a]
Proguanil	Safe for long-term use No limit[a]
Mefloquine	Safe for long-term use No limit (UK: up to 3 y)
Atovaquone/proguanil	Safe for long-term use No limit in US; up to 3–6 mo in most European countries[b] Issue of cost
Doxycycline	Safe for long-term use Advised between 4 mo (US) to 2 y (most other countries)
Primaquine	Safe for long-term use No limit or no specific recommendation

[a] Chloroquine and proguanil should always be used in combination; there are considerable concerns about the efficacy of this combination in most of endemic areas.
[b] Post-licencing experience needed.
Adapted from Chen LH, Wilson ME, Schlagenhauf P. Prevention of malaria in long-term travelers. JAMA 2006;296(18):2234–44; and Chiodini P, Hill D, Lalloo D, et al. Guidelines for malaria prevention in travellers from the United Kingdom 2007. Health Protection Agency. Available at: http://www.hpa.org.uk/Publications/InfectiousDiseases/TravelHealth/0701Malariapreventionfortravellersfromthe UK/. Accessed December 23, 2011.

and repeated use of repellents, the use of barriers such as windows screen and indoor residual spraying of houses with pyrethroid. A clear message that a prompt response to the development of any febrile symptoms should be made repeatedly so that a delayed presentation of malaria does not lead to an avoidable fatality.

Pregnancy

Pregnant women are at increased risk of severe malaria. The WHO and other organizations recommend that women should not travel to malaria endemic regions during pregnancy. If travel can not be avoided chemoprophylaxis must be recommended for pregnant women visiting any malaria-endemic area. Mefloquine is the only chemoprophylactic agent which has, through indirect observational studies, been shown not to have led to any foetal damage or loss and it remains effective throughout pregnancy. Alternatively atovaquone/proguanil can be discussed, as both atovaquone and proguanil have been used separately during pregnancy, without any evidence of toxicity but in combination has there is limited safety data.

Travelers with Chronic Diseases

Cardiac disease

Mefloquine should be avoided as it can affect cardiac conduction particular if used with similar types of drug. Atovaquone/proguanil is preferred. Patients on beta-blockers can be prescribed mefloquine when there is not concomitant arrhythmia.

Severe renal disease
Atovaquone/proguanil is contraindicated in patients with a creatinine clearance of less than 30 mL/min. Mefloquine and doxycycline can be safely given as they are metabolized by the liver.

Severe liver disease (ASAT and ALAT double the norm)
Proguanil, doxycycline and mefloquine are metabolized in the liver and these chemoprophylactic agents should therefore be avoided. Travellers with severe liver disease should be advised not to travel to malaria-endemic areas.

Epilepsy
Mefloquine and chloroquine are contraindicated as they lower the epileptogenic threshold. Atovaquone/proguanil or doxycycline can be used. Phenobarbitone and phenytoin may increase the metabolism of doxycyline and reduce its half life.

HIV infection
Protease inhibitors can influence mefloquine and atovaquone/proguanil plasma concentrations. Doxycycline is usually preferred since no interactions are expected with protease inhibitors and NNRTI. Details on interactions with antiretroviral therapies can be checked on the website www.hiv-druginteraction.org.

Organ transplants
The plasma concentration of several medications, e.g. cyclosporine A, can be reduced by malaria medication. The advantage of SBET versus chemoprophylaxis should be balanced with the risk of malaria in this instance. It is possible to start chemoprophylaxis earlier, before departure, and check plasma drug concentrations and adapt the dose if necessary.

A case history revisited

The family visiting the Serengeti Park in Tanzania and the North East coast of Zanzibar should be assessed and advised as follows:

Exposure assessment: moderate risk in the Serengeti Park; hardly any risk in Zanzibar in December.

Host assessment: the woman is not pregnant but could be at the time of travel; doxycycline is contraindicated for the two children; the husband prefers not to take chemoprophylaxis.

Advice:

- Inform the family about mosquito bite avoidance and propose repellent suitable for the whole family, such as one containing DEET.

- Chemoprophylaxis is recommended, mainly for the Tanzanian mainland, even if the risk is quite low.
  - Mefloquine or atovaquone/proguanil are options for chemoprophylaxis. Doxycycline is contraindicated in children and not advised for the mother who wants to become pregnant. Mefloquine would be the best option, because (i) it can be given to all family members, (ii) the weekly intake improves adherence and is easy to administer in small children, (iii) it is the cheapest option (using the generic form).

- For the husband, insist on protective measures to avoid mosquito bites, and if he will not take chemoprophylaxis suggest SBET with atovaquone/proguanil. The latter could be used by the wife or children, should any side effects occur with mefloquine during travel.

- Explain clearly what should be done if a fever develops. Providing the address and phone number of a reliable health facility in Dar es Salaam is helpful.

REFERENCES

1. Public Health Agency of Canada. Canadian recommendations for the prevention and treatment of malaria among international travellers. CCDR 2008;34S3:1–45. Available at: http://www.phac-aspc.gc.ca/publicat/ccdr-rmtc/09vol35/35s1/index-eng.php. Accessed December 21, 2011.
2. Steffen R, Heusser R, Mächler R, et al. Malaria chemoprophylaxis among European tourists in tropical Africa: use, adverse reactions, and efficacy. Bull World Health Organ 1990;68(3):313–22.
3. Phillips-Howard PA, Radalowicz A, Mitchell J, et al. Risk of malaria in British residents returning from malarious areas. BMJ 1990;300(6723):499–503.
4. Askling HH, Nilsson J, Tegnell A, et al. Malaria risk in travelers. Emerg Infect Dis 2005;11(3):436–41.
5. Leder K, Black J, O'Brien D, et al. Malaria in travelers: a review of the GeoSentinel surveillance network. Clin Infect Dis 2004;39(8):1104–12.
6. WHO. World malaria report 2010. Available at: http://www.who.int/malaria/world_malaria_report_2010/en/index.html. Accessed January 10, 2012.
7. D'Acremont V, Lengeler C, Genton B. Reduction in the proportion of fevers associated with *Plasmodium falciparum* parasitaemia in Africa: a systematic review. Malar J 2010;9:240.
8. Behrens RH, Bisoffi Z, Björkman A, et al. Malaria prophylaxis policy for travellers from Europe to the Indian subcontinent. Malar J 2006;5:7.
9. Behrens RH, Carroll B, Beran J, et al. The low and declining risk of malaria in travellers to Latin America: is there still an indication for chemoprophylaxis? Malar J 2007;6:114.
10. Seringe E, Thellier M, Fontanet A, et al. Severe imported *Plasmodium falciparum* malaria, France, 1996-2003. Emerg Infect Dis 2011;17(5):807–13.
11. Lobel HO, Baker MA, Gras FA, et al. Use of malaria prevention measures by North American and European travelers to East Africa. J Travel Med 2001;8(4):167–72.
12. Landry P, Iorillo D, Darioli R, et al. Do travelers really take their mefloquine malaria chemoprophylaxis? Estimation of adherence by an electronic pillbox. J Travel Med 2006;13(1):8–14.
13. Chen LH, Wilson ME, Schlagenhauf P. Controversies and misconceptions in malaria chemoprophylaxis for travelers. JAMA 2007;297(20):2251–63.
14. Schlagenhauf P, Tschopp A, Johnson R, et al. Tolerability of malaria chemoprophylaxis in non-immune travellers to sub-Saharan Africa: multicentre, randomised, double blind, four arm study. BMJ 2003;327(7423):1078.
15. Schlagenhauf P, Adamcova M, Regep L, et al. The position of mefloquine as a 21st century malaria chemoprophylaxis. Malar J 2010;9:357.
16. Schlagenhauf P. Cochrane Review highlights the need for more targeted research on the tolerability of malaria chemoprophylaxis in travellers. Evid Based Med 2010;15(1):25–6.
17. Kuhn S, Gill MJ, Kain KC. Emergence of atovaquone-proguanil resistance during treatment of *Plasmodium falciparum* malaria acquired by a non-immune north American traveller to West Africa. Am J Trop Med Hyg 2005;72(4):407–9.
18. Osei-Akoto A, Orton L, Owusu-Ofori SPO. Atovaquone-proguanil for treating uncomplicated malaria. Cochrane Database Syst Rev 2005;(4):CD004529.
19. Taylor WRJ, White NJ. Antimalarial drug toxicity: a review. Drug Saf 2004;27(1):25–61.

20. Tan KR, Magill AJ, Parise ME, et al. Doxycycline for malaria chemoprophylaxis and treatment: report from the CDC expert meeting on malaria chemoprophylaxis. Am J Trop Med Hyg 2011;84(4):517–31.

21. Griffith KS, Lewis LS, Mali S, et al. Treatment of malaria in the United States: a systematic review. JAMA 2007;297(20):2264–77.

22. Baird JK, Fryauff DJ, Hoffman SL. Primaquine for prevention of malaria in travelers. Clin Infect Dis 2003;37(12):1659–67.

23. WHO. International travel and health. Available at: http://www.who.int/ith/chapters/en/index.html. Accessed December 22, 2011.

24. Jacquerioz FA, Croft AM. Drugs for preventing malaria in travellers. Cochrane Database Syst Rev 2009;(4):CD006491.

25. Senn N, D'Acremont V, Landry P, et al. Malaria chemoprophylaxis: what do the travelers choose, and how does pretravel consultation influence their final decision. Am J Trop Med Hyg 2007;77(6):1010–4.

26. Hatz C, Soto J, Nothdurft HD, et al. Treatment of acute uncomplicated falciparum malaria with artemether-lumefantrine in nonimmune populations: a safety, efficacy, and pharmacokinetic study. Am J Trop Med Hyg 2008;78(2):241–7.

27. Nothdurft HD, Jelinek T, Pechel SM, et al. Stand-by treatment of suspected malaria in travellers. Trop Med Parasitol 1995;46(3):161–3.

28. Jelinek T, Amsler L, Grobusch MP, et al. Self-use of rapid tests for malaria diagnosis by tourists. Lancet 1999;354(9190):1609.

29. Chen LH, Wilson ME, Schlagenhauf P. Prevention of malaria in long-term travelers. JAMA 2006;296(18):2234–44.

Insect Bite Prevention

Sarah J. Moore, PhD[a,b],
Anne Jennifer Mordue (Luntz), PhD, FRES, FSB[c,]*,
James G. Logan, PhD, FRES[a]

KEYWORDS

- Insect bites • Protection • Disease-endemic countries

KEY POINTS

- Travellers are strongly advised to protect themselves from the bites of arthropod vectors of disease as the first line of defence against disease transmission.
- A variety of protection measures should be used including insect repellents, mosquito nets, mosquito coils, aerosol sprays, protective clothing, screening and air conditioning for both day and night protection.
- Travellers should select protection measures and active ingredients based on knowledge of the vectors concerned and their distribution in the area of travel.
- Travellers should be advised to fully comply with the manufacturers' instructions to gain full protection from bites.
- An overview of the worldwide distribution of insect vectors and the pathogens they transmit is provided as a basis of advice for protection from bites.

INTRODUCTION

Many biting arthropods have specialized to feed on humans and, as a result, transmit a variety of pathogens in addition to causing significant distress or discomfort. This article provides an overview of the worldwide distribution of different vectors, the pathogens they carry and their behavioral activity, in terms of seasonality and time of day, which should be used when giving advice to travelers for protection from arthropod bites (**Fig. 1, Table 1**). Three vector-borne diseases (malaria transmitted by anopheline mosquitoes, dengue transmitted by *Stegomyia* [formally *Aedes*] mosquitoes, and rickettsial infections [eg, typhus] transmitted by ticks) account for half of all systemic febrile illness in returned travelers attending travel or tropical medicine clinics.[1] Of the remaining illnesses, the mosquito-borne arbovirus diseases West Nile fever in the United States and chikungunya, which is now entering Europe, are

---

The authors have nothing to disclose.
[a] Department of Disease Control, London School of Hygiene and Tropical Medicine, Keppel Street, London WC1E 7HT, UK; [b] Ifakara Health Institute, Bagamoyo Research and Training Centre, Bagamoyo, Tanzania; [c] School of Biological Sciences, University of Aberdeen, Tillydrone Avenue, Aberdeen AB24 2TZ, UK
* Corresponding author.
E-mail address: a.j.mordue@abdn.ac.uk

Infect Dis Clin N Am 26 (2012) 655–673
http://dx.doi.org/10.1016/j.idc.2012.07.002
0891-5520/12/$ – see front matter © 2012 Elsevier Inc. All rights reserved.

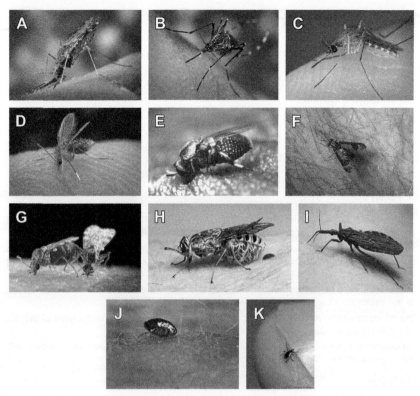

Fig. 1. Arthropod vectors of disease. Numbers relate to those in **Table 1** and link disease agent with each vector type, their bionomics, and recommended methods of bite prevention. (*A*) *Anopheles* mosquito (*A. albimanus*). (*B*) *Stegomyia* (*Aedes*) mosquito (*S. aegypti*). (*C*) *Culex* mosquito (*C. quinquefasciatus*). (*D*) Sandfly (*Phlebotomus papatasi*). (*E*) Blackfly (*Simulium damnosum*). (*F*) Deerfly (*Chrysops* sp). (*G*) Midge (*Culicoides imicola*). (*H*) Tsetse fly (*Glossina morsitans*). (*I*) Reduviid bug (*Rhodnius prolixus*). (*J*) Oriental rat flea (*Xenopsylla cheopis*). (*K*) Hard tick (*Ixodes scapularis*). Photographs are of vector type and not necessarily the main vector species of disease. Indication of scale is given by presence of human skin in each photograph.

increasing in frequency. Several epidemics of yellow fever, West Nile fever, Rift Valley fever and chikungunya have occurred in the last decade, largely as a result of climate anomalies associated with climate change.[2]

Insect bites can be avoided through careful use of appropriate personal protection methods, and bite protection methods should be considered as the first line of prevention against vector-borne disease in addition to the use of preventative drugs and vaccines where appropriate.

Travelers are usually at lower risk of exposure to vector-borne diseases in urban areas where vector breeding sites are limited, especially if they sleep in screened or air-conditioned rooms. However, the vectors of dengue are abundant in many tropical urban centers and bite mostly during the day. Therefore, all travelers should heed local epidemic warnings. Travelers to rural areas and long-term travelers living in areas where sanitation is poor are usually at higher risk of exposure to disease vectors than those traveling to urban regions or for shorter periods of time.[3] Personal protection is therefore essential not only in the early evening and during the night when most

Table 1
Overview of insect vectors of disease, their behavior, and means of preventing bites

Vector	Disease	Location	Time of Biting	Indoors/ Outdoors	Transmission Season	Recommendation	Incidence in Travelers[a]	References
1. *Anopheles* mosquitoes (**Fig. 1A**)	Malaria	SSA	Dusk to dawn with late-night peak	Indoors and outdoors	All year with peak during and following the rainy season	Avoid mosquito bites, especially after sunset, by using insect repellents containing DEET or PMD and long clothing. Sleep beneath insecticide-impregnated bed nets. Sleep in air-conditioned/screened rooms if possible and use mosquito coils containing transfluthrin, d-allethrin, or metofluthrin if possible outdoors after dark.	622	1
		SA	Dusk to dawn with early evening peak	Mainly outdoors	During and following the rainy season		133	
		CA		Indoors and outdoors			CA 133, Caribbean 65 130 139	
		SEA SCA						
	Lymphatic filariasis	Mainly SSA (75% of cases) some SCA, CA, SA, mainly in long-term travelers >1 mo	Dusk to dawn with late-night peak	Indoors and outdoors			1.5	55

(continued on next page)

Table 1
(continued)

Vector	Disease	Location	Time of Biting	Indoors/Outdoors	Transmission Season	Recommendation	Incidence in Travelers[a]	References
2. *Stegomyia* mosquitoes (**Fig. 1B**)	Dengue fever	SSA SCA SEA CA CAR SA	Daytime and early evening	Indoors and outdoors	All year round, but especially following the rainy season and during epidemics	Prevention of mosquito bites during daytime using a repellent with DEET or PMD is essential during epidemics. Use of mosquito coils or heated mats indoors and sleeping in screened accommodation is advised.	7 142 315 123 238 137	1
	Rift Valley fever	SSA, ME			During epidemics related to very high rainfall		<0.001	56
	Chikungunya	SSA, NAf and ME, SEA, EU			Chikungunya entering EU with climate change		1.7	57
	Yellow fever	SSA, SA			Can occur year round, but mainly during and following the rainy season and during epidemics	Ensure vaccination for yellow fever before traveling to endemic areas.	<0.02	1

3. Culex mosquitoes (Fig. 1C)	Japanese encephalitis	SEA	Mainly outdoors	All year round, risk mainly among travelers to rural areas	Ensure vaccination for JE before traveling to endemic areas. Avoid mosquito bites especially after sunset by using insect	<0.02	1
	Lymphatic filariasis	SSA, SCA, SEA, SA (Haiti, the Dominican Republic, Guyana, and Brazil)	Dusk to dawn, with early evening peak	Indoors and outdoors	All year round, risk mainly among long-term travelers	repellents containing DEET or PMD and long clothing. Sleep beneath insecticide-impregnated bed nets.	1.5	55
	West Nile fever	SSA, NAf and ME, SCA, NA, EU			All year round in tropics, warmer months in Northern Hemisphere	Sleep in screened rooms where possible and use mosquito coils containing transfluthrin, d-allethrin or metofluthrin if possible outdoors after dark	0.002	58

(continued on next page)

Table 1
(continued)

Vector	Disease	Location	Time of Biting	Indoors/Outdoors	Transmission Season	Recommendation	Incidence in Travelers[a]	References
4. Sandflies (Fig. 1D)	Leishmaniasis	SSA, SCA, CA, SA 90% of visceral leishmaniasis cases occur in India, Bangladesh, Nepal, Sudan, Ethiopia, and Brazil 90% of cutaneous leishmaniasis cases occur in Afghanistan, Algeria, Iran, Saudi Arabia, Syria, Brazil, Bolivia, Colombia, and Peru	Most species are active at dawn and dusk and during the night, but in forests and dark room they may also attack in the daytime	Most species feed outdoors but a few feed indoors	All year round	Use long clothing in areas where sandflies are common, because their short mouthparts cannot bite through clothes. Avoid sandfly bites, particularly after sunset, by using insect repellents containing DEET or PMD and by wearing long clothing. Sleep under insecticide-impregnated bed nets (small mesh) and in screened accommodation if possible	CA 64 SA 143 SSA 14 SCA 19	[1]
5. Blackflies (Fig. 1E)	River blindness	Mainly SSA (West Africa), also CA, SA, mountainous wet areas, and southern Yemen	Daytime	Outdoors	All times of the year but more common in long-term travelers >3 mo	Avoid areas where blackflies are active: near large and fast-flowing rivers. Wear long, light-colored clothing. Treat clothing with permethrin if habitat cannot be avoided.	2.3	[55]

6. Deer flies (**Fig. 1F**)	Loiasis	SSA (West and Central Africa) in rainforested areas	Daytime	Outdoors	All times of the year but especially the rainy season, and more common in long-term travelers	Avoid areas where deer flies are active: near muddy rivers. Deer flies are attracted to wood smoke so avoid campfires. Wear long clothing. Treat clothing with permethrin if habitat cannot be avoided.	1.5	55
7. Biting midges (**Fig. 1G**)	No disease, but severe nuisance	AU, NA, CA, EU Most northerly temperate regions	Crepuscular but, for most species, biting activity peaks in the early evening. Biting in the daytime if conditions are humid, still, and cloudy	Outdoors	Spring, summer, and autumn when adults are present	Avoid areas where midges are active: breeding grounds are acid, boggy soils, or coastal salt marsh. Use repellents of choice. Wear midge hoods. Wear long, light-colored clothing. Treat clothing with permethrin if habitat cannot be avoided.	—	—

(continued on next page)

Table 1
(continued)

Vector	Disease	Location	Time of Biting	Indoors/ Outdoors	Transmission Season	Recommendation	Incidence in Travelers[a]	References
8. Tsetse flies (**Fig. 1H**)	African sleeping sickness	SSA mainly Tanzania, Uganda, Malawi, and Zambia (East African form) Democratic Republic of Congo, Angola, Sudan, Central African Republic, Chad, and northern Uganda (West African form)	Daytime. East African tsetse prefers wooded thickets, and West African tsetse is found in forests and vegetation along streams	Outdoors	All times of year	Avoid wearing dark blue or black clothing. Keep car windows closed when traveling through areas of woodland. Wear long permethrin-treated clothing if outdoors in tsetse habitat.	0.06	1
9. Triatomine bugs (**Fig. 1I**)	Chagas disease	CA and SA, mainly Bolivia	Night	Indoors in rural forested areas, especially in poor housing (mud walls and thatched roofs)	All times of year	Sleep under insecticide-impregnated bed nets. Move the bed away from the wall.	13.5	57

Vector	Disease	Regions	Day or night	Indoors or outdoors	Time of year	Prevention	Per 1000[a]	Ref
10. Fleas (Fig. 1J)	Plague	SSA, SCA, NA	Day or night	Indoors or outdoors	All times of year	Avoid areas of high rodent density (primary host). Wear a repellent containing DEET and tuck trousers into socks to avoid bites around the ankles. Use an insecticide-treated bed net if sleeping in endemic areas.	<0.02	1
11. Hard ticks (Fig. 1K)	Tick-borne encephalitis	SCA, EU, SEA (China and Korea)	Day and night	Outdoors	Tropics: any time Temperate: spring and summer, although season extending because of climate change	Vaccine available in Europe and Canada, but not licensed for use in the United States.	0.00015	57
	Rickettsial diseases including spotted fevers and Q fever	SSA SCA, SEA, NA, EU,			—	Avoid areas where ticks are abundant: woody and bushy areas with high grass and leaf litter. Walk in the center of trails. Examine clothes and skin for ticks regularly (at least daily) and remove ticks with forceps. Wear long clothing and tuck clothing into boots.	56 (SSA) 10 (SCA) 16 (SEA)	1
	Tularemia Lyme borreliosis	SSA, NA, EU			—	Use repellent containing DEET or permethrin on clothing.	<0.02	1
Soft ticks	Relapsing fever, borreliosis	SSA, SCA, SEA, NA, EU			—		0.1	57
12. Chigger mites	Scrub typhus	SEA	Any time	Outdoors	All times of year	As for ticks	0.1	57

Abbreviations: AU, Australia; CA, Central America; CAR, Caribbean; EU, Europe; ME, Middle East; NA, North America; NAf, North Africa; SA, South America; SCA, south central Asia; SEA, southeast Asia; SSA, sub-Saharan Africa.
[a] Per 1000 with syndrome attending travel clinics on return.

malaria vectors are active but also during the day, when vectors of dengue are active. Those planning travel that involves walking in vegetated areas should use precautions to avoid tick bites.

MECHANISM OF BITING

The mouthparts of blood-feeding arthropods (insects and acarines) form feeding tubes that penetrate the skin and suck up blood. Mosquitoes and triatomine bugs are capillary feeders with feeding tubes that deeply penetrate the skin. Other arthropods, like sandflies and *Culicoides* midges, are known as pool feeders and have penetrating mouthparts that cut into the soft tissue. All have an arsenal of chemicals in their saliva that are injected into the host before uptake of blood and that serve to prevent blood coagulation, initiate digestion, and, in some cases, to anesthetize the local area. These chemicals act as allergens to the host and cause a skin reaction to bites (see the article by Rachael Morris-Jones and Steve Morris-Jones elsewhere in this issue). Vectors of disease transmit disease agents to vertebrate hosts via the mouthparts during feeding. Pathogens multiply in the arthropod host, with the infective stage traveling to the salivary glands where they are passed to the host in the saliva during feeding. The one exception to this is the triatomine bug, in which transmission of trypanosomes occurs through the insect feces via skin lesions caused by scratching.

MEANS OF BITE PREVENTION

The World Health Organization (WHO) has recommended that all travelers to disease-endemic areas should minimize exposure to insect bites by selecting a combination of personal protection methods including insect repellents, mosquito nets, mosquito coils, aerosol sprays, protective clothing, screening, and air-conditioning (**Box 1**).[4] The methods described in **Box 1** have been deemed safe for use by children and pregnant and lactating women although research is ongoing for pyrethroid treated clothing. The effectiveness of all these methods depends on their appropriate usage and users' continued compliance.[5]

Topical or Skin Repellents

Skin-applied repellents are one of the most common and effective ways of preventing insect bites and are often considered as the first line of defense against vectors of disease. Although the benefits of using topically applied repellents as a personal protection measure have been accepted for decades, the evidence base for reducing disease transmission is only now being recognized. For example, it has been shown in a clinical trial in the Bolivian rainforest that the use of the skin repellent *p*-menthane-3,8-diol (PMD) from lemon eucalyptus (see **Box 1**) can reduce malaria transmission.[6] Further investigations are taking place to determine whether the use of repellents can control dengue fever, which is vectored by day-biting *Stegomyia* mosquitoes, when bed nets are of little use. A detailed review regarding the evidence base of repellents is provided by Goodyer and colleagues[7] (2010).

There are many commercially available repellent products that contain several different active ingredients (AIs). Some repellents are synthetic in origin and these tend to be more effective than their natural counterparts that, with the exception of PMD, usually require frequent reapplication. Topically applied repellents come in many different forms including sprays, lotions, creams, sticks, wipes, roll-ons, and sun care products. Despite the many different products available, the AIs are few and it is important to advise purchasers of the correct active ingredient and the appropriate strength for different arthropod pests.

Box 1
Means of bite prevention

Topical or skin repellents

The most commonly used means of preventing bites by arthropods consist of the application of lotions, oils, creams, and wipes to the skin. The active ingredients (AI) slowly evaporate because of body heat and release molecules that either cause the arthropods to move away or prevent them from feeding. The 3 most highly recommended repellents for disease prevention are the synthetic repellent *N,N*-dimethyl-*m*-toluamide (DEET), an amide developed in the 1950s in the United States; the plant-derived terpene repellent *p*-menthane-3,8-diol (PMD) from lemon eucalyptus and the piperidine Icaradin, an effective synthetic alternative to DEET that is not a plasticizing agent. Of other repellents, the synthetic amide compound, ethyl butylacetylaminopropionate (IR3535), shows excellent repellent activity with evidence increasing to show good protection against several vectors of disease. The essential oil of citronella (*Cymbopogon nardus*), a botanic repellent, shows protection times of less than 2 hours without careful formulation, because of its high volatility, and is therefore not recommended for disease-endemic areas.

Pyrethroid-treated clothing

There is strong evidence from numerous authorities and reports of expert committees supporting the use of impregnated insecticides (permethrin) on clothing as an important method of personal protection against arthropod bites from all disease vectors. When used according to instructions, permethrin-treated clothing presents no risk to health. There is limited evidence that wearing untreated long clothing is also protective against malaria in travelers and should be recommended because it carries no risks.

Bed nets

Mosquito nets can be made from cotton, polyethylene, polyester, or nylon hung over a bed to prevent bites from arthropods at night. A mesh size of 1.2 mm stops mosquitoes, and smaller mesh, such as 0.6 mm, stops other biting insects such as midges and sandflies. Intact bed nets treated with insecticide prevent almost 100% of mosquito bites. It is recommended that travelers use polyethylene bed nets pretreated with pyrethroid insecticide, because these are the most hardwearing and most highly protective nets.

Spatial or area repellents and aerosols

These are insecticides that are evaporated through gentle heat using a mosquito coil or a vaporizer mat, or sprayed into a space using an aerosol. There is consistent evidence that insecticide vaporizers prevent insect bites. Because mosquito coils generate smoke, to prevent chest complaints it is recommended that mosquito coils are used only outdoors. The most effective and safe molecules for spatial protection from mosquitoes and sandflies include metofluthrin (<0.01%), transfluthrin (<0.05%), D-allethrin (<2%), prallethrin (<0.2%), and esbiothrin (<1%). Coils containing DDT and lindane, which are often on sale in low-income to middle-income countries, should be avoided.

Sleeping in screened rooms

There is good evidence that sleeping in screened accommodation (which includes air-conditioned rooms) prevents exposure to vectors of malaria, filariasis, leishmaniasis, and dengue. Wherever possible, travelers should sleep in improved accommodation and use insect knock-down sprays to clear rooms after windows have been open, to avoid many vector-borne diseases.

There is now robust scientific evidence to support claims of high levels of efficacy for 3 main AIs and, for a fourth (ethyl butylacetylaminopropionate [IR3535]), evidence is accumulating for use in disease-endemic countries.

1. *N,N*-dimethyl-*m*-toluamide (DEET)
2. 2-(2-Hydrocyethyl)-piperidinecarboxylic acid 1-methyl ester (Icaridin)

3. PMD
4. IR3535

Other repellents, including those based on plant essential oils, are generally not as effective as those mentioned earlier and can therefore not be recommended for use in disease-endemic areas.

DEET

On the strength of available evidence, DEET (chemical name N,N-diethyl-3-methylbenzamide, Chemical Abstracts Service [CAS] no. 134-62-3) is the first-line choice recommended for disease prevention in concentrations between 20% and 50%, and is safe for use on children more than 6 months old and in pregnant and lactating women.[7] It is classified as toxicity category IV (practically nontoxic) for acute inhalation toxicity and primary dermal irritation and toxicity category III (slightly toxic) for acute oral, acute dermal, and primary eye irritation.[8]

DEET is the best-studied and most widely used active ingredient and there is good reason for this. Countless studies have proved that this compound can provide high levels of protection over long periods of time, and it is recommended by the WHO as the gold standard against which to compare new repellent products.[9] DEET has a broad spectrum of activity and protects against Stegomyia, Anopheles, and Culex mosquitoes, although reapplication rates need to be greater for Anopheles mosquitoes.[10] Its efficacy, in terms of longevity, is dose dependent, with higher concentrations lasting longer than lower concentrations. Efficacy also depends on formulation, with some DEET microencapsulated formulations lasting up to 8 to 12 hours.[11] Efficacy decreases at higher doses, and 50% is the recommended dose for malarial areas.

DEET has also been tested for protection against other arthropods including Culicoides biting midges, bed bugs, and ticks; however, the levels of protection against these arthropods is not always clear. For example, studies on some DEET formulations revealed minimal protection against ticks. However, a more recent study using 33% DEET extended-duration formulation showed adequate protection for up to 12 hours.[12]

Icaridin

Icaridin (formerly picaridin; trade name Bayrepel, Saltadin; development reference code KBR 3023; chemical name 2-(2-hydroxyethyl)-piperidinecarboxylic acid 1-methyl ester; CAS no. 119515-38-7) was developed as an alternative to DEET and is more pleasing in odor and feel. It needs to be used at 20% or reapplied frequently to get protection similar to that provided by DEET. However, it is often sold in low concentrations requiring frequent reapplication. It is classified as toxicity category IV (practically nontoxic) for acute inhalation toxicity and primary dermal irritation, and toxicity category III (slightly toxic) for acute oral, acute dermal, and primary eye irritation.[13]

Icaridin at 20% has similar levels of protection as 20% DEET against Anopheles and culicine mosquitoes. Although data are limited to a few field trials, the evidence for efficacy against African malaria mosquitoes shows excellent protection, similar to that of DEET over 10 hours.[14] Low levels of protection were seen against ticks using 20% lotions,[15] whereas, in another study, 20% Icaridin lotion gave high levels of protection for up to 12 hours in simulated field-contact conditions against Amblyomma.[12]

PMD

A plant-based insect repellent derived from lemon eucalyptus, PMD (CAS no. 42822-86-6 at 30% is a repellent of equal efficacy and longevity as DEET for Stegomyia, Anopheles, Culex, and Ochlerotatus mosquitoes,[16] as well as ticks, stable flies, and biting midges.[17] It may be used on children more than 6 months old. PMD is the only plant-based repellent that has been advocated for use in disease-endemic areas by the Centers for Disease Control and Prevention, because of its proven clinical efficacy to prevent malaria transmission,[6] and it is considered to pose no risk to human health provided it is used according to the instructions on the label.[18] It has a strong fresh-lemon scent and does not possess the plasticizing properties of DEET, which makes it more desirable to users. It may, therefore, be recommended at concentrations of greater than 20% PMD (60% Citriodiol) as a repellent for use in disease-endemic areas.

IR3535
For IR3535 (chemical name 3-[N-butyl-N-acetyl]-aminopropionic acid, ethyl ester) the evidence for effectiveness against Anopheles is incomplete, consisting of a few field trials and laboratory studies.[7] However, it is approved by the WHO Pesticide Evaluation Scheme and commercially available in the United States, but IR3535 should not be recommended for use in malaria-endemic regions.

Other repellents
There are other natural AIs used in repellent products. Extracts of neem, citronella, thyme, geraniol, peppermint, patchouli, and clove tend to provide low levels of protection or require frequent reapplication and can irritate the skin when used in high concentrations.[19] Oils, or compounds derived from oils, such as Skin So Soft bath oil, act by providing a physical barrier to landing and feeding on the skin.[20]

Impregnated Clothing
There are several clothing products available to travelers that are impregnated with an insecticide rather than a repellent. Protective clothes are usually impregnated with permethrin, which is one of the most repellent of the pyrethroid insecticides. The repellent and insect-irritant properties of insecticides at very low concentrations are essential in these personal protection strategies.[21] Insecticide is absorbed through the skin when using impregnated clothing and, although this is less than the no-observed-effect level,[22] impregnated clothing use is still being researched for pregnant women and children.

Evidence for efficacy
There is good evidence for the protective effect of treated clothing and it is recommended by WHO as a means of personal protection for travelers.[4] Permethrin-treated clothing is effective against a variety of biting arthropods including Stegomyia, Anopheles, and Culex mosquitoes[23–25]; chigger mites[26,27]; ticks[28–30]; tsetse flies, body lice[31]; and sandflies.[32,33]

For disease control, the picture is unclear. A significant impact on disease transmission has been shown in some studies. A randomized controlled trial of 172 Colombian soldiers patrolling a malaria-endemic area for a mean of 4.2 weeks found that permethrin-impregnated uniforms significantly reduced the incidence of malaria and cutaneous leishmaniasis by 75% compared with nonimpregnated uniforms.[32] For malaria control, the potential of using impregnated clothing and bedding was shown in Pakistan[23] and Kenya.[34] However, other studies have shown impregnated clothing to have no effect.[35]

AI and application methods
Permethrin, a natural pyrethroid, is one of the most commonly used AIs in impregnated clothing because of its proven efficacy, persistence, low toxicity to users, and lack of irritancy to wearers of treated garments.[26]

Other chemicals that have been used for impregnation of materials include dibutyl phthalate, which can be effective against chiggers[27]; bifenthrin, which has been shown to protect against *Anopheles* and *Aedes* mosquitoes; organophosphates such as pirimiphos[21] and *N,N*-diethyl phenylacetamide[36]; and pyrethroids such as deltamethrin, λ-cyhalothrin, α-cypermethrin, cyfluthrin, and etofenprox (WHO Web site, 2010). Studies have shown that impregnated clothing worn alongside a topically applied repellent, such as DEET, can provide better protection than impregnated clothing or repellent alone.[21,37–39]

There is some concern over the safety of using impregnated clothing. For example, impregnated garments worn by Desert Storm personnel are implicated in causing Gulf War syndrome. However, the evidence for adverse effects is sparse. Most studies have shown that maximum permethrin uptake from impregnated clothing is less than the acceptable daily intake (ADI) and therefore health impairments are unlikely.[22,40,41]

Mosquito Nets

Mosquito nets provide a physical means of preventing contact with night-biting insects provided the net has a sufficiently small mesh size: 1.2-mm mesh prevents mosquitoes from passing through, and a smaller mesh size, such as 0.6 mm, is effective against other biting insects such as sandflies. Travelers to high-risk areas for leishmaniasis should be advised to use small-mesh nets that are more protective[42] than conventional nets[43] against leishmaniasis, as shown from clinical trials, even though conventional nets with larger mesh size are preferred because they maximize air circulation. There is evidence that the use of insecticide-treated bed nets is protective against malaria among residents of malarious areas[44,45] and should be strongly recommended for all travelers to the rural tropics. It is important that bed nets are used correctly and are well maintained, because torn or holed nets offer significantly reduced protection. However, even torn nets retain excellent protective efficacy when treated with a pyrethroid insecticide because these compounds prevent insects from feeding even when the nets are damaged.[46] The best nets are those that are termed long-lasting insecticide-treated nets (LLINs). Those with full WHO recommendation are Permanet 2.0 (Vestergaard), Olyset (Sumitomo), and Interceptor (BASF).[47] These are available in most tropical countries. All are durable and have insecticide incorporated into the fibers that remains effective for 3 years after purchase.[48] It is recommended that LLINs be purchased, although well-maintained, untreated nets provide equivalent protection to treated nets.[49] Therefore, if treated nets are unavailable, it is recommended that travelers frequently check their untreated nets for holes and repair them using a needle and thread. Mosquito nets may be made from cotton, polyethylene, polyester, or nylon, although polyethylene nets are the most durable and provide the most reliable protection.

Coils, Vaporizers, Spatial Repellents

Insecticide vapor is useful to prevent insect bites, especially in areas where vectors and nuisance insects are active outside sleeping hours. Several methods are used to release the insecticide: using gentle heat from mosquito coils through burning, through a heating device that plugs into the wall for vaporizing mats and liquid vaporizers, or through air movement from ambient emanators. Insecticides of the pyrethroid group have been approved for use in this format because they have low mammalian toxicity. The evidence that spatial repellents prevent disease is less strong than that for bed nets or topical repellents.[35] However, they may be recommended because of the strong demonstration of their efficacy at reducing insect bites against mosquito vectors of malaria, filariasis, and dengue,[50] and sandfly vectors of leishmaniasis[51]; in addition, an unpublished randomized controlled trial of transfluthrin mosquito coils showed a clinical reduction in malaria episodes among users of the coils.[52] Travelers are advised only to use mosquito coils outdoors or in well-ventilated rooms to avoid chest problems[53] and to purchase vaporizing mats and liquid vaporizers before travel to ensure that they are using approved insecticides dispensed from safe electrical evaporating devices.

DEBUNKING THE MYTHS ON BITE PREVENTION

There is anecdotal evidence that food can affect a person's attraction to biting insects. There is no doubt that personal smell is affected by certain foods. For example, even the human olfactory system, which is inferior to that of insects, can detect someone who has eaten garlic the night before. Because the main way that insects find humans is through their sense of smell, it is plausible that an alteration in body odor may make humans unappealing. However, the key questions are whether insects detect the chemicals that change in body odor as a result of eating such foods, and whether these chemicals elicit repellent or attractant behavioral effects in the insects? It would be appealing to gain protection from insects by eating a certain type of food; however, the scientific evidence to support this is lacking.

One of the most common anecdotes is that vitamin B complex supplements protect against biting insects, and some early studies suggested that they may have a small effect. Recent, scientifically robust evidence has revealed that vitamin B has no effect on mosquito biting rates,[54] and the taking of vitamin B should not be suggested as a bite prevention measure even though many pharmacists who give travel advice still recommend its use to protect against mosquito bites.

Other anecdotal remedies include the taking of garlic, marmite, vegemite, brewer's yeast tablets, blood pressure medication, and alcohol. However, there is no robust scientific evidence that any of these prevent mosquito bites and none of these purported remedies should ever be recommended as a method of bite protection, especially in disease-endemic countries.

SUMMARY

It is recommended that highly effective repellents only should be used when traveling to vector-borne disease–endemic countries. The most reliable repellents include those that contain the active ingredient DEET (20%–50%), followed by Icaridin (20%), and PMD (30%), and these are broadly effective. Consumers should look at the AI and dosage before buying, and also the vectors they wish to be protected from, because different AIs are effective against different vectors. They should also follow the instructions on application rates and the simple rules listed later, but sweating, swimming, and rubbing can remove the repellent and frequent reapplication is necessary to ensure continuous levels of protection. There are several useful factors that can affect the efficacy of any repellent product and these should be taken into consideration when giving advice to travelers.[7]

- Concentration: the greater the concentration, the longer the efficacy, although this tends to plateau at around 50% for DEET.
- Application: travelers tend to apply low doses onto their skin, probably lower than those recommended by manufacturers, so there is a need for adequate and frequent reapplication.
- Exercise: sweat can wash off the repellent.
- Weather: rain can wash the repellent off the skin. Wind and high temperatures increase evaporation and reduce longevity of repellents.

- Attractiveness: people differ in their level of attractiveness to biting insects and therefore repellents have different levels of protection for different users. Users should reapply repellents when they notice that insects have resumed biting, because labels are only a guideline.
- Biting density: the more mosquitoes there are, the greater chance of being bitten, so greater vigilance is needed.

It is recommended that consumers avoid using natural remedies, such as vitamin B and garlic, as well as repellents based on essential oils of plants (with the exception of PMD) when in countries with high risk of vector-borne disease. However, in regions where there is no risk of disease, such as certain parts of Europe where insects are simply a nuisance, and where the user does not show adverse reaction to bites, it might be acceptable for consumers to use whatever product they think works best for them, when safe to do so.

A strong evidential basis exists for the use of insecticide-treated bed nets for protection against vectors of disease and these are to be recommended as essential tools to travelers visiting disease-endemic areas. Permethrin-treated clothing, another scientifically proven method of bite control, should be considered in areas of high risk of disease transmission. Of the other methods, coils are effective and may help to reduce the risk of malaria; however, care must be taken on their use. Insecticide vaporizers and essential oil candles may help to reduce nuisance biting but there is little evidence to support prevention of disease. Overall, travelers should be encouraged to take seriously methods of bite protection as a means of preventing disease.

ACKNOWLEDGMENTS

SJM is supported by The Bill & Melinda Gates Foundation award 51431.The authors thank Graham Hickling for allowing us to use his image of a tick.

REFERENCES

1. Freedman DO, Weld LH, Kozarsky PE, et al. Spectrum of disease and relation to place of exposure among ill returned travelers. N Engl J Med 2006;354:119–30.
2. Powers AM. Overview of emerging arboviruses. Future Virol 2009;4(4):391–401.
3. Chen LH, Wilson ME, Davis X, et al. Illness in long-term travelers visiting GeoSentinel clinics. Emerg Infect Dis 2009;15(11):1773–82.
4. WHO. International travel and health. Geneva (Switzerland): World Health Organization; 2011. Available at: http://www.who.int/ith/chapters/en/index.html. Accessed November 15, 2011.
5. Sagui E, Resseguier N, Machault V, et al. Determinants of compliance with antivectorial protective measures among non-immune travellers during missions to tropical Africa. Malar J 2011;10(32). http://dx.doi.org/10.1186/1475-2875-1110-1232.
6. Hill N, Lenglet A, Arnez AM, et al. Randomised, double-blind control trial of p-menthane diol repellent against malaria in Bolivia. BMJ 2007;335:1023.
7. Goodyer LI, Croft AM, Frances SP, et al. Expert review of the evidence base for arthropod bite avoidance. J Travel Med 2010;17(3):182–92.
8. EPA. Reregistration eligibility decision RED DEET. 1998. Available at: http://www.epa.gov/oppsrrd1/REDs/0002red.pdf. Accessed November 15, 2011.
9. WHOPES. Guidelines for efficacy testing of mosquito repellents for human skin WHO/HTM/NTD/WHOPES/2009.4. Available at: http://whqlibdoc.who.int/hq/2009/WHO_HTM_NTD_WHOPES_2009.4_eng.pdf. 2009. Accessed September 2, 2011.

10. Frances SP, Waterson DG, Beebe NW, et al. Field evaluation of repellent formulations containing DEET and picaridin against mosquitoes in Northern Territory, Australia. J Med Entomol 2004;41(3):414–7.

11. Rutledge LC, Gupta RK, Mehr ZA, et al. Evaluation of controlled-release mosquito repellent formulations. J Am Mosq Control Assoc 1996;12(1):39–44.

12. Carroll JF, Benante JP, Klun JA, et al. Twelve-hour duration testing of cream formulations of three repellents against Amblyomma americanum. Med Vet Entomol 2008;22(2):144–51.

13. EPA. New pesticide fact sheet. Picaridin. Washington, DC: United States Environmental Protection Agency: Prevention, Pesticides and Toxic Substances; 2005.

14. Costantini C, Badolo A, Ilboudo-Sanogo E. Field evaluation of the efficacy and persistence of insect repellents DEET, IR3535, and KBR 3023 against Anopheles gambiae complex and other Afrotropical vector mosquitoes. Trans R Soc Trop Med Hyg 2004;98(11):644–52.

15. Pretorius AM, Jensenius M, Clarke F, et al. Repellent efficacy of DEET and KBR 3023 against Amblyomma hebraeum (Acari: Ixodidae). J Med Entomol 2003; 40(2):245–8.

16. Carroll SP, Loye J. PMD, a registered botanical mosquito repellent with DEET-like efficacy. J Am Mosq Control Assoc 2006;22(3):507–14.

17. Trigg JK, Hill N. Laboratory evaluation of a eucalyptus-based repellent against four biting arthropods. Phytother Res 1996;10(4):313–6.

18. EPA. Menthane-3,8-diol (011550) Biopesticide registration eligibility document. 1998. Available at: http://www.epa.gov/oppbppd1/biopesticides/ingredients/tech_docs/tech_011550.htm. Accessed August 20, 2011.

19. Maia MF, Moore SJ. Plant-based insect repellents: a review of their efficacy, development and testing. Malar J 2011;10(Suppl 1):S11.

20. Magnon GJ, Robert LL, Kline DL, et al. Repellency of two DEET formulations and Avon Skin-So-Soft against biting midges (Diptera: Ceratopogonidae) in Honduras. J Am Mosq Control Assoc 1991;7(1):80–2.

21. Pennetier C, Chabi J, Martin T, et al. New protective battle-dress impregnated against mosquito vector bites. Parasit Vectors 2010;3:81.

22. Rossbach B, Appel KE, Mross KG, et al. Uptake of permethrin from impregnated clothing. Toxicol Lett 2010;192(1):50–5.

23. Rowland M, Durrani N, Hewitt S, et al. Permethrin-treated chaddars and top-sheets: appropriate technology for protection against malaria in Afghanistan and other complex emergencies. Trans R Soc Trop Med Hyg 1999;93(5):465–72.

24. Sholdt LL, Schreck CE, Qureshi A, et al. Field bioassays of permethrin-treated uniforms and a new extended duration repellent against mosquitoes in Pakistan. J Am Mosq Control Assoc 1988;4(3):233–6.

25. Schreck CE, Kline DL. Personal protection afforded by controlled-release topical repellents and permethrin-treated clothing against natural populations of Aedes taeniorhynchus. J Am Mosq Control Assoc 1989;5(1):77–80.

26. Breeden GC, Schreck CE, Sorensen AL. Permethrin as a clothing treatment for personal protection against chigger mites (Acarina: Trombiculidae). Am J Trop Med Hyg 1982;31(3 Pt 1):589–92.

27. Frances SP, Yeo AE, Brooke EW, et al. Clothing impregnations of dibutylphthalate and permethrin as protectants against a chigger mite, Eutrombicula hirsti (Acari: Trombiculidae). J Med Entomol 1992;29(6):907–10.

28. Evans SR, Korch GW Jr, Lawson MA. Comparative field evaluation of permethrin and DEET-treated military uniforms for personal protection against ticks (Acari). J Med Entomol 1990;27(5):829–34.

29. Deblinger RD, Rimmer DW. Efficacy of a permethrin-based acaricide to reduce the abundance of *Ixodes dammini* (Acari: Ixodidae). J Med Entomol 1991; 28(5):708–11.

30. Vaughn MF, Meshnick SR. Pilot study assessing the effectiveness of long-lasting permethrin-impregnated clothing for the prevention of tick bites. Vector Borne Zoonotic Dis 2011;11(7):869–75.

31. Sholdt LL, Rogers EJ Jr, Gerberg EJ, et al. Effectiveness of permethrin-treated military uniform fabric against human body lice. Mil Med 1989; 154(2):90–3.

32. Soto J, Medina F, Dember N, et al. Efficacy of permethrin-impregnated uniforms in the prevention of malaria and leishmaniasis in Colombian soldiers. Clin Infect Dis 1995;21(3):599–602.

33. Fryauff DJ, Shoukry MA, Hanafi HA, et al. Contact toxicity of permethrin-impregnated military uniforms to *Culex pipiens* (Diptera: Culicidae) and *Phlebotomus papatasi* (Diptera: Psychodidae): effects of laundering and time of exposure. J Am Mosq Control Assoc 1996;12(1):84–90.

34. Kimani EW, Vulule JM, Kuria IW, et al. Use of insecticide-treated clothes for personal protection against malaria: a community trial. Malar J 2006;5:63.

35. Croft A. Malaria prevention in travellers. Clin Evid 2010;7(903):1–34.

36. Rao KM, Prakash S, Kumar S, et al. *N,N*-diethylphenylacetamide in treated fabrics as a repellent against *Aedes aegypti* and *Culex quinquefasciatus* (Diptera: Culicidae). J Med Entomol 1991;28(1):142–6.

37. Gupta RK, Sweeney AW, Rutledge LC, et al. Effectiveness of controlled-release personal-use arthropod repellents and permethrin-impregnated clothing in the field. J Am Mosq Control Assoc 1987;3(4):556–60.

38. Schreck CE, Haile DG, Kline DL. The effectiveness of permethrin and DEET, alone or in combination, for protection against *Aedes taeniorhynchus*. Am J Trop Med Hyg 1984;33(4):725–30.

39. Harbach RE, Tang DB, Wirtz RA, et al. Relative repellency of two formulations of *N,N*-diethyl-3-methylbenzamide (DEET) and permethrin-treated clothing against *Culex sitiens* and *Aedes vigilax* in Thailand. J Am Mosq Control Assoc 1990; 6(4):641–4.

40. Snodgrass HL. Permethrin transfer from treated cloth to the skin surface: potential for exposure in humans. J Toxicol Environ Health 1992;35(2):91–105.

41. Appel KE, Gundert-Remy U, Fischer H, et al. Risk assessment of Bundeswehr (German Federal Armed Forces) permethrin-impregnated battle dress uniforms (BDU). Int J Hyg Environ Health 2008;211(1–2):88–104.

42. Ritmeijer K, Davies C, van Zorge R, et al. Evaluation of a mass distribution programme for fine-mesh impregnated bednets against visceral leishmaniasis in eastern Sudan. Trop Med Int Health 2007;12(3):404–14.

43. Picado A, Singh SP, Rijal S, et al. Longlasting insecticidal nets for prevention of *Leishmania donovani* infection in India and Nepal: paired cluster randomised trial. BMJ 2010;341:c6760.

44. Lengeler C. Insecticide-treated bednets and curtains for preventing malaria. Cochrane Database Syst Rev 2004;(2):CD000363.

45. Lim SS, Fullman N, Stokes A, et al. Net benefits: a multicountry analysis of observational data examining associations between insecticide-treated mosquito nets and health outcomes. PLoS Med 2011;8(9):e1001091.

46. Corbel V, Chandre F, Brengues C, et al. Dosage-dependent effects of permethrin-treated nets on the behaviour of *Anopheles gambiae* and the selection of pyrethroid resistance. Malar J 2004;3(1):22.

47. WHO. WHO recommended long-lasting insecticidal mosquito nets. Updated July 2011. 2009. Available at: http://www.who.int/entity/whopes/Long_lasting_insecticidal_nets_Jul_2011.pdf. Accessed November 11, 2011.
48. WHO. Guidelines for monitoring the durability of long-lasting insecticidal mosquito nets under operational conditions. Geneva (Switzerland): World Health Organization; 2011.
49. Clarke SE, Bogh C, Brown RC, et al. Do untreated bednets protect against malaria? Trans R Soc Trop Med Hyg 2001;95(5):457–62.
50. Lawrance CE, Croft AM. Do mosquito coils prevent malaria? A systematic review of trials. J Travel Med 2004;11(2):92–6.
51. Alten B, Caglar SS, Simsek FM, et al. Field evaluation of an area repellent system (Thermacell) against *Phlebotomus papatasi* (Diptera: Psychodidae) and *Ochlerotatus caspius* (Diptera: Culicidae) in Sanliurfa Province, Turkey. J Med Entomol 2003;40(6):930–4.
52. Hill N. Clinical evaluation of plant-based insect repellents against malaria in the Bolivian Amazon and coils in China. Paper presented at: XXIII International Congress of Entomology. Durban, July 6–12, 2008.
53. Tang L, Lim WY, Eng P, et al. Lung cancer in Chinese women: evidence for an interaction between tobacco smoking and exposure to inhalants in the indoor environment. Environ Health Perspect 2010;118(9):1257–60.
54. Ives AR, Paskewitz SM. Testing vitamin B as a home remedy against mosquitoes. J Am Mosq Control Assoc 2005;21(2):213–7.
55. Lipner EM, Law MA, Barnett E, et al. Filariasis in travelers presenting to the GeoSentinel surveillance network. PLoS Negl Trop Dis 2007;1:e88. http://dx.doi.org/10.1371/journal.pntd.0000088.
56. Beeching NJ, Fletcher TE, Hill DR, et al. Travellers and viral haemorrhagic fevers: what are the risks? Int J Antimicrob Agents 2010;36S:S26–35.
57. Field V, Gautret P, Schlagenhauf P, et al. Travel and migration associated infectious diseases morbidity in Europe, 2008. BMC Infect Dis 2010;10:330.
58. CDC. West Nile virus disease and other arboviral diseases–United States, 2010. MMWR Morb Mortal Wkly Rep 2011;60:1009–13.

Travel-Associated Skin Disease

Rachael Morris-Jones, FRCP, PhD, PCME[a],*,
Stephen Morris-Jones, MRCP, FRCPath, DTM&H[b]

KEYWORDS

- Skin • Infection • Rash • Tropical • Bite • Sting

KEY POINTS

- Taking a thorough travel history is essential to making an accurate and rapid diagnosis in travel related skin disease.
- Widespread rashes usually represent endogenous disease whereas localised skin lesions usually result from exogenous assault from bites/stings/trauma or portal of entry for infection.
- Widespread travel associated rashes with fever are usually investigated through serology whereas localised lesions are usually investigated through skin biopsy for culture/PCR and histopathology.

INTRODUCTION

Skin abnormalities are one of the commonest reasons for travelers to seek medical attention on their return home. Such cutaneous manifestations may represent a spectrum of disease from localized infections, penetrating injuries, bites or stings from insects or an animal, or be a marker of an underlying systemic disease acquired while traveling. Sound knowledge of the geographic distribution and epidemiology of infectious diseases may be invaluable in focusing the list of differentials and leading to a clinical diagnosis; however, sometimes skin biopsies for histology, mycobacterial/ bacterial, and fungal cultures may be required to provide a definitive diagnosis. A logical approach by health care practitioners ensures rapid as well as accurate diagnosis and provides optimal management of patients with travel-related skin disease, which is best achieved through comprehensive clinical history taking, thorough examination of physical signs, and focused investigations.

When assessing a patient with a cutaneous disease, which develops after travel, essential questions should ascertain where the patient has been (both country and region), whether the setting was rural or urban, the type of accommodation used (luxury or budget hotels, bush-camping), and any activities undertaken that might have led to

No conflicts of interest and no financial support from outside organizations declared.
[a] Dermatology Department, Kings College Hospital, Kings College London, Normanby Building, London SE5 9RS, UK; [b] Department of Clinical Microbiology, University College London Hospitals, 65 Whitfield Street, London W1 T 4EU, UK
* Corresponding author.
E-mail address: Rachael.morris-jones@nhs.net

Infect Dis Clin N Am 26 (2012) 675–689
http://dx.doi.org/10.1016/j.idc.2012.05.010
0891-5520/12/$ – see front matter © 2012 Elsevier Inc. All rights reserved.

id.theclinics.com

the direct exposure of the skin to infectious agents (fresh/seawater, animal contact, etc). Similarly, travel may provide opportunities for new sexual encounters, with associated risks for infections with both local and systemic manifestations. Other important clues may be gained by establishing when the skin changes appeared, while away or on return, and whether the lesions are fixed or fluctuating, deteriorating or improving? Is there recollection of any skin trauma, bites or stings, and were others affected similarly? Have any treatments been used, and if so did they help? The most important pointers are presence or absence of systemic symptoms, and the nature of skin abnormalities, focal or generalized. Any investigations indicated depends on the patient's clinical history and signs; however, skin biopsies for histology and culture are usually needed for localized lesions/nodules/ulcers, whereas for diffuse rashes serologic investigations are more frequently indicated to confirm the underlying systemic diagnosis.

The global epidemiology of travelers' infections is described in more detail elsewhere in this issue; keeping up to date with ongoing infectious disease alerts worldwide ensures a heightened awareness of trends in disease prevalence. At present, the most common cutaneous manifestations in travelers (in descending order) are cutaneous larva migrans, insect bites, skin abscesses, infected insect bite reactions, allergic rashes, dog bites, superficial fungal infections, dengue, cutaneous leishmaniasis, rickettsial spotted fevers, and scabies.[1] This article describes typical presentations and management of some of these most common skin diseases, predominantly of infectious origin, that are acquired while traveling. Rare cutaneous manifestations of parasitic infections and other potentially travel related global infections such as meningococcemia are not discussed in this chapter.

LOCALIZED SKIN DISEASE
Insect Bite Reactions

Insects that bite are present worldwide, each with their own unique habitat and preferred species of animal host that may include humans. Most common insects that bite include mosquitoes, fleas, bed bugs, midges, tsetse, and sand flies. Some individuals seem to be more susceptible to insect bites, and some to severe allergic bite reactions. Skin reactions result from chemical/immunologic assault on the skin by the saliva injected when a blood meal is taken. Only a small number of insects that bite humans also transmit infectious diseases, some of which can result in more prolonged cutaneous reactions. Chapter 8 provides more details on insect bites and their prevention.

Clinical history

Most individuals affected by bites are usually unaware of the bite event. The notable exceptions include the bites of the tsetse fly or midges, which are painful and therefore usually recalled. Useful markers in the clinical history that point to insect bite reactions include travel abroad to rural areas, camping, contact or close association with animals, several members of a group being affected, and intense itching of the resultant lesions. Some patients develop severe allergies to insect bite reactions with rapid swelling from local histamine release in their skin. Most bite reactions usually last a few days to weeks. Current trends in travel dermatology demonstrate a high frequency of severe reactions to mosquito bite (**Fig. 1**), attributed in part to the northward geographic spread of the mosquito *Aedes albopictus* into Europe.[2]

Examination

Exposed skin is generally most vulnerable to insect bites, especially the ankles, feet and wrists. Bites from flying insects are clustered on the skin, whereas bites from crawling insects exhibit a linear pattern (**Fig. 2**). The morphology of individual bites

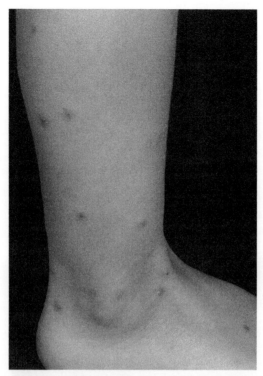

Fig. 1. Mosquito bite reactions on the lower leg showing urticated papules and vesicles with associated erythema and crusting.

is highly variable, but characteristically they have a central erythematous urticated papule/nodule/vesicle with a paler erythematous halo surrounding it. Diameters of bite reaction are usually less than 1 cm but can reach up to 5 cm in severe reactions. Excoriations are frequently seen around these intensely pruritic lesions.

Investigations

These are usually not required because the diagnosis is made based on the clinical history and signs. If the diagnosis is inconclusive then a skin biopsy of the affected skin for histopathological analysis, characteristically showing marked epidermal spongiosis and an acute inflammatory response with lymphocytes and eosinophils in the dermis and periadnexal structures. Consideration should be made of possible transmission of underlying infection such as malaria, dengue fever, and chikungunya.

Management

Oral antihistamines and application of a potent topical steroid, such as betamethasone ointment (Betnovate, GlaxoSmithKline), twice daily to the affected skin are involved in management. To remove secondary colonization or infection of staphylococci, a cleansing wash with dilute chlorhexidine should be used daily. Oral antistaphylococcal agents are rarely required. Most insect bite reactions should settle within a few weeks. Future bites should be prevented using insect repellents, insecticides, clothing, bed nets, and so forth.

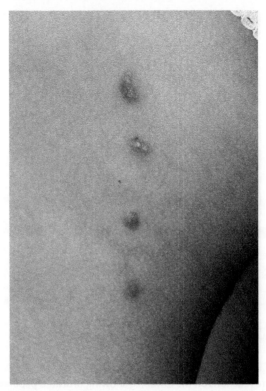

Fig. 2. Linear distribution of erythematous papular insect bites up the posterior thigh caused by a crawling insect.

Tsetse Fly Bites

Tsetse flies are large horseflylike insects found in riverine Western and savannah central and Eastern Africa. Feeding on humans as well as domestic and large wild animals, these flies are medically important for transmitting the protozoan *Trypanosoma brucei sp*, the causative agent of African trypanosomiasis. Although uncommon, there are increasingly frequent reports of African trypanosomiasis reflect the rising popularity of African game park safaris and the consequent exposure of tourists to these insects. Infected bites develop into a characteristic chancre—a relatively painless area of induration and often with marked edema associated with regional lymphadenopathy. Because of the significant mortality rate associated with the consequent systemic spread of trypanosomes into the bloodstream and cerebrospinal fluid, appropriate expert management is required as an emergency.

Abscesses

The ability to maintain adequate skin hygiene is often compromised by budget travelers, and minor skin infections, often secondary to insect bites or apparently insignificant trauma, are frequently reported. More recently, however, increasing numbers of individuals are presenting with severe, multiple, and recurrent skin abscesses that develop after travel (**Fig. 3**). The increased clinical virulence of these infections has been attributed to the acquisition of strains of *Staphylococcus aureus* that carry a gene encoding the Panton-Valentine leucocidin (P-VL) toxin.[3] Patients with

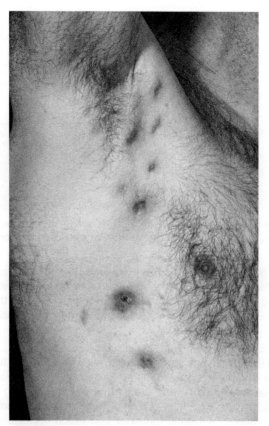

Fig. 3. Multiple necrotic abscesses on the trunk secondary to Panton-Valentine leukocidin toxin producing *Staphylococcus aureus*.

P-VL-positive staphylococcal infections can be managed by incision and drainage, but many only respond to additional prolonged oral antimicrobial therapy and attempts to reduce skin and nasal carriage.[4]

Myiasis

Often mistaken for boils, myiasis is the infection of larvae of dipteran flies in humans. The commonest forms of myiasis are caused by the maggots of the African tumbu fly, *Cordylobia anthropophaga*, or the South and Central American human botfly, *Dermatobia hominis*. The tumbu fly lays eggs on sandy soil or clothing, and eggs hatch on contact with human skin, allowing penetration of the larva directly. The toes, feet, lower legs, buttocks and trunk are commonly affected skin sites. In *Dermatobia* infections, the large botfly traps a smaller fly such as a mosquito and attaches its eggs to the abdomen; when the mosquito subsequently takes a blood meal from a human, the eggs hatch out, stimulated by the body warmth, and the larvae burrow into the skin. Hair-bearing sites (such as the scalp) are particularly affected in Latin Amercian myiasis. Larvae of both flies develop and mature by feeding on the flesh of the host before dropping to the ground to complete their life cycle.

Patients present on return from travel with persistent boils that exude serous fluid (**Fig. 4**A) and sometimes report sensations of movement or pain in their skin. Close

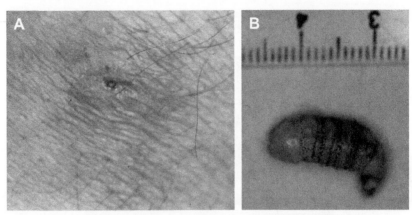

Fig. 4. (*A*) Boil-like lesion on the trunk discharging serosanginous fluid secondary to botfly myiasis infestation. (*B*) Botfly larva after removal from the boil-like lesion.

inspection of the boil reveals the diagnostic moving spiracles of the larvae. The lesions should be occluded with paraffin for 2 hours (this blocks the larval air supply and thus forces them to the surface); lidocaine can then be infiltrated around the lesions before larvae (see **Fig. 4**B) are removed with forceps and by gentle squeezing.

Tungiasis

Tunga penetrans (jigger, chigger, and chigoe) is a tiny parasitic flea found in the West Indies, South and Central America, West and East Africa. The gravid female burrows into broken skin on contact and lives there for 2 weeks until her eggs are ready to be shed. Patients may notice initial itching at the site of the lesions and then over a few weeks callous formation. A typical tungiasis skin lesion appears as a pale/white, annular blisterlike papule with a central black punctum (the spiracles of the flea) on the toes (**Fig. 5**), plantar feet, or hands (children playing with soil). After shedding

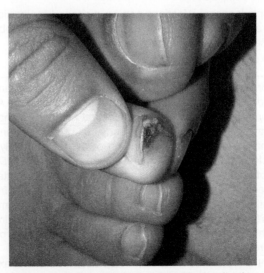

Fig. 5. *Tunga penetrans* parasitic flea with her eggs inside the distal toe pulp.

her eggs the female dies in the skin and therefore lesions are self-resolving and frequently require no intervention. If active lesions are painful, the engorged female flea can be excised under local anesthetic after suffocation with paraffin. Prevention programs have concentrated on wearing protective footwear, and providing concrete flooring in dwelling places. More recently, a repellent (Zanzarin; Zecken Schutz Bio) applied twice daily to the feet has been shown to reduce infestation rates to zero in 98% of participants.[5]

Tick Bites

Ticks are indiscriminate and voracious feeders biting wild and domesticated mammals. Humans are bitten when staying in areas endemic to ticks (forest, bush, and grassland regions) or working with livestock. Hard ticks (which transmit the majority of diseases) take a blood meal over several hours and at the end of that may transmit disease through saliva; soft ticks more rarely transmit disease but within minutes of feeding, which usually lasts an hour. Most tick bites are painless and therefore patients are usually unaware of it. Diseases transmitted by ticks that particularly affect travelers include Lyme disease with local cutaneous manifestations, and the variety of spotted fevers, including Rocky Mountain spotted fever (RMSF), fievre boutonneuse, and African tick fever (see section on Generalized skin manifestations).

Lyme disease caused by the bacteria *Borrelia burgdorferi* is transmitted by deer ticks (*Ixodes*) in the United States (Northern, Central, mid-Atlantic, Pacific coastal), Australia, and Europe. Patients may remain asymptomatic or within a few days exhibit flulike symptoms and develop an erythematous mark at the site of the bite that spreads out (1 cm/d) in a ring-shape over days to weeks called erythema chronicum migrans.[6] The annular lesion is classically erythematous with a raised (indurated) circumference and normal skin centrally (**Fig. 6**). Occasionally, a series of concentric erythematous and white rings appear at the bite site termed as bulls eye. If the disease is untreated, months/years later patients may develop systemic symptoms such as headache, nerve palsies, arthritis, carditis, and allergic skin rashes. The diagnosis is made based on the history (endemic area traveled, activities undertaken during the trip, and known tick bite) and examination (presence of tick and presence of erythema chronicum migrans); serology for *Borrelia burgdorferi* should be requested, and treatment is started promptly with doxycycline (Vibramycin; Pfizer), amoxicillin

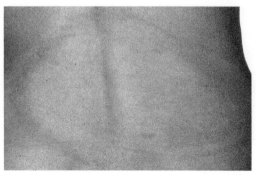

Fig. 6. Indurated annular spreading eruption of erythema chronicum migrans associated with Lyme disease.

(Amoxil; GlaxoSmithKline), erythromycin (Erythrocin; Abbott), or azithromycin (Zithromax; Pfizer).[7] Promptly remove any ticks still attached to the patient.

Mites

Mites are tiny arthropods that feed on insects, birds, and mammals. Most mites have a preferred host (mice, rats, dogs, chickens, etc) and feed on them intermittently in the wild. If a host animal dies or comes into contact with humans then mites can alternatively feed on human skin causing itching and irritation. Oral antihistamines and a application of a potent topical steroid (such as betamethasone ointment [Betnovate; GlaxoSmithKline]) twice daily to the affected skin can help alleviate the symptoms.

Scabies is caused by an infestation with the human mite *Sarcoptes scabiei*, which burrows in the skin causing an intense itching that characteristically keeps patients awake at night. The mites are transmitted by prolonged skin-to-skin contact. Pruritus takes 4 to 6 weeks to develop as a result of delayed-type hypersensitivity allergic reactions in the skin to the feces and egg proteins of the mite. Itching can, however, be almost immediate on re-infestation. Hints in the clinical history to the diagnosis of scabies include intense itching, which is worse at night, and more than 1 affected family member. Clinical signs in adults are typically seen as small linear burrows in the finger webs and multiple excoriated papules around the wrists, genitalia, and trunk. In babies and young children, the lesions are papular (**Fig. 7**) or even vesicular and clustered on the soles of their feet, axillae, and trunk. Clinical signs of crusted scabies (skin infested with hundreds of mites) include confluent plaques of crusting on the trunk and limbs with very limited erythema and minimal pruritus in the elderly or immunocompromised individuals. The diagnosis of scabies is usually made on clinical grounds; however, with a fine sterile needle, mites can be extracted from their burrows (or in the crust from crusted scabies) for confirmatory microscopy. Management is usually with aqueous topical preparations of permethrin 5% cream (Lyclear; Chefaro) or malathion 0.5% lotion (Prioderm, or Derbac-M; SSL International) applied simultaneously to all family members (even if asymptomatic) from the neck downwards, left overnight and rinsed in the morning. The treatment should be repeated 7 days later as the chemicals are not ovicidal. In crusted scabies or where systemic preparations are easier to administer (ie, control of scabies in large populations) oral ivermectin 200 mcg/kg (Stromectol/Ivomec/Mectizan; Merck) as a single dose (or 2 doses 7 days apart) is as effective as 5% permethrin.[8] Ivermectin should be avoided in children younger than 2 years and in pregnant women. Bedding and underclothing should be washed. Patients must be warned about severe pruritus, which will not settle until about 4 to 6 weeks after successful treatment. Skin itching can be soothed with bland emollients, aqueous with menthol, and mild topical steroids, such as

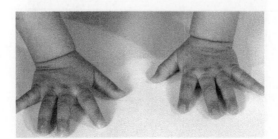

Fig. 7. Erythematous and flesh-colored papules on the hands of a child with a scabies infestation.

hydrocortisone or clobetasone butyrate (Betnovate; GlaxoSmithKline). Treatment failure usually results from incorrect application of topical preparations,[9] such as not treating all family members, not treating everyone at the same time, washing hands after chemical application (highest concentration of burrows between the fingers), not leaving the treatment on long enough, and not repeating the treatment after 7 days. Babies and young children with extensive disease need treatment to be applied to their head/neck area in addition to their body.

Cutaneous larva migrans (creeping eruption) results from the inadvertent penetration by the larval stage of hookworms into human skin, most commonly the parasitic nematode of dogs *Ancylostoma braziliense*. Dogs shed immature hookworm eggs in their feces. On maturation the larvae hatch and come into contact with human skin, most typically on tropical sandy beaches. The larvae penetrate through skin that is in direct contact with the ground, such as the feet, buttocks and knees. The parasite is unable to complete its life cycle (as it cannot penetrate through the human basement membrane) and is therefore confined to wander through the skin leaving its characteristic pruritic and serpiginous tracts (**Fig. 8**) until it dies. Rarely a brisk local

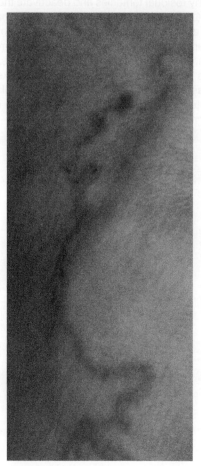

Fig. 8. Erythematous and serpiginous migrating tract caused by the dog hookworm larva in human skin, cutaneous larva migrans.

inflammatory reaction can lead to blistering. The diagnosis is usually made on clinical grounds. Treatment is highly effective with oral albendazole 400 mg (Albenza; Amedra Pharmaceuticals) for 3 consecutive days, or ivermectin (Stromectol/Ivomec/Mectizan; Merck) 200 mcg/Kg on 2 to 3 days. Application of 15% thiabendazole (Mintezol/Tresaderm/Arbotect) paste can be applied topically to an area 10 cm in diameter around the leading end of the tract. However, if a conservative approach to treatment is indicated (young child, pregnancy) then waiting for spontaneous resolution may be reasonable. An oral antihistamine plus a moderately potent topical steroid (such as betamethasone valerate) may relieve the pruritus. Rarely a sufficient local reaction causes blistering.

Jellyfish (jellies/sea jelly) stings are relatively common in individuals who swim/wade in the sea or in those who touch beached/dying jellies on the shore. However, the most stings are minor and settle rapidly with little need for medical intervention. However, severe cutaneous reactions to the stinging tentacles can arise (after encounters with Portuguese man-of-war, lion's mane jellyfish, sea nettle, and moon jellyfish) or even lead to death (Box jellyfish and Irukandji). Immediate management of stings from jellies includes washing the skin thoroughly with seawater (not freshwater) in an attempt to remove any residual tentacles and deactivate the nematocysts (stinging cells). Washing with 3%to 5% vinegar or applying a paste made from baking soda/shaving foam can help alleviate stings; however, they may not be immediately available. Antihistamines can relieve some of the immediate symptoms. Skin reactions can be severe (**Fig. 9**) leading to marked inflammation, blisters, erosions and eventual scarring. Skin reactions can last from hours or days to weeks. Super potent topical steroid such as clobetasol propionate 0.05% (Dermovate; GlaxoSmithKline) applied twice daily to the affected skin can reduce symptoms more rapidly and reduce the risk of permanent scarring.

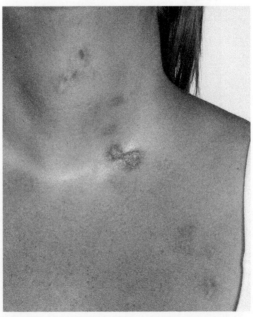

Fig. 9. Eroded erythematous acute inflammatory areas on the neck as a result of a jellyfish sting.

Leeches are blood-sucking worms found mainly in freshwater areas around the world. Usual hosts include fish and invertebrates but humans may be affected when traveling through wet/high humidity regions. Leaches have a mouth and 2 suckers and readily attach to human skin; they inject anesthetic and anticoagulant to aid in feeding, which may last up to 2 hours. The leeches will then spontaneously drop off leaving behind bleeding, cutaneous erosions. Leeches can be prised-off the skin using a finger nail to release each suckered end and then be flicked away. The skin should then be washed, and a pressure dressing applied to limit the bleeding. Rarely anaphylaxis to leech bites can occur.

Snakebites occur in most parts of the world affecting the unwary traveler or local inhabitant who is usually bitten when the reptile is accidentally disturbed or feels threatened. Interestingly 40% of snakebites reported in the United States occurred after individuals deliberately tried to capture wild snakes or while handling pets.[10] In the United States 99% of snakebites result from the pit viper family (rattlesnakes, cotton mouths, copperheads, and water moccasins).[11] Globally snakebites are divided into 2 main categories: venomous and nonvenomous (dry snakebites). The latter are usually painful and may become secondarily infected and are rarely serious, whereas the former are fatal through hematogenous or neurologic effects. The severity of a venomous bite depends on the species of snake, the body site affected, amount of venom injected and whether the victim is otherwise healthy (**Fig. 10**). Identification of the biting snake through a description or direct observation (after biting, snakes usually retire into the undergrowth within 20 ft of the victim) is very helpful in the management of snakebites. Clinically, all snakebites present with erythema at the bite site, broken/punctured skin from the fangs, edema, and occasionally rapid onset blisters and tissue necrosis. The onset of systemic symptoms, including fainting, weakness, nausea/vomiting, headache and hallucinations can be rapid. In fatal cases tachycardia, internal bleeding and multi-organ failure progress over the subsequent hours. Children are usually more severely affected than adults. Immediate care in the field includes immobilization/splinting of the bite site and lymphatic constriction (not too tight) and rapid access to a health care post/hospital if possible. Where is it clinically indicated/available anti-venom should be administered to the victim as soon as possible after the venomous snake bite.

Scorpion stings usually occur in humans when they inadvertently disturbed in their daytime hiding places amongst rocks. Most stings are uncomfortable but rarely fatal. Children are usually more severely affected than adults. Immediate symptoms and

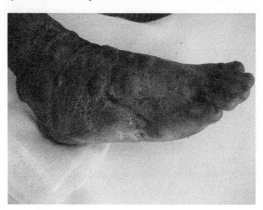

Fig. 10. Severe localized blistering reaction with necrosis as a result of a Red Spitter snake bite. (*Courtesy of* Dr V.M. Yates, Mr B.J. Bale.)

signs of scorpion stings include pain, erythema, and swelling at the site. Other symptoms vary but may include tachycardia, paresthesia or numbness, weakness, muscle twitching, sweating, and a high respiratory rate. The mainstay of treatment for most scorpion stings is with analgesia, ice packs, and reassurance. In severe cases, victims should be taken to a health post/hospital as they may require equine anitvenom (Anascorp) to be administered.

GENERALIZED SKIN DISEASE
Arboviral Infection

Returning travelers may describe generalized symptoms and display nonlocalized cutaneous exanthemata. Many of these rashes are due to nontropical viral infections, which are only coincidentally associated with the recent travel. However, a knowledge of some of the more common causes of generalized infectious rashes improves diagnostic rates.

Most important of the arthropod-borne viral illnesses (arboviral infections) is dengue fever. The global distribution of this infection is increasing because of the inability to contain the spread of the *Aedes* mosquito vector. Able to lay its eggs and complete its life cycle in tiny bodies of water, *Aedes* have successfully outmaneuvred control efforts and are now found throughout South East Asia, East and West Africa, the Caribbean, South and Central America, and the Pacific basin. Reports monitoring its progression up into the southern United States are concerning. Dengue is characterized in travelers (who are usually encountering the infection for the first time) with the sudden onset of high fevers, headache (often retro-orbital), and severe myalgia and arthralgia (break-bone fever). A pronounced generalized dense petechial rash typically appears after about 3 days, usually starting with the trunk and chest and moving peripherally. Dramatic blanching of the petechial rash is often displayed (**Fig. 11**). Leucopenia and thrombocytopenia are standard and may be profound. As symptoms subside, the confluence of the rash may give way to characteristic areas of normal skin "islands in a sea of red." In nonendemic areas, resolution following supportive care is the usual outcome. However, in endemic areas even though the majority of cases are not severe, the mortality rate associated with dengue is high because transmission and prevalence is so high, and subsequent exposures have been shown to induce more severe disease, presumably through some form of immune priming mechanism.

Reflecting the success of the *Aedes* vector, recent years have seen a resurgence of another arboviral infection, chikungunya fever.[12,13] This fever has occurred primarily in

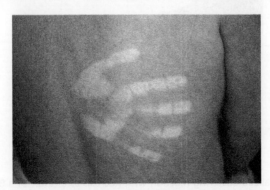

Fig. 11. Widespread macular erythematous blanching rash of early stage Dengue fever.

South-East Africa and South Asia, and has even led to initiation of a European focus of transmission. Similar to dengue, there may be a skin eruption, accompanied by fever and often very profound arthralgia.

Spotted Fevers

Tick-borne spotted fevers are not at all infrequent in more adventurous travelers who venture into rural and forested areas. In the United States, RMSF caused by *Rickettsia rickettsii* and transmitted by ticks is the commonest rickettsial illness. The infection is endemic in South America through North America and into Canada. Globally, similar tick-borne rickettsial diseases, such as fievre boutonneuse in Europe and African tick fever, are seen. Asian scrub typhus, caused by *Orientia tsutsugamushi*, is rare amongst travelers because the trombiculid mite vector is limited to very focal ecological islands in jungle plantations. The other tick-borne rickettsial spotted fevers display similar clinical features. Patients become rapidly unwell with severe headache, fever, and muscle pains. Subsequently (2–5 days later) 80% of patients develop a macular rash initially on palms/soles, wrists, and ankles, which spreads centripetally and evolves into papules, which may become classically petechial (**Fig. 12**). In the African

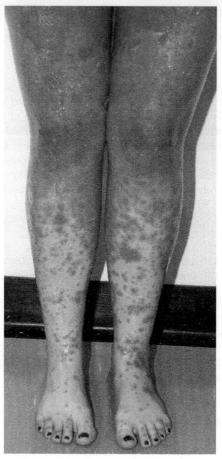

Fig. 12. Centripetally spreading macular and papular erythematous rash of Rickettsia becoming petechial on the lower legs.

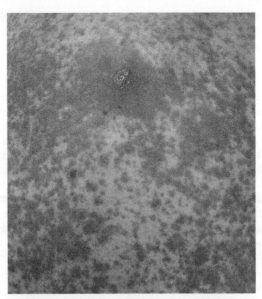

Fig. 13. Rickettsial infection leading to a maculopapular eruption on the back with a central necrotic area where the tick bite occurred.

and European forms, but not in RMSF, an eschar with a necrotic scab may develop at the site of the tick attachment (**Fig. 13**). Early diagnosis and prompt treatment are essential to prevent fatalities (reportedly 3%–5% of cases of RMSF).[14] Blood tests may show a low platelet count, low sodium and increased liver function levels. Serology can be requested. There is a worse prognosis in elderly patients, men, Afro-caribbeans, those with glucose-6-phosphate dehydrogenase deficiency, and in chronic alcohol use. Patients should be treated without delay using doxycycline 100 mg (Vibramycin; Pfizer) twice daily (children 4 mg/kg/d in divided doses) for 5 to 10 days.

REFERENCES

1. Lederman ER, Weld LH, Elyazar IR, et al. Dermatologic conditions of the ill returned traveler: an analysis from the GeoSentinel Surveillance Network. Int J Infect Dis 2008;12(6):593–602.
2. Lambrechts L, Scott TW, Gubler DJ. Consequences of the expanding global distribution of *Aedes albopictus* for dengue virus transmission. PLos Negl Trop Dis 2010;4(5):e646.
3. Raisigade JP, Laurent F, Lina G, et al. Global distribution and evolution of Panton-Valentine leukocidin-positive methicillin-susceptible *Staphylococcus aureus*, 1981-2007. J Infect Dis 2010;201(10):1589–97.
4. Fogo A, Kemp N, Morris-Jones R. Easily missed? Panton Valentine Leukocidin *Staphylococcus aureus* infections. BMJ 2011;343:d5343.
5. Buckendahl J, Heukelbach J, Ariza L, et al. Control of tungiasis through intermittent application of a plant-based repellent: an intervention study in a resource-poor community in Brazil. PLos Negl Trop Dis 2010;4(11):e879.
6. Bhate C, Schwartz RA. Lyme disease: part I. Advances and perspectives. J Am Acad Dermatol 2011;64(4):619–36.

7. Massarotti EM, Luger SW, Rahn DW, et al. Treatment of early lyme disease. Am J Med 1992;92(4):396–403.

8. Sharma R, Singal A. Topical permethrin and oral ivermectin in the management of scabies: a prospective, randomized, double blind, controlled study. Indian J Dermatol Venereol Leprol 2011;77(5):581–6.

9. Wolf R, Davidovici B. Treatment of scabies and pediculosis: facts and controversies. Clin Dermatol 2010;28(5):511–8.

10. Kurecki B, Brownlee H. Venomous snakebites in the United States. J Fam Pract 1987;25(4):386–92.

11. Juckett G, Hancox JG. Venomous snakebites in the United States: management review and update. Am Fam Physician 2002;65(7):1367–75.

12. Sane J, Kurkelas S, Vapalahti O, et al. Chikungunya, a new global epidemic? Duodecim 2011;127(5):457–63.

13. Pialoux G, Gauzere BA, Jaurequiberry S, et al. Chikungunya, an epidemic arbovirosis. Lancet Infect Dis 2007;7(5):319–27.

14. Chen LF, Sexton DJ. What's new in rocky mountain spotted fever? Infect Dis Clin North Am 2008;22:415.

Traveler's Diarrhea

Herwig Kollaritsch, MD, Maria Paulke-Korinek, MD, MSc, PhD,
Ursula Wiedermann, MD, PhD*

KEYWORDS

- Traveler's diarrhea • Enterotoxigenic *Escherichia coli* • Vaccination • Prophylaxis

KEY POINTS

- Usually, TD occurs within the first two weeks of a trip; in expatriates the risk of TD is decreases with the length of the stay.
- Most episodes of TD have bacterial etiology, and besides from oral rehydration, loperamide is the first-line treatment for TD, antibiotics are administered in febrile illnesses.
- "Boil it, cook it, peel it" has limited effects in preventing TD.
- An oral vaccine against cholera is available, which offers limited protection against diarrhea form ETEC.
- In travelers with special mission such as politicians, athletes, or persons with underlying disease at risk of aggravating during diarrhea, the use of prophylactic antibiotics should be considered.

EPIDEMIOLOGY

Traveler's diarrhea (TD) continues to be the most common travel-associated disease. The first systematic description of disease prevalence was in 1983, and, by 2011, similar TD rates remain in some areas, as reported in a recent study of Dutch travelers to destinations outside highly industrialized regions of the world.[1,2] At least 1 episode of diarrhea occurs in 40% to 50% of travelers during their stay abroad, and the incidence of TD is influenced by various global factors.[3–6] They can be classified as travel-related risk factors and traveler-related factors.[7]

Financial disclosure/conflict of interest: HK received research grants, fees for giving lectures and consultancy, as well as support for attending advisory boards and international conferences from Baxter and Novartis. MPK has received fees for speaking and consultancy, and support for advisory boards and attending international conferences from Novartis, GSK, and Pfizer. UW received research grants from Baxter and Nestlé and attended advisory boards organized by Novartis, Pfizer, and GSK.

Institute of Specific Prophylaxis and Tropical Medicine, Center for Pathophysiology, Infectiology and Immunology, Medical University of Vienna, Kinderspitalgasse 15, A-1090 Vienna, Austria

* Corresponding author.

E-mail address: ursula.wiedermann@meduniwien.ac.at

Infect Dis Clin N Am 26 (2012) 691–706
http://dx.doi.org/10.1016/j.idc.2012.06.002
0891-5520/12/$ – see front matter © 2012 Published by Elsevier Inc.

id.theclinics.com

TRAVEL-RELATED RISK FACTORS

The travel destination has a major influence on the risk of TD, and 3 geographic regions with different risk categories have been defined.[7–10] Low-risk areas where the TD incidence is less than or equal to 8% during a 2-week stay include central and northern Europe, the United States, Canada, Japan, and Australia. Regions with an intermediate risk of more than 8% to 20% during a similar exposure include southern and eastern Europe, Russia, China, Israel, the Caribbean, and South Africa. The areas with highest risk, where TD rates are between 20% and 90% during a 2-week exposure, include countries in the Middle East, southern Asia, Central and South America, and Africa.[6]

However, the regional risk may vary widely, within a country, or even between hotels a few hundred meters apart.[3,6,8,11] In temperate zones, the TD incidence is usually higher in warmer periods, but this remains a controversial concept.[11,12] In addition, in low-standard accommodations and in luxury hotels there seems to be a higher risk of TD than in standard accommodations.[6,8]

The second factor predicting a risk of TD is the duration of exposure of stay. The risk declines with the duration of stay and is highest during the first week.[13,14] In expatriates in high-risk countries, the risk of TD decreases at around 1 year of stay, possibly because of acquired immunity to enteropathogens.[15]

A further recognized risk is the style of travel. Backpackers have a higher risk of TD than individuals visiting resorts, and the incidence increases the more independent the travel is.[8,12] Factors that contribute to this phenomenon include the type of accommodation and food sources (eg, eating food bought from street vendors, which is known to be hazardous).[16,17]

TRAVELER-RELATED RISK FACTORS

The traveler's country of origin is relevant. Individuals from countries with high sanitary standards have higher TD rates than individuals from countries with less developed sanitary and economic infrastructure,[14] highlighting the role of acquired immunity protecting against enteropathogens.

In younger groups, particularly in the third decade, the risk of TD is highest.[1,8,9] Risky behavior and more adventurous travel may contribute to their higher risk. Neither gender nor repeated travel seems to influence the risk of TD. However, the TD rate is lower in individuals who had TD in the preceding year.[12]

Several predisposing risk factors influence diarrhea, including genetic and pathophysiologic factors (eg, individuals with the O blood group are more susceptible to diarrhea from Norovirus and *Shigella*,[18] and immunocompromised travelers such as human immunodeficiency virus [HIV]–positive subjects with decreased immunologic function are at risk of parasitic TD).[19]

Gastric acidity is an important barrier against enteropathogens. Medications that reduce gastric acid secretion, such as proton pump inhibitors or histamine 2 receptor antagonists, are known to increase the risk of TD by a factor of 12.[20,21]

Dietary errors put travelers at risk of infection. Individuals who adhered to strict dietary lists had a lowered incidence of disease.[22] However adherence to the food hygiene advice to boil it, cook it, peel it, or forget it had a marginal benefit.[8,23]

CAUSES OF TD

An infectious pathogen can be identified in 60% to 80% of individuals with TD.[24] Bacteria and their toxins cause 50% to 80% of symptomatic TD episodes. Viruses and protozoa/helminths each can be detected in up to 36% of cases.[24,25] The findings in a review of more than 51 published studies between 1973 and 2008, examining the cause of TD in 30.884 travelers and 57 separate travel groups to Africa, south Asia, southeast Asia and Latin America detailed in **Table 1**.[26] A significant geographic variation was noted for all enteric pathogens in TD, except for Rotavirus and *Cryptosporidium*.

Bacterial Pathogens (and Their Toxins)

Escherichia coli cause up to 60% of TD and is most prevalent in Latin America, south Asia (India), and Africa.[26,27] Among *E coli* isolates, enterotoxigenic *E coli* (ETEC) are most commonly identified.[24,26] However, in Latin America and the Caribbean, one-quarter of travelers with diarrhea had enteroaggregative *E coli* (EAEC) isolated.[26] Other enteropathogenic species of *E coli*, including enteropathogenic, enteroinvasive, enterohemorrhagic, or diffuse-adhering *E coli*, play only a minor role in the causes of TD. *Campylobacter* is identified in 2% to 32% of isolates from patients with TD, and

Table 1
Cause of travelers' diarrhea (mean percentages of isolation rates of different pathogens in various studies)

Pathogen	Latin America/ Caribbean (%)	Africa (%)	South Asia (%)	Southeast Asia (%)
Enterotoxigenic *Escherichia coli*	33.6	31.2	30.6	7.2
Enteroaggregative, enteropathogenic, enteroinvasive, enterohemorrhagic, or diffuse-adhering *E coli*[a]	47.3	11.3	18.9	19.0
Campylobacter	2.5	4.6	7.8	32.4
Shigella spp	6.6	8.6	8.0	2.2
Salmonella spp	4.4	5.5	6.6	9.1
Aeromonas spp	0.8	3.2	2.8	3.3
Arcobacter[b]	7	-	9	-
Enterotoxigenic *Bacteroides fragilis*[b]	5	-	10	-
Plesiomonas	1.3	2.5	5.4	4.8
Noncholera vibrios	0.1	2.3	3.0	9.0
Vibrio cholerae	0	0	0.4	0.2
Rotavirus	7.2	6.7	5.1	3.8
Norovirus	16.9	12.8	-	3.2
Giardia lamblia	1.3	1.6	6.2	5.7
Cryptosporidium	2.0	1.3	2.8	0.6
Entamoeba histolytica	1.1	1.0	3.8	2.5
No pathogen identified	48.8	44.7	39.0	50.2

[a] Cumulative percentages of isolation rates.
[b] Only from Ref.[27]

Adapted from Shah N, DuPont HL, Ramsey DJ. Global etiology of travelers' diarrhea: systematic review from 1973 to the present. Am J Trop Med Hyg 2009;80(4):609–14; and Jiang ZD, Dupont HL, Brown EL, et al. Microbial etiology of travelers' diarrhea in Mexico, Guatemala, and India: importance of enterotoxigenic *Bacteroides fragilis* and *Arcobacter* species. J Clin Microbiol 2010;48(4):1417–9.

in southeast Asia it is found more frequently than ETEC, possibly because of the widespread presence of antimicrobial resistance of *Campylobacter* in this region.[26,28] In early studies on the causes of TD, isolation of *Campylobacter* was rarely undertaken because it was a complex process. *Salmonella* species occur in less than 5% of patients with TD, with the exception of Asia, where it has been identified in up to 10% of cases. *Shigella* spp are detected in between 2% and 9% of travelers, particularly to Africa. In past surveys, a high proportion of studies failed to isolate or identify pathogens, and a high number of samples produced *Salmonella* and *Shigella*. Improved diagnostic testing now produces lower isolation rates of *Shigella* and *Salmonella*, with increased isolation of other pathogens now being made.[3,11,14,26,27,29] *Aeromonas* spp are more common in Asia, but are isolated in less than 4% of patients with TD. Identification of *Plesiomonas*[26] and noncholera vibrios is made in less than 10% of patients with TD in southeast Asia, but *Vibrio cholerae* is rarely detected. In Mexico, Guatemala, and India, *Bacteroides fragilis* and *Arcobacter* spp are recognized in 7% and 8% of persons with TD, respectively.[27]

Viral Pathogens

Norovirus may occur in up to 17% of isolates of diarrheal episodes in travelers from the Caribbean and Africa,[30,31] and is an important cause of acute diarrhea and vomiting outbreaks on cruise ships.[24,30] Rotavirus is uncommon, being found in 4% to 7% of patients with acute TD, but the global rotavirus mass vaccination programs may reduce the circulation of this pathogen and therefore its role in TD may decrease.[32] No other viruses have been associated with a key role in TD; however, in most studies, only astroviruses and enteric adenoviruses are important in childhood diarrhea and seldom affect adults.[24]

Protozoans and Helminths

Entamoeba histolytica and *Giardia lamblia* are well recognized in the cause of TD, with isolation rates of up to 4% and 6%, respectively, in south Asia.[11,26] In a recent study from Nepal, *Giardia* was isolated in 11% of cases.[33] Helminths usually do not play a major role in the cause of acute TD because of their long infection cycle.

However, several factors affect the cause of TD: no pathogens are isolated in more than 40% of TD cases despite state-of-the-art microbiological detection technology.[11,14,26,27,29] Over more than 30 years, studies have been conducted on this subject, and microbiological methods have improved significantly, with highly sensitive methods including polymerase chain reaction. Results of older studies may therefore not be comparable. There is no agreement on the cause of microbiologically negative cases of TD and they may be caused by unknown pathogens or by noninfectious agents such as allergies and excessive food or alcohol consumption.[24] In persons with acute TD, more than 1 potential pathogen can often be identified.[24]

CLINICAL PICTURE

The clinical picture of TD does not allow any association with the cause.[4,34–36] The first symptoms of TD occur within the first 4 to 7 days after arrival, with 90% of episodes presenting during the first 2 weeks of the stay.[34,36] Acute watery diarrhea predominates in 90% and signs of invasive infection, including fever and bloody/mucoid stools, occur in 3% to 30% of those affected.[4,14,34] Most patients report 3 to 5 bowel movements per day, but, in one-fifth, a higher frequency of up to 20 daily stools occurs.[3,4,14,34] Other symptoms such as nausea (10%–70%), vomiting (4%–36%), abdominal cramps/pain, tenesmus (80%), urgency (more than 90%), and nongastrointestinal features including myalgia, arthralgia, and headache are reported.[34] The average episode resolves within 3 to 5 days. Prolonged symptoms of more than 1 week occur in 8% to 15% of cases, and chronic diarrhea (>1 month) in 1% to 3% of episodes.[34] *Giardia* is the most frequent cause of long-lasting TD.[37]

Half of all travelers are incapacitated for at least 1 day, and 1 in 5 are confined to bed for 1 or 2 days. A medical consult results in 5% to 15% of episodes, but hospitalization is rare.[34,36] In children less than 12 years of age, TD tends to be more severe, and medical care is sought 3 to 4 times more frequently than for adults.[38]

Classic TD typically resolves without complications. In prolonged or severe episodes, diarrhea may result in electrolyte imbalance, posing a problem for persons with chronic underlying morbidity such as renal or cardiac insufficiency.[34] Postinfectious irritable bowel syndrome (IBS) can follow a range of infectious diarrhea.[39] A few data suggest an increased moderate risk for IBS after acute TD.[40,41] Reiter syndrome is a well-recognized but rare complication following invasive TD, and Guillain-Barré syndrome has been reported following *Campylobacter* infection.[34]

Differential diagnosis of acute TD includes falciparum malaria and other systemic infections/diseases, for example viral hepatitis, dengue fever, irritable bowel disease, or symptoms of malignancy (**Fig. 1**).[34,36]

SPECIFIC THERAPY AND PREVENTION
Diagnosis and Management of TD

Management of TD is determined by the clinical severity and risk factors, including age, coexisting morbidity, and subsequently the pathogen isolated from the stool.

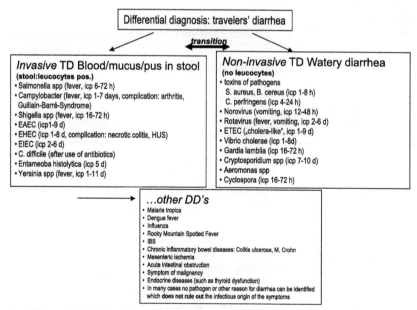

Fig. 1. Differential diagnosis of TD. DD, differential diagnosis; EHEC, enterohemorrhagic *E coli*; EIEC, enteroinvasive *E coli*; icp, incubation period. (*Adapted from* Kollaritsch H, Paulke-Korinek M. Durchfallerkrankungen. In: Löscher T, Burchard GD, editors. Tropenmedizin in Klinik und Praxis mit Reise- und Migrationsmedizin. 4th edition. Georg Thieme Verlag. New York: Stuttgart; 2010; with permission.)

Because TD usually is self-limiting, detailed clinical, laboratory, and diagnostic investigations are neither necessary nor cost-effective.[34,36] The symptoms may mimic other more serious disorders, especially in children, and signs of severe dehydration or symptoms of incipient organ failure (eg, renal failure) should not be missed. Stool samples should be examined through culture and microscopy for protozoa and/or helminths in persons with persistent diarrhea. **Fig. 2** presents a flow chart for the management of acute TD.[36]

Fluid, Electrolyte Therapy, and Diet

TD is not a life-threatening illness in older children and healthy adults. They rarely require oral rehydration therapy, although maintenance of fluid intake during episodes should be encouraged. Small quantities of food are known to support mucosal recovery following infection. Diet does not always enhance clinical recovery, in particular when antibiotics are administered.[42] Children should be continued on their normal diet.

Elderly patients are at risk of dehydration and oral rehydration therapy should be used. Infants less than 1 year old similarly should receive oral rehydration and electrolyte therapy, which can be lifesaving. Breast-feeding should be continued and formula-fed children should continue to receive formula to ensure that they maintain an adequate nutrient intake. Unless recommended by the physician, children less than 1 year should not receive antibacterial therapy.

Symptomatic Treatment: Antisecretory Drugs

In uncomplicated/mild cases of TD (without fever or bloody stools), treatment with antisecretory drugs may control or reduce the symptoms, but does not treat the underlying cause.

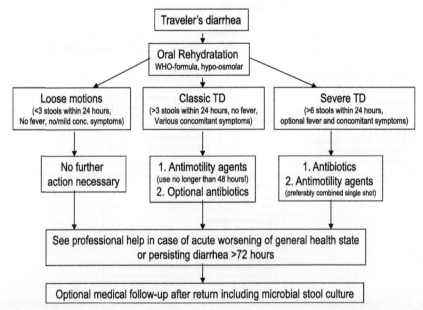

Fig. 2. Management of acute TD. WHO, World Health Organization. (*Adapted from* Kollaritsch H, Paulke-Korinek M. Durchfallerkrankungen. In: Löscher T, Burchard GD, editors. Tropenmedizin in Klinik und Praxis mit Reise- und Migrationsmedizin. 4th edition. Georg Thieme Verlag. New York: Stuttgart; 2010; with permission.)

Bismuth subsalicylate has been widely used in mild forms of TD and has reduced the number of stools by 50%.[43,44]

The most widely used drug in the treatment of TD is loperamide, which elicits both antisecretory as well as antimotility effects.[45] It has been shown to be more efficacious than bismuth subsalicylate, is fast acting, safe, and well tolerated. However, the prolonged (mis)use of loperamide during invasive TD may lead to a paralytic ileus, severe colitis, and/or perforation. It should not be used in patients with bloody stools, fever of more than 38.5°C, or in children, who may develop extrapyramidal signs and hallucinations.[46–48] Despite limited evidence,[49] loperamide should not be used with an antibiotic in suspected invasive diarrhea.[50]

There are other antisecretory drugs available that have been used for the treatment of TD. Zaldaride maleate is an inhibitor of the intestinal calmodulin that inhibits intracellular calcium uptake and transport.[51] Crofelemer acts via blockage of chloride channels, thereby controlling secretion during TD.[52] A third drug with similar effects is racecadotril, an enkephalinase inhibitor of the endogenous peptide enkephalin, which blocks secretion of water and electrolytes into the intestinal lumen. It has been used in children and adults with diarrhea, but has not been explicitly tested against TD.[53,54] In general, the use of opiate-like substances and diphenoxylate are not recommended, because they can elicit reactions (eg, in the central nervous system), particularly in elderly travelers.

In severe cases of TD, a combination of antisecretory treatment and antibacterial chemotherapy should be given. The beneficial effects of the adjunctive treatment with different antibiotics have been well documented in cases of ETEC diarrhea.[50,55,56]

Antibacterial Drugs

In several studies, antibiotics have been shown to reduce the duration of diarrhea by 1 to 2 days. Currently recommended antibiotics are listed in **Table 2**. Sulfonamides, tetracycline, trimethoprim, and trimethoprim/sulfamethoxazole are no longer used because of widespread resistance against most diarrhea-eliciting pathogens.

Table 2
Common treatments for TD

Treatment	Dosage
Symptomatic Treatment	
Bismuth subsalicylate	1 dose of 525 mg (2 tablets of Pepto-Bismol Chewable Tablets) po every 30 min, no more than 8 doses per day
Loperamide	4 mg po, then 2 mg after each loose stool, not to exceed 16 mg per day (for 48 h)
Antibiotic Treatment	
Fluoroquinolones	
Ciprofloxacin	500 mg po, bid
Ofloxacin	200 mg po, bid
Azithromycin	1000 mg po, once
Rifaximin	200 mg po, tid

Abbreviations: bid, twice a day; po, by mouth; tid, 3 times a day.

Adapted from Hill DR, Ericsson CD, Pearson RD, et al. The practice of travel medicine: guidelines by the Infectious Diseases Society of America. Clin Infect Dis 2006;43(12):1499–539; and de Saussure PP. Management of the returning traveler with diarrhea. Therap Adv Gastroenterol 2009;2(6):367–75.

Fluoroquinolones are a first-line therapeutic agent against bacterial pathogens causing TD. They are useful if a patient has a fever and/or bloody diarrhea associated with an invasive pathogen. However, increasing rates of resistance have been observed, mainly in *Campylobacter* species in southeast Asia and India.[57,58] Fluoroquinolones are not recommended during pregnancy and there have been concerns for their use in children (mainly ciprofloxacin use) because of transient musculoskeletal adverse effects.[59] However, there are also studies in children that support the use of ciprofloxacin for short-term treatment.[60] Besides abdominal discomfort and nausea, frequently observed side effects are insomnia and irritability.

Azithromycin, belonging to the macrolide group of antibiotics, is effective against most TD-causing pathogens worldwide, including fluoroquinolone-resistant *Campylobacter* and *Shigella* strains.[33,61] Azithromycin treatment has been preferentially recommended in Southeast Asia because, in this region, the prevalence of invasive bacterial enteropathogens with resistance to fluoroquinolones is increased and the effectiveness of rifaximin might be limited.

The use of azithromycin is safe in pregnancy as well as in children. Frequently observed side effects are pruritus and candida vaginitis.

Rifaximin is a nonabsorbed antibiotic derivative of rifamycin for the treatment of afebrile, nondysenteric TD. It has a good safety profile and can be used in travelers aged more than 12 years. No clinical data exist about the use in pregnant or lactating women. Because of limited absorption, this antibiotic is only used against enteric diseases, predominantly against ETEC. A clinical trial comparing the efficacy of ciprofloxacin and rifaximin in a high-risk area of ETEC inducing TD showed comparable effectiveness for both antibiotics. Rapid improvement and greater overall wellness after TD was recently shown when rifaximin was given in combination with loperamide. This treatment regimen was significantly superior to the treatment with either agent alone.[56] Another study comparing the use of ciprofloxacin and rifaximin in Guatemala, Mexico, and India did not show an advantage of treatment with rifaximin, which might be because invasive illness frequently occurs in these areas too. It therefore needs to be mentioned that rifaximin is not approved for treatment of diarrhea associated with fever, bloody stools, or when *Shigella*, *Salmonella*, or *Campylobacter* are the suspected diarrhea-causing pathogens.

Duration of Treatment

In comparative studies of treatment regimens with absorbed antibiotics, no difference in the efficacy between a single-dose or 3-dose regimen has been shown,[62–65] even though it is generally thought that longer courses of treatment might prove more successful in cases of severe diarrhea. For the nonabsorbed antibiotic rifaximin, most studies have used a 3-day treatment schedule.[66]

Drawbacks of Antibacterial Treatment Regimens and Considerations

The widespread use of antibiotics has led to the development of antibiotic resistance against enteric pathogens. In particular, resistance to fluoroquinolones in southeast Asia and India has been observed in *Campylobacter*,[33,57] *Shigella*,[67] as well as in ETEC.[68] However, in areas with high fluoroquinolone resistance, effective treatment has been shown with azithromycin or, in the case of ETEC, with rifaximin use, thereby providing an adequate alternative treatment.

After treatment with fluoroquinolones, depletion of the gut flora has been shown to predispose to *Clostridium difficile* colitis, causing persistent or chronic diarrhea in some travelers.[69] However, the rare events of posttreatment *C difficile* diarrhea do not warrant abandoning the use of antibiotic treatment in severe cases of TD.

A few studies have raised concerns that antibiotic treatment may lead to prolongation of enteric infections. In particular, with acute salmonellosis by nontyphoid *Salmonella*, ciprofloxacin treatment failed to eradicate the pathogen and resulted in prolonged pathogen carriage. However, this was during a *Salmonella* outbreak in health care workers[70] and not in patients treated for TD.

In cases of Shiga toxin–producing *E coli*, antibiotic treatment with quinolones is thought to increase the risk of complications, for example of hemolytic uremic syndrome, because of enhanced release of Shiga toxin into the gut lumen.[71,72] However, this has not been reported with other antibiotics such as rifaximin. Shiga-producing *E coli* are not common pathogens causing TD and therefore this might be a problem of minor importance.

Prophylaxis of TD

The many causes of TD make it difficult to control using a single approach. There are several preventive actions that can be taken, ranging from food hygiene and prophylactic vaccination to prophylactic antibiotic treatment, but the effectiveness and use of these measures requires detailed evaluation and discussion.

Prophylaxis Using Food Hygiene Measures

For decades, food hygiene was considered one of the most important and effective tools for preventing TD and this was not challenged for a long time. TD usually is transmitted feco-orally and consumption of risky food such as raw meat, oysters, or sauces and dips have been associated with diarrheal outbreaks. However, in a review published in 2005, Shlim[23] described hygiene measures as being less effective than was generally assumed. According to this review, a relationship between the number of dietary mistakes and the frequency of TD was shown in only 1 out of 8 studies. In this study, travelers were asked to adhere to strict dietary lists, and the rates of TD were lower in individuals who followed the lists.[22,23] In contrast, Steffen[6,23] showed that the highest diarrheal rates were among those who paid most attention to consuming low-risk foods. It is evident that travelers either cannot follow dietary restrictions because of limited food choice or they cannot resist the temptation of eating exotic buffet foods and so forth.[7,8] There seems to be a major difference between theory and practice: the risk of TD is reduced in self-prepared food, because travelers tend to be careful when making their own meals, whereas hotel tourists more frequently eat salad, add ice cubes to their drinks, and drink fresh dairy products or tap water. More than 95% of tourists who stayed in hotels in Jamaica were reported to have consumed drinks/and or food in this way.[7,14]

Although it seems to have limited impact, travel health bodies (eg, the Infectious Disease Society of America) consider it prudent to continue educating travelers about food and water hygiene measures.[73] Travelers should be reminded of common-sense precautions such as avoiding raw fish, meat, or oysters.

Prevention by Antibiotics and Nonantibiotic Agents

TD can be effectively prevented by prophylactic intake of antibiotics, although these are currently not routinely recommended. Doxycycline and trimethoprim/sulfamethoxazole have been effective in the prevention of TD, but are no longer recommended because of antimicrobial resistance.[73] Antibiotics that are currently considered for prophylaxis of TD are the fluoroquinolones such as ciprofloxacin, which, in daily doses of 250 to 500 mg, are effective in preventing up to 90% of cases of TD. However, because of limited experience and the potential for adverse events, fluoroquinolone use should be limited to a maximum of 3 weeks.[73–75] Other considerations are antimicrobial resistance and potentially poor efficacy in the prevention of diarrhea due to *Campylobacter* in some regions such as southeast Asia,[58,73] where azithromycin is a reasonable option.[58]

Another option that seems to be safe is rifaximin, which has been shown to be effective in preventing TD in US travelers in Mexico. In the first of these studies, doses of 200 mg, 400 mg, and 600 mg of rifaximin per day were used and were shown to be protective against TD in 72% of cases.[76] A further study showed the effectiveness of a daily dose of 600 mg in up to 58% of TD cases during the summer.[77] However, in a study conducted between July 2009 and January 2010 in Mexico, rifaximin at a daily dose of 550 mg did not protect against TD compared with the placebo group. This finding was explained by generally lower rates of diarrhea during that time of the year. The rate of bacterial diarrhea was noted to be lower during this time of year, with more norovirus infection.[78] This example shows that the efficacy of this antibiotic depends on the epidemiologic situation, and it is therefore not helpful to generalize study results. In regions with a high percentage of bacterial enteropathogens susceptible to rifaximin (with the exception of *Campylobacter*-resistant strains[57,73]), prophylactic use of rifaximin can be expected to be effective.

In conclusion, antibiotic prophylaxis of TD can be considered for certain groups and for a limited period of time (less than 2 to 3 weeks). According to the International Society of Travel Medicine, such groups include athletes or politicians, persons with underlying illnesses in whom TD could complicate the disease (ie, inflammatory bowel disease, advanced cancer, or HIV infection), and individuals with underlying conditions making them more susceptible to TD, for example patients with gastric disease or those on gastric acid–reducing drugs.[75]

Probiotics have frequently been purported to be effective in the prevention of TD, but evidence for their effectiveness is limited[73]: The only species of *Lactobacillus* that showed positive effects in 1 study was *Lactobacillus* GG, which was protective in up to 45% of cases with TD.[73,79] *Saccharomyces boulardii* showed protection in travelers to North Africa, but not in travelers to other destinations.[80] Further research in this area is needed.

Another nonantibiotic agent that can be used for preventing TD is bismuth subsalicylate. It is used in the United States but, because of concerns regarding toxicity (encephalopathy) it is usually not administered in Europe, Australia, or New Zealand. It has antibacterial activity and is effective in preventing TD in up to 65% of cases. However, apart from the adverse effects (blackening of the tongue and dark stools), daily use is hampered by a rigid schedule of administration and it must be taken 4 times a day.[73,75]

PREVENTION BY VACCINES

No universal vaccine exists to prevent TD because of its wide range of causes. Initial results from a study using a vaccine patch containing heat-labile toxin (LT) were promising,[81] but subsequent studies did not confirm the protective efficacy of the vaccine and no further development of the vaccine has been undertaken. Orochol, a live oral cholera vaccine, is not currently produced, another oral cholera vaccine is available only in India, Indonesia, and Vietnam (Shanchol).[82]

The only widely available and licensed vaccine that can, to some extent, prevent TD is therefore Dukoral, but its primary indication is to protect against cholera. In Europe and Australia, it is only licensed for cholera prevention but, in several other countries including Canada, it is also licensed for prevention of TD caused by ETEC.[82] It contains inactivated *V cholerae* and the recombinant B subunit of the cholera toxin, which is 80% homologous to the LT produced by ETEC. The vaccine therefore induces antibodies not only against *V cholerae* but also against LT-producing ETEC.[83] Two doses are required between 1 and 6 weeks. Studies in cholera-endemic regions showed a protective efficacy against cholera of up to 85% within the first 6 months after vaccination,[84] with protection decreasing to about 52% in the second year. No data exist on the prevention of cholera in travelers, but cholera infection is rare in travelers. However, protection against cholera can become an important issue in outbreak situations; for example, large cholera outbreaks have recently been reported from the Republic of Congo and from Sierra Leone.[85] The largest cholera outbreak, with more than 540,000 cases and 7360 deaths, occurred at the end of 2010 in Haiti and the Dominican Republic after an earthquake.[86] Vaccination against cholera is important for individuals such as aid workers visiting outbreak areas.

Dukoral has been reported to provide up to 67% protection against ETEC diarrhea.[83] However, there are limited data on its protective efficacy in travelers. In one study, protection against ETEC persisted for only 3 months.[87] A study in Finnish travelers to Morocco showed protective effects in 60% of the travelers against ETEC diarrhea.[88] A Spanish trial described a protective efficacy of 57% in high-risk travelers,[89] and a recent study not only proved protective in Spanish travelers but also described the vaccine as being cost-effective when administered in travelers to regions endemic for TD.[90] Thus, when recommending vaccination against ETEC-TD, the risk of ETEC-TD in the travel destination must be considered. In general, the proportion of TD caused by ETEC is low, and therefore Dukoral is reported to have a limited protective efficacy, preventing 7% or less cases of TD.[75] However, in individuals going to high-risk areas for TD, and particularly those at greater risk of complications from TD, prophylactic vaccination with Dukoral is justified.

SUMMARY

Although TD is the most important health problem in travelers,[91] measures to control it are still not satisfactory and recommendations on food and water hygiene alone have not proved effective. Bacteria cause most of the episodes of TD, but long-term prophylaxis with antibiotics is not generally recommended because of the risk of increased antimicrobial resistance and their potential for side effects. Most cases of diarrhea are self-limiting and do not need medical attention. In severe cases, TD can be effectively treated with antibiotics such as rifaximin, ciprofloxacin, or azithromycin (alone or in combination with antisecretory drugs). For high-risk travelers, oral cholera vaccines, which provide some cross-protection against TD, might be a valuable option.

REFERENCES

1. Steffen R, van der Linde F, Gyr K, et al. Epidemiology of diarrhea in travelers. JAMA 1983;249(9):1176–80.
2. Belderok SM, van den Hoek A, Kint JA, et al. Incidence, risk factors and treatment of diarrhoea among Dutch travellers: reasons not to routinely prescribe antibiotics. BMC Infect Dis 2011;11(1):295.
3. von Sonnenburg F, Tornieporth N, Waiyaki P, et al. Risk and aetiology of diarrhoea at various tourist destinations. Lancet 2000;356(9224):133–4.
4. Kollaritsch H. Traveller's diarrhea among Austrian tourists to warm climate countries: II. Clinical features. Eur J Epidemiol 1989;5(3):355–62.

5. Guerrant RL, Oria R, Bushen OY, et al. Global impact of diarrheal diseases that are sampled by travelers: the rest of the hippopotamus. Clin Infect Dis 2005; 41(Suppl 8):S524–30.

6. Steffen R. Epidemiology of traveler's diarrhea. Clin Infect Dis 2005;41(Suppl 8): S536–40.

7. Castelli F, Black R. Epidemiology of travelers' diarrhea. In: Ericsson C, DuPont HL, Steffen R, editors. Travelers' diarrhea. 2nd edition. Ontario (Canada): BC Decker; 2008. p. 92–104.

8. Kollaritsch H. Travelers diarrhea among Austrian tourists to warm climate countries: I. Epidemiology. Eur J Epidemiol 1989;5:74–81.

9. Steffen R. Epidemiologic studies of travelers' diarrhea, severe gastrointestinal infections, and cholera. Rev Infect Dis 1986;8(Suppl 2):S122–30.

10. Castelli F, Carosi G. Epidemiology of traveler's diarrhea. Chemotherapy 1995; 41(Suppl 1):20–32.

11. Steffen R, Tornieporth N, Clemens SA, et al. Epidemiology of travelers' diarrhea: details of a global survey. J Travel Med 2004;11(4):231–7.

12. Cobelens FG, Leentvaar-Kuijpers A, Kleijnen J, et al. Incidence and risk factors of diarrhoea in Dutch travellers: consequences for priorities in pre-travel health advice. Trop Med Int Health 1998;3(11):896–903.

13. Cavalcanti A, Clemens SA, Von Sonnenburg F, et al. Traveler's diarrhea: epidemiology and impact on visitors to Fortaleza, Brazil. Rev Panam Salud Publica 2002; 11(4):245–52.

14. Steffen R, Collard F, Tornieporth N, et al. Epidemiology, etiology, and impact of traveler's diarrhea in Jamaica. JAMA 1999;281(9):811–7.

15. Hoge CW, Shlim DR, Echeverria P, et al. Epidemiology of diarrhea among expatriate residents living in a highly endemic environment. JAMA 1996;275(7):533–8.

16. Estrada-Garcia T, Lopez-Saucedo C, Arevalo C, et al. Street-vended seafood: a risk for foodborne diseases in Mexico. Lancet Infect Dis 2005;5(2):69–70.

17. Jones TF, Angulo FJ. Eating in restaurants: a risk factor for foodborne disease? Clin Infect Dis 2006;43(10):1324–8.

18. Al-Abri SS, Beeching NJ, Nye FJ. Traveller's diarrhoea. Lancet Infect Dis 2005; 5(6):349–60.

19. Brink AK, Mahe C, Watera C, et al. Diarrhea, CD4 counts and enteric infections in a community-based cohort of HIV-infected adults in Uganda. J Infect 2002;45(2): 99–106.

20. Giannella RA, Broitman SA, Zamcheck N. Influence of gastric acidity on bacterial and parasitic enteric infections. A perspective. Ann Intern Med 1973;78(2): 271–6.

21. Bavishi C, Dupont HL. Systematic review: the use of proton pump inhibitors and increased susceptibility to enteric infection. Aliment Pharmacol Ther 2011; 34(11–12):1269–81.

22. Kozicki M, Steffen R, Schar M. 'Boil it, cook it, peel it or forget it': does this rule prevent travellers' diarrhoea? Int J Epidemiol 1985;14(1):169–72.

23. Shlim DR. Looking for evidence that personal hygiene precautions prevent traveler's diarrhea. Clin Infect Dis 2005;41(Suppl 8):S531–5.

24. Wilder-Smith A, Belkind-Gerson J. Relative importance of pathogens and noninfectious courses. In: Ericsson CD, Steffen R, DuPont HL, editors. Travelers' diarrhea. 2nd edition. Ontario (Canada): BC Decker; 2008.

25. DuPont HL, Ericsson C, Steffen R. Historical perspectives of travelers diarrhea. In: Ericsson C, Steffen R, DuPont HL, editors. Travelers' diarrhea. 2nd edition. Ontario (Canada): BC Decker; 2008.

26. Shah N, DuPont HL, Ramsey DJ. Global etiology of travelers' diarrhea: systematic review from 1973 to the present. Am J Trop Med Hyg 2009; 80(4):609–14.
27. Jiang ZD, Dupont HL, Brown EL, et al. Microbial etiology of travelers' diarrhea in Mexico, Guatemala, and India: importance of enterotoxigenic *Bacteroides fragilis* and *Arcobacter* species. J Clin Microbiol 2010;48(4):1417–9.
28. Luangtongkum T, Jeon B, Han J, et al. Antibiotic resistance in *Campylobacter*: emergence, transmission and persistence. Future Microbiol 2009; 4(2):189–200.
29. Jiang ZD, Lowe B, Verenkar MP, et al. Prevalence of enteric pathogens among international travelers with diarrhea acquired in Kenya (Mombasa), India (Goa), or Jamaica (Montego Bay). J Infect Dis 2002;185(4):497–502.
30. Koo HL, Ajami N, Atmar RL, et al. Noroviruses: the leading cause of gastroenteritis worldwide. Discov Med 2010;10(50):61–70.
31. Koo HL, Ajami NJ, Jiang ZD, et al. Noroviruses as a cause of diarrhea in travelers to Guatemala, India, and Mexico. J Clin Microbiol 2010;48(5):1673–6.
32. Patel MM, Steele D, Gentsch JR, et al. Real-world impact of rotavirus vaccination. Pediatr Infect Dis J 2011;30(Suppl 1):S1–5.
33. Pandey P, Bodhidatta L, Lewis M, et al. Travelers' diarrhea in Nepal: an update on the pathogens and antibiotic resistance. J Travel Med 2011;18(2):102–8.
34. Löscher T. Clinical presentation and management of travelers' diarrhea. In: Keystone JS, Kozarsky PE, Freedman DO, et al, editors. Travel medicine. 2nd edition. Philadelphia: Mosby Elsevier; 2008.
35. Kaufmann GR, Mattila L, Gyr K. Travelers' diarrhea: clinical features and syndromes. In: Ericsson CD, Steffen R, DuPont HL, editors. Travelers' diarrhea. 2nd edition. Ontario (Canada): BC Decker; 2008.
36. Kollaritsch H, Paulke-Korinek M. Durchfallerkrankungen. In: Löscher T, Burchard GD, editors. Tropenmedizin in Klinik und Praxis mit Reise- und Migrationsmedizin. 4th edition. Georg Thieme Verlag. New York: Stuttgart; 2010.
37. Ortega YR, Adam RD. *Giardia*: overview and update. Clin Infect Dis 1997;25(3): 545–9 [quiz: 550].
38. Hill DR. Occurrence and self-treatment of diarrhea in a large cohort of Americans traveling to developing countries. Am J Trop Med Hyg 2000;62(5):585–9.
39. Hungin AP, Chang L, Locke GR, et al. Irritable bowel syndrome in the United States: prevalence, symptom patterns and impact. Aliment Pharmacol Ther 2005;21(11):1365–75.
40. Ilnyckyj A, Balachandra B, Elliott L, et al. Post-traveler's diarrhea irritable bowel syndrome: a prospective study. Am J Gastroenterol 2003;98(3):596–9.
41. Okhuysen PC, Jiang ZD, Carlin L, et al. Post-diarrhea chronic intestinal symptoms and irritable bowel syndrome in North American travelers to Mexico. Am J Gastroenterol 2004;99(9):1774–8.
42. Huang DB, Awasthi M, Le BM, et al. The role of diet in the treatment of travelers' diarrhea: a pilot study. Clin Infect Dis 2004;39(4):468–71.
43. Steffen R. Worldwide efficacy of bismuth subsalicylate in the treatment of travelers' diarrhea. Rev Infect Dis 1990;12(Suppl 1):S80–6.
44. DuPont HL, Sullivan P, Pickering LK, et al. Symptomatic treatment of diarrhea with bismuth subsalicylate among students attending a Mexican university. Gastroenterology 1977;73(4 Pt 1):715–8.
45. Epple HJ, Fromm M, Riecken EO, et al. Antisecretory effect of loperamide in colon epithelial cells by inhibition of basolateral K+ conductance. Scand J Gastroenterol 2001;36(7):731–7.

46. DuPont HL, Flores Sanchez J, Ericsson CD, et al. Comparative efficacy of loperamide hydrochloride and bismuth subsalicylate in the management of acute diarrhea. Am J Med 1990;88(6A):15S–9S.
47. Palmer KR, Corbett CL, Holdsworth CD. Double-blind cross-over study comparing loperamide, codeine and diphenoxylate in the treatment of chronic diarrhea. Gastroenterology 1980;79(6):1272–5.
48. van Loon FP, Bennish ML, Speelman P, et al. Double blind trial of loperamide for treating acute watery diarrhoea in expatriates in Bangladesh. Gut 1989;30(4):492–5.
49. DuPont HL, Hornick RB. Adverse effect of lomotil therapy in shigellosis. JAMA 1973;226(13):1525–8.
50. Riddle MS, Arnold S, Tribble DR. Effect of adjunctive loperamide in combination with antibiotics on treatment outcomes in traveler's diarrhea: a systematic review and meta-analysis. Clin Infect Dis 2008;47(8):1007–14.
51. DuPont HL, Ericsson CD, Mathewson JJ, et al. Zaldaride maleate, an intestinal calmodulin inhibitor, in the therapy of travelers' diarrhea. Gastroenterology 1993;104(3):709–15.
52. DiCesare D, DuPont H, Mathewson J, et al. A double blind, randomized, placebo-controlled study of SP-303 (Provir) in the symptomatic treatment of acute diarrhea among travelers to Jamaica and Mexico. Am J Gastroenterol 2002;97(10):2585–8.
53. Salazar-Lindo E, Santisteban-Ponce J, Chea-Woo E, et al. Racecadotril in the treatment of acute watery diarrhea in children. N Engl J Med 2000;343(7):463–7.
54. Wang HH, Shieh MJ, Liao KF. A blind, randomized comparison of racecadotril and loperamide for stopping acute diarrhea in adults. World J Gastroenterol 2005;11(10):1540–3.
55. Ericsson CD, DuPont HL, Okhuysen PC, et al. Loperamide plus azithromycin more effectively treats travelers' diarrhea in Mexico than azithromycin alone. J Travel Med 2007;14(5):312–9.
56. Dupont HL, Jiang Z, Belkind-Gerson J, et al. Treatment of travelers' diarrhea: randomized trial comparing rifaximin, rifaximin plus loperamide, and loperamide alone. Clin Gastroenterol Hepatol 2007;5(4):451–6.
57. Ruiz J, Marco F, Oliveira I, et al. Trends in antimicrobial resistance in *Campylobacter* spp. causing traveler's diarrhea. APMIS 2007;115(3):218–24.
58. Tribble DR, Sanders JW, Pang LW, et al. Traveler's diarrhea in Thailand: randomized, double-blind trial comparing single-dose and 3-day azithromycin-based regimens with a 3-day levofloxacin regimen. Clin Infect Dis 2007;44(3):338–46.
59. Chalumeau M, Tonnelier S, D'Athis P, et al. Fluoroquinolone safety in pediatric patients: a prospective, multicenter, comparative cohort study in France. Pediatrics 2003;111(6):e714–9.
60. Grady R. Safety profile of quinolone antibiotics in the pediatric population. Pediatr Infect Dis J 2003;22(12):1128–32.
61. Gomi H, Jiang ZD, Adachi JA, et al. In vitro antimicrobial susceptibility testing of bacterial enteropathogens causing traveler's diarrhea in four geographic regions. Antimicrob Agents Chemother 2001;45(1):212–6.
62. Ericsson CD, DuPont HL, Mathewson JJ. Single dose ofloxacin plus loperamide compared with single dose or three days of ofloxacin in the treatment of traveler's diarrhea. J Travel Med 1997;4(1):3–7.
63. Ericsson CD. Rifaximin: a new approach to the treatment of travelers' diarrhea. Conclusion. J Travel Med 2001;8:s40.

64. DuPont HL, Ericsson CD, Mathewson JJ, et al. Five versus three days of ofloxacin therapy for traveler's diarrhea: a placebo-controlled study. Antimicrob Agents Chemother 1992;36(1):87–91.

65. Kuschner RA, Trofa AF, Thomas RJ, et al. Use of azithromycin for the treatment of *Campylobacter* enteritis in travelers to Thailand, an area where ciprofloxacin resistance is prevalent. Clin Infect Dis 1995;21(3):536–41.

66. DuPont HL, Ericsson CD, Mathewson JJ, et al. Rifaximin: a nonabsorbed antimicrobial in the therapy of travelers' diarrhea. Digestion 1998;59(6):708–14.

67. Haukka K, Siitonen A. Emerging resistance to newer antimicrobial agents among *Shigella* isolated from Finnish foreign travellers. Epidemiol Infect 2008;136(4): 476–82.

68. Vila J, Vargas M, Ruiz J, et al. Quinolone resistance in enterotoxigenic *Escherichia coli* causing diarrhea in travelers to India in comparison with other geographical areas. Antimicrob Agents Chemother 2000;44(6):1731–3.

69. Norman FF, Perez-Molina J, Perez de Ayala A, et al. *Clostridium difficile*-associated diarrhea after antibiotic treatment for traveler's diarrhea. Clin Infect Dis 2008;46(7):1060–3.

70. Neill MA, Opal SM, Heelan J, et al. Failure of ciprofloxacin to eradicate convalescent fecal excretion after acute salmonellosis: experience during an outbreak in health care workers. Ann Intern Med 1991;114(3):195–9.

71. Zhang X, McDaniel AD, Wolf LE, et al. Quinolone antibiotics induce Shiga toxin-encoding bacteriophages, toxin production, and death in mice. J Infect Dis 2000; 181(2):664–70.

72. Rogers TJ, Paton JC. Therapeutic strategies for Shiga toxin-producing *Escherichia coli* infections. Expert Rev Anti Infect Ther 2009;7(6):683–6.

73. Hill DR, Ericsson CD, Pearson RD, et al. The practice of travel medicine: guidelines by the Infectious Diseases Society of America. Clin Infect Dis 2006;43(12): 1499–539.

74. Rendi-Wagner P, Kollaritsch H. Drug prophylaxis for travelers' diarrhea. Clin Infect Dis 2002;34(5):628–33.

75. DuPont HL, Ericsson CD, Farthing MJ, et al. Expert review of the evidence base for prevention of travelers' diarrhea. J Travel Med 2009;16(3):149–60.

76. DuPont HL, Jiang ZD, Okhuysen PC, et al. A randomized, double-blind, placebo-controlled trial of rifaximin to prevent travelers' diarrhea. Ann Intern Med 2005; 142(10):805–12.

77. Martinez-Sandoval F, Ericsson CD, Jiang ZD, et al. Prevention of travelers' diarrhea with rifaximin in US travelers to Mexico. J Travel Med 2010;17(2): 111–7.

78. Flores J, Dupont HL, Jiang ZD, et al. A randomized, double-blind, pilot study of rifaximin 550 mg versus placebo in the prevention of travelers' diarrhea in Mexico during the dry season. J Travel Med 2011;18(5):333–6.

79. Hilton E, Kolakowski P, Singer C, et al. Efficacy of *Lactobacillus* GG as a diarrheal preventive in travelers. J Travel Med 1997;4(1):41–3.

80. Kollaritsch H, Holst H, Grobara P, et al. Prophylaxe der Reisediarrhoe mit *Saccharomyces boulardii*. [Prevention of travelers' diarrhea by *Saccharomyces boulardii*: results of a placebo-controlled double-blind study]. Fortschr Med 1993;11:153–6 [in German].

81. McKenzie R, Bourgeois AL, Frech SA, et al. Transcutaneous immunization with the heat-labile toxin (LT) of enterotoxigenic *Escherichia coli* (ETEC): protective efficacy in a double-blind, placebo-controlled challenge study. Vaccine 2007; 25(18):3684–91.

82. Centers for Disease Control and Prevention. Cholera - general information. Available at: http://www.cdc.gov/cholera/general/#vaccine. Accessed March 14, 2012.

83. Hill DR, Ford L, Lalloo DG. Oral cholera vaccines: use in clinical practice. Lancet Infect Dis 2006;6(6):361–73.

84. Jelinek T, Kollaritsch H. Vaccination with Dukoral against travelers' diarrhea (ETEC) and cholera. Expert Rev Vaccines 2008;7(5):561–7.

85. Health Map. Global outbreaks. Available at: http://healthmap.org/en/. Accessed March 14, 2012.

86. Periago MR, Frieden TR, Tappero JW, et al. Elimination of cholera transmission in Haiti and the Dominican Republic. Lancet 2012;379(9812):e12–3.

87. Clemens JD, Sack DA, Harris JR, et al. Cross-protection by B subunit-whole cell cholera vaccine against diarrhea associated with heat-labile toxin-producing enterotoxigenic Escherichia coli: results of a large-scale field trial. J Infect Dis 1988; 158(2):372–7.

88. Peltola H, Siitonen A, Kyrönseppä H, et al. Prevention of travellers' diarrhoea by oral B-subunit/whole-cell cholera vaccine. Lancet 1991;338:1285–9.

89. Torrell JM, Aumatell CM, Ramos SM, et al. Reduction of travellers' diarrhoea by WC/rBS oral cholera vaccine in young, high-risk travellers. Vaccine 2009; 27(30):4074–7.

90. Lopez-Gigosos R, Garcia-Fortea P, Calvo MJ, et al. Effectiveness and economic analysis of the whole cell/recombinant B subunit (WC/rbs) inactivated oral cholera vaccine in the prevention of traveller's diarrhoea. BMC Infect Dis 2009;9:65.

91. Steffen R, Amitirigala I, Mutsch M. Health risks among travelers–need for regular updates. J Travel Med 2008;15(3):145–6.

Environmental Hazards, Hot, Cold, Altitude, and Sun

Sundeep Dhillon, MBE, MA, BM BCh, MRCGP, Dip IMC, RCSEd, DCh, FRGS, FAWM

KEYWORDS

- Extreme environments • Heat • Cold • High altitude

KEY POINTS

- There has been an increase in both recreational and adventure travel to areas where the environmental conditions are extremely harsh.
- Short-term visitors can adjust to these austere environments provided they have the knowledge and time to acclimatize sufficiently.
- This chapter deals with disorders related to extremes of temperature (Heat and Cold); and High altitude.

EXTREME ENVIRONMENTS

Humans have colonized most areas of the planet, including areas where the environmental conditions are extremely harsh. Native populations to these areas have developed strategies that include clothing, shelter, technology, and behavior, as well as physiologic adaptation, over generations. Short-term visitors can adjust to these austere environments provided they have the knowledge and time to acclimatize sufficiently. There has been an increase in both recreational and adventure travel to extreme environments.[1]

HEAT-RELATED DISORDERS

Humans are well adapted to hot climates but require a period of acclimatization from cold/temperate climates, especially in humid conditions. There is considerable variability of thermal tolerance between individuals, but ultimately everyone will succumb if the duration and intensity of exposure are sufficiently challenging.

Heat Balance

Core body temperature must be maintained around 37°C—failure to maintain this leads to decreased mental and physical performance and, if severe/prolonged, may

The author has nothing to disclose.

Institute of Human Health and Performance, Centre for Aviation Space and Extreme Environment Medicine, University College London, London, United Kingdom

E-mail address: DrSDhillon@aol.com

Infect Dis Clin N Am 26 (2012) 707–723

http://dx.doi.org/10.1016/j.idc.2012.07.001

id.theclinics.com

eventually result in death. Eighty percent of metabolic energy is produced as heat, which is transferred to and from the body via 1 or more of 4 processes: radiation, conduction, convection, or evaporation.[2]

Radiation is the direct transfer of heat between the body surface and other sources of radiant energy, mainly the sun. Conduction is the direct transfer of heat between the body and any solid in contact with it, particularly the ground. Conduction will stop when the 2 solids in contact reach thermal equilibrium. Convection is the removal of heat by the flow of one substance over another, particularly air or water, but also blood from muscles. Convection augments conductive heat transfer, but thermal equilibrium does not develop due to the constant flow of the medium, which prevents thermal equilibrium. The rate of heat transfer depends on the difference in temperature between the body surface and the materials or radiating surfaces in the environment and the air or water velocity.[1]

Heat can be lost indirectly via evaporation of sweat produced by eccrine sweat glands. Each liter of sweat evaporated from the body removes approximately 580 kcal of energy.[3] Sweat that falls off the body without evaporating has not changed state and removes a fraction of this energy (<15%).

During exercise (and at rest in hot environments), heat is produced in muscles and conducted directly to the skin (also via convection by the circulation of blood), where it is dissipated to the environment. Usually the skin is in contact with air, which is a poor conductor, and therefore conductive losses are small. At rest at 20°C, conduction and convection account for only 10% to 20% of our heat loss, with the majority occurring through radiation.[4]

Once the environmental temperature is greater than 35°C, it is impossible to lose heat through conduction, convection, and radiation. Our ability to function and survive in these conditions depends on sweating. Sweating allows the body to lose heat at any environmental temperature through evaporation. Evaporative heat loss can occur only if the air is not saturated with water vapor. It is therefore most efficient in hot, dry conditions and least efficient in hot, humid conditions. Humidity has a greater effect on the ability to lose heat than the absolute temperature.[1,2,4]

The relative importance of various modes of heat transfer is summarized in **Table 1**.

Measurement of Environmental Heat Stress

Assessment of environmental heat stress is necessary to determine the risk to an individual. There are 4 environmental characteristics that influence heat stress:

1. Air temperature—insufficient on its own for determining risk of heat illness
2. Solar (or radiant heat) load
3. Absolute humidity—contributes 70% to calculation
4. Wind speed

Table 1 The relative importance of various modes of heat transfer		Contribution		
Environment	Mode of Heat Transfer	25°C	30°C	35°C
Hot, still air	Radiation	67%	41%	4%
Hot, moving air	Conduction and convection	10%	33%	6%
Hot, moving air, humid	Evaporation	23%	26%	90%

Data from Morimoto T. Heat loss mechanisms. In: Blatteis CM, editor. Physiology and pathophysiology of temperature regulation. Singapore: World Scientific Publishing; 1998. p. 81.

The gold standard measurement is the wet bulb globe temperature (WBGT) index, which measures the first 3 of these characteristics. The American College of Sports Medicine provides guidelines for exercise in hot environments and recommends canceling sporting events if the WBGT is greater than 28°C.[5]

Thermoregulation

Temperature is sensed centrally by the anterior hypothalamus, peripherally by receptors in the skin and via deep body receptors along the great vessels. The anterior hypothalamus contains specialized heat- and cold-sensitive neurons in a 3:1 ratio (reflecting the importance of losing heat effectively) that can detect temperature fluctuations of 0.01°C. Conversely, cold-sensitive receptors dominate the deep and peripheral receptors. Signals from these are evaluated centrally in combination with the central receptors and pain signals and result in involuntary and voluntary (ie, behavioral) changes.[6]

Involuntary responses to a change in core temperature are mediated via skeletal muscles (shivering), smooth muscles (vasoconstriction/vasodilatation and piloerection), eccrine sweat glands (sweating), and the adrenal medulla (norepinephrine and epinephrine increase metabolic rate).[1]

Injuries Caused by Heat

Heat illness occurs predominantly in nonacclimatized individuals in hot, humid environments but can occur with prolonged activity (and inappropriate clothing/equipment) in temperate or cold environments. Several risk factors for heat illness have been identified (**Box 1**).

The most important individual factors are reduced physical fitness, lack of acclimatization, dehydration, and concurrent illness. Exercise time to exhaustion is reduced when either the temperature or humidity (or both) is increased. Dehydration (>2% of

---

Box 1
Risk factors for heat illness

- High temperature and humidity
- Insufficient shade
- Inappropriate clothing and heavy equipment
- Low physical fitness/unaccustomed activity
- Obesity
- Lack of acclimatization
- Inadequate hydration/nutrition
- Previous history of heat-related illnesses
- Heat-related skin conditions (sunburn, miliaria rubra)
- Sleep deprivation/jet lag
- Concurrent illnesses (fever, respiratory infection, diarrhea, vomiting)
- Sweat gland dysfunction
- Extremes of age
- Alcohol/recreational drug use (amphetamines, cocaine, ecstasy)
- Medication (anticholinergics, antihistamines, atropine, β-blockers, diuretics, major tranquillizers, phenothiazines, scopolamine, theophylline, tricyclic antidepressants)

total body water) decreases exercise performance, time to exhaustion, and the ability to dissipate heat. Hyperthermia occurs when the rate of heat production by the muscles exceeds the body's ability to transfer this to the ambient environment. Heat production during heavy exercise may be 15 to 20 times that at rest. Heat illness must be excluded or treated whenever a previously well individual collapses in a hot environment (or during heavy exercise in a temperate/cold environment).[1]

Clinical Presentations

Heat exhaustion is the most commonly encountered form of heat illness. It occurs when the cardiac output is insufficient to meet the demands of increased blood flow to the skin, working muscles, and vital organs. This is compounded due to a decreased effective plasma volume (redistribution of blood), dehydration, and salt loss caused by sweating. Heat exhaustion does not result in any organ damage, and some individuals may be fit to resume activities after 24 to 48 hours.

Classic heatstroke typically occurs when humans are left in hot, unventilated environments such as mines or prisons, when a human is a stowaway, and when children are left in cars during heat waves. It tends to affect those individuals with impaired thermoregulation (children, the elderly, people with underlying medical conditions, or people taking drugs known to interfere with thermoregulation).

Exertional Heatstroke

Exertional heat stroke (EHS) is defined as a core body temperature greater than 40°C as a result of strenuous exercise and/or environmental heat exposure associated with central nervous system dysfunction and multiple system organ failure (usually cardiovascular collapse). Heat shock proteins and cytokines contribute to the systemic inflammatory response syndrome.[2] This is most often associated with pale, sweaty skin as apposed to the hot, dry, flushed skin seen in classic heat stroke.[7] As tissue temperatures increase, cell membranes and enzyme-dependent energy systems are disrupted, leading to variable cell and organ dysfunction and death. The exact effects are unpredictable but are directly related to the duration and degree of elevation of core temperature. Most patients recover fully if cooled rapidly enough to allow core temperature and cognitive function to return to normal within 1 hour of onset of symptoms. Recognition and prompt treatment are therefore paramount.[2,5]

Pathophysiology of Heat Stroke

The brain is acutely sensitive to hyperthermia (cognitive function and level of consciousness are important diagnostic and prognostic factors). Autoregulation of blood flow and pressure is disrupted, leading to collapse. Cardiac tissue is directly suppressed by hyperthermia, which contributes to collapse by reducing cardiac output and therefore oxygen delivery and heat transfer. Gastrointestinal blood flow is reduced at the expense of peripheral vasodilatation, which impairs splanchnic heat exchange, especially if the person is dehydrated. Disruption of skeletal muscle membranes may lead to rhabdomyolysis and consequent renal tubular dysfunction and obstruction. Coagulopathy from disseminated intravascular coagulation secondary to vascular endothelial damage may occur. Hepatic injury is manifested by raised transaminase levels and sometimes jaundice.[2]

Prevention of Heat Illness

Heat illness is largely preventable following a sufficient period of acclimatization provided that sufficient water and electrolytes are available to maintain euhydration. A strategy to reduce heat illness is given in **Box 2**.

Box 2
Prevention of heat illness

- Identify individuals at risk.
- Monitor environmental heat stress (ideally WBGT).
- Adjust activity accordingly.
- Educate about heat illness (prevention, early recognition and treatment).
- Provide adequate, clean, palatable drinking water; shade; and latrines.
- Ensure a robust medical treatment and evacuation system is in place.

Acclimatization to Heat

Acclimatization involves repeated exposure to heat, sufficient to raise the core body temperature by at least 1°C for at least 60 min/d, ideally around 100 min/d. The degree and rate of acclimatization depend on the thermal stress to which the individual is exposed and its duration. Full heat acclimatization takes 10 to 14 days with carefully supervised exercise for 2 to 3 h/d. The intensity of exercise should be gradually increased every day, working up to an appropriate physical training schedule adapted for the environment. Physical training should be conducted in the morning or evening, avoiding the hottest part of the day, noting that humidity is often highest in the morning.[3,6]

Acclimatization results in blood vessels opening wider and sooner, increasing conductive/convective heat transfer. Sweat rates increase from around 0.5 L/h in the acclimatized to greater than 2 L/h with full acclimatization. The net result is large increase in the rate of heat loss (up to 20-fold). The benefits of acclimatization are lost during 20 to 40 days after returning to a temperate environment. The overall effects of acclimatization are summarized in **Box 3**.[1,6]

Fluid and Electrolyte Replacement

Sweating can remove heat only if there is sufficient fluid to spare for evaporation. A reduction in total body water of 1% affects thermoregulation, and losses of 2% significantly impair physical and mental performance. Thirst is a poor stimulus to drink, and total body water losses of 5% to 10% have been tolerated in experiments. Fluid must be consumed before, during, and after physical activity to maintain normal (eu-) hydration. This is most easily assessed by measuring the specific gravity of the first urine of the day (a specific gravity of ≤1.020 can be considered as euhydrated), along with

---

Box 3
Physiologic responses to heat acclimatization

- Increased sweat production
- Decreased salt concentration of sweat
- Sweating initiated at a lower temperature
- Decreased heart rate
- Increased blood volume
- Decreased glycogen consumption
- Increased renal salt conservation

changes in daily body weight performed at the same time (and before and after activity). There are considerable variations between heat tolerance, sweating rates, and water and electrolyte losses between individuals and between different activities.[8]

Dehydration predisposes the individual to heat exhaustion, heat stroke, and muscle cramps. Hyponatremia may be life threatening and results from excess sodium losses in sweat or rehydration with water alone. Women tend to have lower sweating rates than do men but may be more prone to exercise-induced hyponatremia. Children have lower sweating rates than do adults. The elderly have a reduced thirst sensation and slower water and sodium homeostatic mechanisms, which predispose them to dehydration and exercise-induced hyponatremia.[8,9]

Approximately 1.5 L of fluid needs to be consumed for each liter of fluid lost in sweat (or each 1-kg difference between pre- and post-activity body weight). Food should be consumed as soon as possible after activity to replenish glycogen stores and provide electrolytes, which in many cases will be sufficient to replace those lost in sweat. Fluids should be consumed slowly several hours before the commencement of activity. Sudden ingestion of a large amount of water leads to an inappropriate diuresis, even if dehydrated. Current recommendations are to imbibe 150 to 300 mL every 15 minutes. During exercise, gastric emptying limits fluid absorption to around 1200 mL/h. If the activity is prolonged (45–60 minutes or longer), fluid should be consumed during the activity. Commercially available sports drinks may provide some advantages over water alone under certain conditions. The drinks are rarely isotonic and should not be used them for the first time in a hot environment or during exercise without first getting used to them. Current recommendations are that they should contain around 20 to 30 mmol sodium, 2 to 5 mM potassium, and 5% to 10% carbohydrate.[3,9,10]

Recognition of Heat Illness

The signs and symptoms of heat illness are varied and nonspecific. Any change in personality or performance, especially in a hot, humid environment, must be assumed to be EHS until proved otherwise. A core temperature must be measured (rectal remains the gold standard, but tympanic temperature measurement, if performed correctly, is quicker and easier). Hypoglycemia must be excluded by blood glucose estimation. The systolic blood pressure is commonly less than 100 mm Hg. The main features of heat illness are listed in **Box 4**.[7,11]

Box 4
Signs and symptoms of heat illness

Weakness	Confusion
• Lethargy	• Irrational/unusual behavior
• Fatigue (may be profound)	• Irritability
• Muscle cramps	• Impaired judgment
• Nausea	• Increased respiratory/heart rate
• Vomiting	• Inability to walk
• Diarrhea	• Loss of balance
• Headache	• Collapse
• Dizziness	• Convulsions
• Disorientation	• Coma

Treatment of Heat Illness

EHS is a life-threatening medical emergency that requires immediate cooling to reduce the severity of heat exposure. Individuals must be removed from the activity into a cool, shaded treatment facility. The most rapid cooling (with lowest morbidity and mortality) is achieved with ice/cold water immersion. Aggressive cooling using ice water–soaked towels in combination with ice packs to the head, neck, axillae, and groin also achieves reasonable cooling. Evaporative cooling using wet towels and fanning is less effective, especially in humid conditions. Intravenous fluid replacement is rarely required and may contribute to hyponatremia. Normal saline at 5°C has been used to successfully treat Hajj pilgrims. Usually less than 1 liter is required, reflecting that the primary effect is by cooling rather than rehydration. Occasionally, individuals with deranged thermoregulation present with shivering. They are acutely unwell and the shivering results in excessive and continuing heat production. Core temperature, heart rate, and blood pressure should be measured as soon as possible but not at the expense of rapid cooling.[5,7,11,12]

Patients may exhibit a lucid interval and all patients except those with the most trivial cases must be observed and transferred to hospital for further assessment. Blood should be taken for hematology (including clotting) and serum biochemistry (including liver enzymes and creatinine kinase). Prolonged elevation of liver and muscle enzymes is a poor prognostic marker. Urine should be checked for myoglobin. Hospital treatment is largely supportive and involves administration of oxygen, correction of abnormalities, and provision of the right thermal environment (thermoregulation will be impaired). Laboratory and clinical signs and renal function should guide fluid and electrolyte replacement. If intensive therapy is required, the prognosis is usually poor.[2,7,12]

Patients may remain heat intolerant for more than 1 year (especially if hepatic damage has occurred), but patients with a minor case may resume activities in a hot environment after about 1 month, providing they have 2 weeks of supervised reacclimatization.[5,7]

Sunburn

Sunburn reduces the thermoregulatory capacity of skin and affects central thermoregulation. Sunburn should be prevented by insisting on the use of adequate sun protection. When sunburn does occur, affected individuals should be kept from significant heat strain until the burn has healed. Repeated exposure to the sun increases the risk of skin cancer and photoaging. A high-protection sun cream, ideally water resistant, should be applied before exposure to the sun and at regular intervals during the day. If possible, exposure to the sun should be avoided between 10:00 AM and 2:00 PM.[13]

Miliaria Rubra

Miliaria rubra is an inflammatory skin eruption that appears in actively sweating skin in humid conditions (or skin covered by clothing in dry environments). Each lesion represents a blocked sweat gland, which cannot function efficiently. The risk of heat illness is increased in proportion to the amount of skin surface involved. Sleeplessness due to itching and secondary infection of occluded glands may further affect thermoregulation. Miliaria is treated by cooling and drying affected skin, avoiding sweating, controlling infection, and relieving itching. Sweat gland function recovers with replacement of the damaged skin, which takes 7 to 10 days.[12]

Heat Edema

Mild swelling of the limbs may be experienced during the first few days' exposure to heat, during which the plasma volume increases to allow for the increased blood flow to the skin. Cutaneous vasodilatation and pooling of increased interstitial fluid in dependent extremities result in swelling of the hands and feet. It is self-limiting, resolving in a few days.[14]

Heat Syncope

Heat syncope is a vasovagal faint due to dependent blood pooling in the legs. Although most cases of heat syncope are harmless, the potential for heat illness (especially dehydration) should be considered, especially following physical work in the heat, or after the acclimatization period. It is more common in the elderly and the poorly acclimatized. Treatment is rest and oral fluids.[14]

Exercise-Associated Muscle (Heat) Cramps

These are painful skeletal muscle spasms following prolonged exercise, often in the heat. They usually occur in the arms, legs, or abdomen as a result of prolonged exercise and are thought to be caused by dilutional hyponatremia, but they also occur in cool conditions, such as during swimming. Treatment is rest, prolonged stretches of affected muscle groups, and oral sodium replacement. If the individual is otherwise well, there is no association with heat illness, but a raised core temperature should be treated promptly.[14]

COLD-RELATED DISORDERS
Accidental Hypothermia

Hypothermia occurs when the core temperature decreases to less than 35°C and can be classified as mild (35°–32°C), moderate (32°–28°C), or severe (<28°C).[15,16] The Swiss classification should be used in the field by rescuers.[17] Risk factors for hypothermia include extremes of age, homelessness, trauma, poor nutrition, exhaustion, mental illness, and alcohol and drug abuse.

Hypothermia affects almost every organ system. Cerebral metabolism increases initially but then declines by 6% for each 1°C decrease in core temperature. At 28°C, oxygen consumption is reduced by about 50%, and at 22°C, by about 75%.[18] This offers some cerebral protection. The electroencephalogram is abnormal at less than 33.5°C and undetectable at less than 25°C.[15] Cold causes peripheral vasoconstriction to reduce skin blood flow. At less than 10°C, vasoconstriction is alternated with transient periods of vasodilatation. This is known as cold-induced vasodilatation, or the "hunting response."[19] Initial increases in heart rate and blood pressure due to catecholamines decline progressively, resulting in a bradycardia of 50% at 28°C, at which temperature spontaneous pacemaker depolarization may occur. The myocardium become increasingly irritable and any dysrhythmias can occur, classically atrial fibrillation with a slow ventricular rate followed by ventricular fibrillation. Characteristic Osborn (J waves) are seen at less than 32°C.[20] Following initial hyperventilation, there is a progressive decrease in respiratory rate and depth leading to carbon dioxide retention and respiratory acidosis. At extreme temperatures, central control of respiration may be lost. The chest wall becomes increasingly stiff. These factors combine to produce noncardiogenic pulmonary edema. Cough and gag reflexes are lost. There may be profound disorders of coagulation. A cold-induced diuresis leads to intravascular volume depletion.[15]

Accidental hypothermia may be underdiagnosed, particularly in temperate climes. Hypothermia may be suspected from the history or clinical examination of a collapsed patient. Measurement of the core temperature using a low-reading thermometer is essential. Shivering eventually gives way to rigor. Subtle changes in behavior deteriorate into loss of consciousness and deep reflexes.[16]

Resuscitation should be performed in accordance with international guidelines. Careful handling is essential in order to not irritate the fragile myocardium. Wet clothing should be removed, and the casualty is dried and insulated. Endotracheal intubation and mechanical ventilation are needed to secure the airway and ventilate the noncompliant chest. Electrocardiograph monitoring is mandatory. If there is any doubt about a pulse, cardiopulmonary resuscitation (CPR) should be commenced, noting that the myocardium is refractory to standard resuscitation drugs and defibrillation until the patient has been warmed to about 30°C and should be withheld until this has been achieved. Passive or active warming techniques may be used depending on the degree of hypothermia, skill and availability of staff and facilities, and distance to a hospital with more advanced capabilities. There should be early liaison with units with cardiopulmonary bypass and extracorporeal membrane oxygenation facilities.[21,22] Death should not be declared until the patient is "warm and dead." Good-quality survival has been reported after cardiac arrest and a core temperature of 13.7°C after immersion in cold water with prolonged CPR.[23] In another case, a severely hypothermic patient was resuscitated successfully after 6.5 hours of CPR.[24] The likelihood of survival following avalanche has recently been established and depends on the time of burial, initial core temperature, and initial serum potassium level. Survival is unlikely if, on finding the victim, he or she has been buried for longer than 35 minutes, has an obstructed airway (snow), has a core temperature of less than 32°C, and has an initial serum potassium level of greater than 12 mM.[25]

Cold Water Immersion

A water temperature of 33° to 35°C is required for a nude person to remain thermally neutral.[26] At less than this temperature, hypothermia will eventually occur, with the greatest risk in water less than 25°C. Cold-water immersion may also result in near drowning.[27]

Sudden immersion in cold water leads to skin cooling, which initiates shivering thermogenesis—increases in heart rate, ventilation, cardiac output, mean arterial pressure, and metabolism. There is an increased diuresis secondary to the hydrostatic pressure of water, which together with fluid shifts compromises tissue perfusion. The initial cold shock response (0–2 minutes) is manifested by a gasp response and hyperventilation with an inability to breath-hold. This may cause drowning if the head is submerged. Hypocapnia ensues, which may cause confusion, altered consciousness, and drowning. Arrhythmias and myocardial ischemia may be triggered by the increased cardiac demand.[28]

Cold incapacitation dominates the second phase: peripheral cooling continues rapidly and neuromuscular activity is severely compromised after about 30 minutes.[29] Fine motor control is lost rapidly so survival tasks (eg, getting into a life raft) become extremely difficult.[30] Many strong swimmers have drowned during this phase while trying to reach safety. The heat escape lessening position, where arms are crossed in front of the chest and knees are drawn up, minimizes heat loss, as does huddling together if in a group.[31]

Most deaths in cold water are due to drowning in the first 2 phases. In the third phase, hypothermia can result if immersion time exceeds 30 to 60 minutes. Small children will cool faster than obese adults.[28]

Rescue is particularly hazardous and associated with circum-rescue collapse. Cardiovascular collapse can occur just before rescue (decreased sympathetic drive and catecholamine release) or during or immediately after rescue. Removal from water results in decreased hydrostatic pressure, sudden pooling of blood in the legs, and a compromised cerebral and cardiac circulation. Ideally, victims who have been submerged should be removed from water in a horizontal position.[32]

Afterdrop is the continued decrease in core temperature after removal from cold water. Drops of 5° to 6°C have been observed in humans, and this has been suggested as an explanation for the postrescue deaths observed between 20 minutes and 24 hours after rescue.[28] Once successfully rescued, the victims should be handled carefully, dried, and managed as for hypothermia.

Frostnip

Frostnip is a superficial reversible nonfreezing cold injury associated with intense vasoconstriction. By definition, tissue does not freeze and therefore tissue loss and long-term damage do not occur provided the affected area is rewarmed and frostbite does not develop. Numbness and pallor usually resolve quickly (<30 minutes) after covering the skin with appropriate clothing, warming the skin with direct contact, breathing with cupped hands over the nose, or gaining shelter that protects from the elements. In some cases, paresthesia can persist for weeks.[33]

Frostbite (Freezing Cold Injury)

Frostbite is a thermal injury that occurs when tissue freezes. It is also known as freezing cold injury (FCI) to distinguish it from nonfreezing cold injury (NFCI), which it can often follow, particularly in the military environment.[34] The severity is related to the temperature and duration of exposure with additional tissue damage occurring during rearming. Wet skin, high humidity, and wind chill increase the chances of frostbite.[35] A 12-year study from Canada found that alcohol consumption was the most important predisposing factor (46%), followed by psychiatric illness. Ninety percent of frostbite cases involved the feet or hands.[36] The pathophysiology of frostbite involves 4 overlapping phases (**Table 2**):

Traditionally, frostbite has been classified by numerical degree, but this is not particularly helpful in the prehospital setting.[37] In the field, frostbite can be described as superficial (no/minimal expected tissue loss) corresponding to first- and second-degree injury or as deep with expected tissue loss (third- and fourth-degree injury). The severity can vary within a digit.[33] The classification proposed by Cauchy relies on ^{99m}TC isotope imaging to provide a prediction of outcome within 48 hours of the injury.[38]

Symptoms and signs of frostbite are initially benign with an insidious onset. Sensation is lost to the affected area, which is cold with markedly reduced function. The skin

Table 2	
The pathophysiology of frostbite	
Phase	**Pathophysiology**
Prefreeze	Tissue cooling and vasoconstriction result in ischemic hyperesthesia/paresthesia
Freeze-thaw	Ice crystal formation disrupts proteins and lipids, causing electrolyte shifts, dehydration, lysis, and cell death
	Thawing produces ischemia-reperfusion injury and triggers the inflammatory response
Vascular stasis	Alternating vasoconstriction and dilation leads to coagulation within vessels or extravascular leak
Late ischemia	Progressive tissue ischemia and infarction resulting in destruction of the microcirculation mediated by thromboxane A_2, prostaglandin $F_{2\alpha}$, bradykinins, and histamine

Data from Imray C, Grieve A, Dhillon S. The Caudwell Xtreme Everest Research Group. Cold damage to the extremities: frostbite and non-freezing cold injuries. Postgrad Med J 2009;85(1007):481–8.

seems waxy, becoming mottled-blue or yellowish-white. Rewarming causes a reactive hyperemia and pain, which can persist for months, even following amputation.

Once frozen, tissue damage is inevitable, so prevention is paramount. Tissue exposure to the cold must be minimized and peripheral perfusion maintained. The risk increases at less than −15°C. Skin should be protected from moisture, wind, and cold, including perspiration and wet extremities. Emollients may increase the risk. Appropriate clothing should be worn in layers supplemented by chemical or electrical hand and feet warmers. Alcohol, tobacco, immersion, exhaustion, hypoxia, carbon monoxide (from poorly ventilated cooking stoves), and drugs affecting judgment must be avoided. Peripheral perfusion must be maintained with adequate hydration. Footwear and clothing should not be constrictive, and immobility should be avoided. Exercise increases the frequency and degree of cold-induced peripheral vasodilatation protecting the extremities but requires adequate energy. Supplemental oxygen should be considered at greater than 7500 m.[33]

Education and prompt recognition are vital with a buddy-buddy system used rigorously to actively enquire and look for frostnip and frostbite, with immediate rewarming. Frozen tissue must be protected from further harm. Jewelry and tight-fitting clothing should be removed. Most tissue will gradually rewarm, but if conditions allow for rapid rewarming, this is preferable because it limits both the temperature and duration of exposure. Refreezing must be avoided at all costs because the freeze-thaw process releases prostaglandins and thromboxane, resulting in significant vasoconstriction, microcirculatory stasis, thrombosis, and cellular injury. If refreezing cannot be prevented in the field, frozen tissue is best left frozen, accepting that some gradual passive thawing is likely to occur. Tissue that is thawed and then frozen almost always dies.[33]

Treatment of frostbite includes actively seeking and managing hypothermia and replacement of fluids. If the frostbitten tissue is associated with a fracture, the limb should be realigned to improve distal perfusion. Frostbitten tissue must be handled gently. It should not be rubbed, nor should ice or snow be applied. Blisters should be left intact. Ibuprofen (12 mg/kg/d in 2 doses) is useful for its antiprostaglandin effect and should be continued for 4 to 6 weeks. Cold water should not be used to thaw the tissues, and high temperatures, such as from a stove, should be avoided.[39] Field rewarming should be carried if adequate facilities exist, definitive medical care is more than 2 hours away, and refreezing can be avoided. The affected tissue is placed in a hot water bath at 37° to 39°C. The tissue should not touch the sides or bottom of the vessel. The water should be circulated around the affected area and temperature retained using additional water of the same temperature. The vessel should not be directly heated and should be insulated from the ground. Flushing of the distal tissue and pain indicate successful rewarming. The tissue should then be air-dried (not rubbed) and topical aloe vera applied if available (reduces prostaglandin and thromboxane formation). Considerable post-thaw edema should be anticipated and bulky dressings should be loosely applied, with sterile pads between affected digits. The affected tissue should be elevated above the level of the heart to reduce edema formation. The casualty must now be considered nonambulatory except when the life of the patient or rescuer is in danger.[33]

Hospital care should be undertaken by someone experienced in the care of frostbite. Tetanus toxoid and opiate analgesia are indicated. Early surgery should be limited to escharotomy or fasciotomy to preserve circulation or if a compartment syndrome develops. Moist gangrene is a nidus for infection, which can become systemic and may necessitate early amputation, but most morbidity from frostbite results from early amputation at the hands of inexperienced surgeons. ^{99m}TC scans allow early predication of devitalized tissues. There has been considerable success with iloprost infusions.[40] Telemedicine services are available to patients worldwide (http://www.christopherimray.co.uk/).

NFCI

NFCI typically occurs after prolonged exposure (hours to days) to temperatures between 0° and 15°C, often associated with wet conditions.[41] Historically, it has been a scourge of the military and typically affects the feet. The main feature is of a local sensory vasoneuropathy, which may be unreported and undiagnosed. Afro Caribbeans have a reduced cold-induced vasodilatory response compared with Caucasians. They are more vulnerable to both NFCI and FCI. Repeated exposure to cold increases cold-induced vasodilatation (CIVD) with shorter intervals between dilatations. This phenomenon has been recorded in high-latitude native populations and cold-water fishermen.[42]

Treatment follows the guidelines for FCI except slower rewarming is advocated. There is a transient pale cyanosis during rewarming, later replaced by hyperemia, edema, erythema, and pain. Pain is the main presenting complaint, which is both more severe and prolonged (months) than that seen in FCI. This may require early use of tricyclic antidepressants. Pain specialists should be consulted early and sympathectomy avoided due to long-term deterioration. In severe cases, a chronic picture resembling reflex sympathetic dystrophy develops, leading to ulceration, hyperhidrosis, edema, and susceptibility to fungal infections. Amputations are sometimes performed. There is permanently increased sensitivity to cold, which is some cases renders the individual unfit to work outdoors.[19]

In the absence of internationally accepted criteria for the diagnosis and management of this disabling condition, prevention through education is paramount.

Altitude-Related Disorders

An increasing number of people travel to high altitudes for recreation. The speed of ascent to greater than 2500 m (1 m = 3.281 ft) is the most important factor in determining the likelihood of the development of altitude illness. The proportion of oxygen in the habitable atmosphere is 21%, but barometric pressure declines in a nonlinear way, with increasing altitude resulting in hypobaric hypoxia, so that at Everest Base Camp (5800 m), there is approximately half the oxygen available compared with sea level. The temperature decreases by 6.5°C for every 1000 m of altitude gained and the air becomes very dry, further adding to the physiologic burden.[43] High altitude can be conveniently described by the physiologic effect on the body (**Table 3**)

Acclimatization

Acute exposure to the summit of Mt Everest would result in loss of consciousness within a few minutes, followed rapidly by death. This is equivalent to sudden aircraft cabin depressurization. Yet, some people have managed to climb Mt Everest without the use of supplemental oxygen. This is only possible due to several changes in human physiology, which are collectively known as acclimatization. The main effects noticed by the individual are an increase in resting heart and respiratory rates accompanied by a decrease in exercise capacity (maximum heart rate). The proportion of red blood cells, which carry oxygen, increases along with a raft of other biochemical adjustments, which aim to improve oxygen delivery and use. Unlike adaptation, where favorable characteristics are genetically selected over many generations, the effects of acclimatization are rapidly lost on descent to low altitudes.[44]

Table 3		
Physiologic effects of high altitude		
Description	**Altitude**	**Physiologic Effects on the Body**
Low altitude	<1500 m	None if otherwise healthy
Intermediate altitude	1500–2500 m	Arterial oxygen saturation (Sao_2) remains >90%. Altitude illness is rare but possible.
High altitude	2500–3500 m	Altitude illness commonly occurs with rapid ascent
Very high altitude	3500–5800 m	Sao_2 falls <90%, especially on exertion/exercise. Altitude illness common, even with gradual ascent.
Extreme altitude	>5500 m	Sao_2 <90% even at rest. Marked hypoxemia with exertion. High-altitude deterioration eventually outstrips acclimatization. Limit of permanent human habitation

Data from Hackett PH, Roach RC. High-altitude medicine & physiology. In: Auerbach PS, editor. Wilderness medicine. 6th edition. Philadelphia: Elsevier; 2012. p. 2–33; and Pollard AJ, Murdoch DR. The high altitude medicine handbook. 3rd edition. Abingdon (Oxfordshire): Radcliffe Publishing; 2003. p. 193.

Altitude-related illnesses usually occur when the rate of ascent exceeds the body's ability to acclimatize to the hypoxia. At greater than 3000 m, the sleeping altitude should be increased by no more than 500 m per day with a rest day every 3 to 4 days. This will not protect everyone as considerable individual variation occurs. There are no reliable sea-level predictors (eg, age, sex, fitness) of susceptibility to altitude disorders.[45] Awareness, early recognition, and prompt treatment of high-altitude illnesses are thus paramount. The rate of ascent is probably the most important modifiable factor in preventing high-altitude illness. In Nepal, 50% of trekkers who reach 4000 m in 5 days suffered from acute mountain sickness (AMS), compared with 84% of those who flew directly to 3860 m.[46,47]

AMS

The symptoms of AMS are headache, nausea, vomiting, lethargy, fatigue, loss of appetite, and poor sleep. None of the symptoms are specific, and other conditions such as dehydration, hypothermia, exhaustion, and viral infections, are also common, but AMS must be excluded in the mountains, particularly if there has been a recent height gain. The mechanism is unknown, but it is thought to involve increased permeability of blood vessels leading to swelling (edema) of the brain. Swelling of the limbs and face are risk factors for altitude illness.[48]

Treatment involves avoiding any further ascent until symptoms have resolved, simple painkillers (paracetamol/acetaminophen or ibuprofen) for headache, and acetazolamide. With severe AMS (or if the symptoms do not improve with the acetazolamide), dexamethasone should be used along with supplemental oxygen.[45]

Descending to a lower altitude is the most effective and definitive treatment of all forms of altitude illness.

High-Altitude Cerebral Edema

High-altitude cerebral edema (HACE) lies at the opposite end of the spectrum of altitude disorders from AMS. It is a life-threatening form of altitude illness. Fortunately, it is rare, affecting around 1% to 2% of people ascending to 4500 m. It is usually preceded by AMS but can occur without warning. The cardinal feature is ataxia (best tested by heel–toe walking with the eyes closed). HACE is often accompanied by strange and inappropriate behavior (eg, removing one's gloves). Almost any neuro-logic sign and symptom may be seen, including strokes, but the most common are confusion, disorientation, hallucinations, and an inability to pass urine. Untreated, it can rapidly lead to unconsciousness, coma, and death.[48]

The main treatment is immediate descent. Dexamethasone and supplemental oxygen (if available) should be given immediately. A portable hyperbaric chamber may also be beneficial and should be considered by all teams ascending to very high/extreme altitudes. Other altitude illnesses commonly occur along with HACE, and both acetazolamide and nifedipine may be required.

High-Altitude Pulmonary Edema

High-altitude pulmonary edema (HAPE) is an independent altitude illness and the most common cause of death related to high altitude. It results from an increased pulmo-nary artery pressure coupled with increased vascular permeability leading to a noncar-diogenic pulmonary edema. The incidence may be 10% with rapid ascents to 4500 m, but 1% to 2% is more likely with a sensible ascent profile.[48] HAPE typically occurs among fit young men on the second night after ascending to high altitude and is more common following a viral upper respiratory tract infection. It may be preceded by AMS and is manifested by decreased exercise tolerance with increased recovery time.

The symptoms progress to dyspnea (initially exertional, but later at rest), fatigue, and lethargy, Symptoms are often worse lying down, with tachycardia, tachypnea, and orthopnea. Peripheral cyanosis is usually present. AMS symptoms are found in 50% of cases and HACE in 14%. Treatment is immediate descent and nifedipine. Supplemental oxygen and a portable hyperbaric chamber may be used if available. HAPE tends to recur at the same altitude and the individual should be advised about the risks of re-ascent.[44] A dry cough is common at altitude due to the dry air and, if not symptomatic, is not related to HAPE.

A summary of the medical management of altitude-related disorders is presented in **Table 4**.

Table 4
Summary of medical management of altitude-related disorders

Medication	Indication	Adult Dose	Pediatric Dose	Route
Acetazolamide	Prevention of AMS and HACE	125 mg q 12 h	2.5 mg/kg bid	Oral
	Treatment of AMS	250 mg q 12 h	2.5 mg/kg bid	Oral
Dexamethasone	Prevention of AMS and HACE	2 mg q 6 h or 4 mg q 12 h	Not recommended	Oral
	Treatment of AMS	4 mg q 6 h		Oral, IV, IM
	Treatment of HACE	8 mg stat followed by 4 mg q 6 h	0.15 mg/kg q 6 h	Oral, IV, IM
Nifidepine	Prevention and treatment of HAPE	60 mg SR daily (30 mg SR bid or 20 mg SR q 8 h)	Not recommended	Oral

Data from Luks AM, McIntosh SE, Grissom CK, et al. Wilderness Medical Society consensus guide-lines for the prevention and treatment of acute altitude illness. Wilderness Environ Med 2010;21:146–55.

SUMMARY

Humans can successfully acclimatize to and perform reasonably well in extreme environments, provided that sufficient time is given for acclimatization (where possible) and if they use appropriate behavior. This is aided by a knowledge of the problems likely to be encountered and their prevention, recognition, and treatment.

REFERENCES

1. Johnson C, Anderson S, Dallimore J, et al. Oxford handbook of expedition and wilderness medicine. Oxford (UK): Oxford University Press; 2010.
2. Leon LR, Kenefick RW. Pathophysiology of heat-related illnesses. In: Auerbach PS, editor. Wilderness medicine. 6th edition. Philadelphia: Elsevier; 2012. p. 215–31.
3. Sawka MN, Burke LM, Eichner ER, et al. American College of Sports Medicine position stand. Exercise and fluid replacement. Med Sci Sports Exerc 2007; 39(2):377–90.
4. Morimoto T, Yoda T, et al. Heat loss mechanisms. In: Blatteis C, editor. Physiology and pathophysiology of temperature regulation. Singapore: World Scientific Publishing; 1998. p. 87–90.
5. Armstrong LE, Casa DJ, Millard-Stafford MM, et al. American College of Sports Medicine position stand. Exertional heat illness during training and competition. Med Sci Sports Exerc 2007;39(3):556–72.
6. Crawshaw LI, Nagashima K, Yoda T, et al. Thermoregulation. In: Auerbach PS, editor. Wilderness medicine. 6th edition. Philadelphia: Elsevier; 2012. p. 104–16.
7. O'Connor FG, Casa DJ, Bergeron MF, et al. American College of Sports Medicine Roundtable on exertional heat stroke–return to duty/return to play: conference proceedings. In: Current Sports Medicine Reports. vol. 9. 2010. p. 314–21.
8. Kenefick RW, Cheuvront SN, Leon LR, et al. Dehydration, rehydration and hyperhydration. In: Auerbach PS, editor. Wilderness medicine. 6th edition. Philadelphia: Elsevier; 2012. p. 1393–405.
9. Noakes TD. Fluid and electrolyte disturbances in heat illness. Int J Sports Med 1998;19(Suppl 2):S146–9.
10. Maughan RJ, Leiper JB, Shirreffs SM. Factors influencing the restoration of fluid and electrolyte balance after exercise in the heat. Br J Sports Med 1997;31(3): 175–82.
11. O'Brien KK, Leon LR, Kenefick RW. Clinical management of heat-related illnesses. In: Auerbach PS, editor. Wilderness medicine. 6th edition. Philadelphia: Elsevier; 2012. p. 232–40.
12. Dallimore J, Dhillon S, Richards P, et al. Hot environments: deserts and tropical forests. In: Warrell DA, Dallimore J, Johnson C, et al, editors. Oxford handbook of expedition and wilderness medicine. Oxford (UK): Oxford University Press; 2010.
13. Kraakowski AC, Kaplan LA. Exposure to radiation from the Sun. In: Auerbach PS, editor. Wilderness medicine. 6th edition. Philadelphia: Elsevier; 2012. p. 294–313.
14. Lugo-Amador NM, Rothenhaus T, Moyer P. Heat-related illness. Emerg Med Clin North Am 2004;22(2):315–27.
15. Danzl DF. Accidental hypothermia. In: Auerbach PS, editor. Wilderness medicine. 6th edition. Philadelphia: Elsevier; 2012. p. 116–42.
16. Leikin SM, Korley FK, Wang EE, et al. The spectrum of hypothermia: from environmental exposure to therapeutic uses and medical simulation. Dis Mon 2012; 58(1):6–32.

17. Durrer BB, Brugger HH, Syme DD. The medical on-site treatment of hypothermia: ICAR-MEDCOM recommendation. High Alt Med Biol 2003;4(1):99–103.

18. Wood SC. Interactions between hypoxia and hypothermia. Annu Rev Physiol 1991;53:71–85.

19. Imray CH, Richards PP, Greeves JJ, et al. Nonfreezing cold-induced injuries. J R Army Med Corps 2011;157(1):79–84.

20. Mattu A, Brady WJ, Perron AD. Electrocardiographic manifestations of hypothermia. Am J Emerg Med 2002;20(4):314–26.

21. Soar J, Perkins GD, Abbas G, et al. European Resuscitation Council guidelines for resuscitation 2010 section 8. Cardiac arrest in special circumstances: electrolyte abnormalities, poisoning, drowning, accidental hypothermia, hyperthermia, asthma, anaphylaxis, cardiac surgery, trauma, pregnancy, electrocution. Resuscitation 2010;81(10):1400–33.

22. Vanden Hoek TL, Morrison LJ, Shuster M, et al. Part 12: cardiac arrest in special situations: 2010 American Heart Association guidelines for cardiopulmonary resuscitation and emergency cardiovascular care. Circulation 2010;122(18 Suppl 3):S829–61.

23. Gilbert MM, Busund RR, Skagseth AA, et al. Resuscitation from accidental hypothermia of 13.7 degrees C with circulatory arrest. Lancet 2000;355(9201):375–6.

24. Lexow K. Severe accidental hypothermia: survival after 6 hours 30 minutes of cardiopulmonary resuscitation. Arctic Med Res 1991;50(Suppl 6):112–4.

25. Boyd J, Brugger H, Shuster M. Prognostic factors in avalanche resuscitation: a systematic review. Resuscitation 2010;81(6):645–52.

26. Choi JS, Ahn DW, Choi JK, et al. Thermal balance of man in water: prediction of deep body temperature change. Appl Human Sci 1996;15(4):161–7.

27. Marino F, Booth J. Whole body cooling by immersion in water at moderate temperatures. J Sci Med Sport 1998;1(2):73–82.

28. Giesbrecht G, Steinman AM. Immersion into cold water. In: Auerbach PS, editor. Wilderness medicine. 6th edition. Philadelphia: Elsevier; 2012. p. 143–70.

29. Vanggaard L. Physiological reactions to wet-cold. Aviat Space Environ Med 1975; 46(1):33–6.

30. Giesbrecht GG, Bristow GK. Decrement in manual arm performance during whole body cooling. Aviat Space Environ Med 1992;63(12):1077–81.

31. Hayward JS, Eckerson JD, Collis ML. Effect of behavioral variables on cooling rate of man in cold water. J Appl Phys 1975;38(6):1073–7.

32. Golden FS, Tipton MJ, Scott RC. Immersion, near-drowning and drowning. Br J Anaesth 1997;79(2):214–25.

33. McIntosh SE, Hamonko M, Freer L, et al. Wilderness Medical Society practice guidelines for the prevention and treatment of frostbite. Wilderness Environ Med 2011;22(2):156–66.

34. Schneider S. Hypothermia: from recognition to rewarming. Emerg Med Rep 1992; 13:1.

35. Grieve AW, Davis PP, Dhillon SS, et al. A clinical review of the management of frostbite. J R Army Med Corps 2011;157(1):73–8.

36. Boswick JA, Thompson JD, Jonas RA. The epidemiology of cold injuries. Surg Gynecol Obstet 1979;149(3):326–32.

37. Mills WJ. Summary of treatment of the cold injured patient. Alaska Med 1973; 15(2):56–9.

38. Cauchy E, Chetaille E, Marchand V, et al. Retrospective study of 70 cases of severe frostbite lesions: a proposed new classification scheme. Wilderness Environ Med 2001;12(4):248–55.

39. State of Alaska cold injuries guidelines, vol. 60. Department of Health and Social Services, Division of Public Health Section of Community Health and EMS. Juneau (AK); 2005.
40. Imray C, Grieve A, Dhillon S. The Caudwell Xtreme Everest Research Group. Cold damage to the extremities: frostbite and non-freezing cold injuries. Postgrad Med J 2009;85(1007):481–8.
41. Francis TJ, Golden FS. Non-freezing cold injury: the pathogenesis. J R Nav Med Serv 1985;71(1):3–8.
42. Greenfield AD, Shepherd JT, Whelean R. Cold vasoconstriction and vasodilatation. Ir J Med Sci 1951;(309):415–9.
43. West JB, Schoene RB, Milledge JS. High altitude medicine and physiology. 4th edition. London: Hodder Arnold; 2007.
44. Hackett PH, Roach RC. High-altitude medicine & physiology. In: Auerbach PS, editor. Wilderness medicine. 6th edition. Philidelphia: Elsevier; 2012. p. 2–33.
45. Luks AM, McIntosh SE, Grissom CK, et al. Wilderness Medical Society consensus guidelines for the prevention and treatment of acute altitude illness. Wilderness Environ Med 2010;21(2):146–55.
46. Hackett PH, Rennie D, Levine HD. The incidence, importance, and prophylaxis of acute mountain sickness. Lancet 1976;2(7996):1149–55.
47. Murdoch D. Altitude illness among tourists flying to 3740 meters elevation in the Nepal Himalayas. J Travel Med 1995;2(4):255–6.
48. Pollard AJ, Murdoch DR. The high altitude medicine handbook. 3rd edition. Abingdon (Oxfordshire): Radcliffe Publishing; 2003. p. 193.

Mass Gatherings and Infectious Diseases: Prevention, Detection, and Control

Jaffar A. Al-Tawfiq, MD, FACP, FCCP[a],
Ziad A. Memish, MD, FRCP(Can), FACP, FRCP(Edin), FRCP(Lond), FIDSA[b],*

KEYWORDS

- Mass migration • Mass gathering • Infectious diseases • Hajj • Pilgrimage
- Prevention • Travel

KEY POINTS

- Most of the fear during mass gatherings is related to the development of communicable diseases.
- Planning for mass gathering is best to begin before the event and should include the participation of governmental and nongovernmental agencies.
- Collaboration between national, regional, and international laboratories is needed for prompt and accurate identification of organisms causing diseases.
- Control of communicable diseases relies on vaccination and other public health strategies.

INTRODUCTION

The World Health Organization (WHO) defines mass gatherings as "events attended by a sufficient number of people to strain the planning and response resources of a community, state or nation."[1] Mass gathering may be classified into spontaneous and planned gathering. Planned gatherings are usually recurrent and occur at different locations (such as the Olympics or religious celebrations) or at the same location (such as Hajj pilgrimage in Saudi Arabia). Interest in medical threats posed by mass gathering initially was related to musical festivals, and was accompanied by interest in preparation and organization of medical services at those festivals.[2] More recently, mass gathering has attracted the attention of the medical community owing to numerous factors, including the sudden increase in the demand made on existing services and the potential for a public health emergency resulting from changes in population dynamics and behaviors. The first international conference on mass

The authors have nothing to disclose.
[a] Saudi Aramco Medical Services Organization, PO Box 76, Room A-428-2, Building 61, Dhahran Health Center, Saudi Aramco, Dhahran 31311, Kingdom of Saudi Arabia; [b] Ministry of Health, College of Medicine, Al Faisal University, PO Box 54146, Riyadh 11514, Kingdom of Saudi Arabia
* Corresponding author.
E-mail address: zmemish@yahoo.com

Infect Dis Clin N Am 26 (2012) 725–737
http://dx.doi.org/10.1016/j.idc.2012.05.005
0891-5520/12/$ – see front matter © 2012 Elsevier Inc. All rights reserved.

id.theclinics.com

gathering was convened in Jeddah, Saudi Arabia, in 2010.[3,4] This conference was the largest such international convention of experts on the health and biosecurity issues related to mass-gatherings medicine. The meeting addressed the complex health care challenges related to communicable diseases surveillance, vaccination, travel medicine, environmental health, emergency preparedness, crowd management, and national and international security.

INFECTIOUS DISEASES IN MASS GATHERINGS

Infectious diseases are of particular concern in mass gatherings. However, historically such diseases were not a significant cause of adverse health events. It was reported that infectious disease was the cause of fewer than 1% of health care visits during the 1996 Olympic Games in Atlanta and the 2000 Olympic Games in Sydney. In addition, mass gatherings may be associated with outbreaks, which are not well documented during these events. Most information on outbreaks occurring during mass gatherings has been derived from the Hajj pilgrimage in Saudi Arabia. It was suggested that the Islamic Hajj pilgrimage provides an excellent opportunity to research infectious diseases because this pilgrimage occurs every year at the same location.[5] It is interesting that pilgrims had an illness known locally as Yethrib fever during the first Hajj in 632 AD.[6] This febrile illness is thought now to be malaria.[6] The annual Hajj is the greatest assembly of humankind on earth, with about 2 to 3 million Muslims attending (**Figs. 1** and **2**). Between 2006 and 2010 1.5 million of these were overseas visitors, 89% of whom arrived by air.

Today most of the fear during mass gatherings is related to communicable diseases. Thus, there are 2 main activities related to these events: outbreak investigation, and prevention and control of outbreaks. For proper prevention and control of communicable diseases, it is important to carefully address 3 broad aspects: risk assessment of possible events that could occur, surveillance activities with a good system for tracking outbreaks, and coordinated response to combat these outbreaks. Infectious outbreaks could overwhelm the health care system and lead to admission to intensive care units (ICU). Severe sepsis and septic shock has accounted for 25% of admissions to ICU during Hajj.[7]

Mass gatherings are associated with increased transmission of infectious diseases. Multiple routes of infectious disease transmission have been documented during mass gatherings, including respiratory, gastrointestinal, vector-borne, and sexual routes. Common respiratory pathogens include influenza, tuberculosis, meningococcal disease, and measles. Each respiratory disease has a different incubation period but

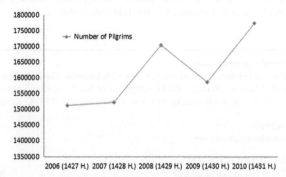

Fig. 1. Number of arriving pilgrims at the Hajj per (2006–2010).

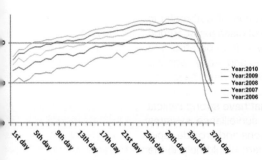

riving pilgrims at the Hajj per day (2006–2010).

siderable morbidity and mortality at mass gatherings. The intense
e created by the limited spaces facilitates the transmission of
   In addition, limited space may compromise food-preparation
ay be served and prepared under suboptimal conditions. In turn,
sufficient food hygiene resulting in food-borne outbreaks. Other
ay be associated with increased frequency of social encounters,
timal needle and shaving behavior, leading to blood-borne infec-
 diseases endemic to the country where the events take place,
alaria, and yellow fever, could cause outbreaks among attendees
if appropriate preventive measures are not taken.

OF INFECTIOUS DISEASES

f risk assessment is to provide an estimate of the likelihood of the
municable diseases at a specific mass gathering. Some of these
ave concentrated on the level of potential attractiveness to terror-
such an assessment is available at the New South Wales Govern-
e WHO specifically assesses the risks of communicable diseases
breaks against 5 benchmarks[1,9]:

gh mortality or morbidity
tional repercussions
al international disease spread
 international travel or trade
istance likely to be needed for disease control

ng for mass gathering is best to begin before the event and should
ation of governmental and nongovernmental agencies. However,
lude 3 phases: before, during, and after the event. In addition, it is
te current surveillance systems at each location hosting a mass
ccess of surveillance depends on a successful system.[10] For the

to have early detection of any outbreaks. The detection of outbreaks in
erings could be enhanced by syndromic surveillance of diseases occurring
es.[13] Such surveillance would be more informative if incorporated into
utine structures for infectious disease surveillance and early warning
Such systems should have already established baseline data based on
itions of the epidemic and/or potentially introduced diseases. However,
surveillance may not add importance in countries that have strong clinical
atory notification systems.[10] The use of electronic surveillance systems
litate the communication between different organizations and provide rapid
he collaboration of all health care sectors in this regard would help in the
ction of unusual patterns of diseases. However, laboratory confirmation of
ould be needed to detect the exact agent causing any outbreak and to
op preventive measures. Local laboratories should be capable of identifying
of local importance. The WHO guidelines stated the following as key
boratory measures that are critical during mass gatherings[1]:

e and identify those pathogens identified as being of particular importance
igh standards of internal and external quality control
rstand the importance of laboratory reporting as it relates to effective
illance
rt test results to the public health surveillance system
de for safe and reliable transport and storage of samples

r collaboration between national, regional, and international laboratories
emphasized for prompt and accurate identification of organisms causing
Moreover, it is important to achieve rapid identification of an outbreak during
gathering. Ten days after an endurance race held in Borneo, Malaysia in
eoSentinel clinic in London reported a patient with symptoms suggestive
irosis, and 2 additional cases were identified in New York and Toronto.
hours of the initial case, a GeoSentinel Alert was distributed, allowing the
on and management of other people at risk.[14,15]

Influenza and Upper Respiratory Diseases

erings pose a risk for outbreaks of influenza and other infectious diseases.
influenza outbreaks during mass gatherings have been described in only 3
[18] In a prospective surveillance for influenza during the 2002 Winter Olym-
t Lake City, influenza A/B was diagnosed in 19% of 188 patients.[18] It was
that "monitoring, postponing, or canceling large public gatherings may
ed close to the epidemic peak but not earlier or later during the epidemic."[19]
ly it was suggested that mass gatherings occurring within 10 days before
nic peak pose a 10% relative increase in the peak prevalence and the total
e of an influenza pandemic.[19] However despite the potential for large
during Hajj, two mass gatherings during the peak of H1N1 infection resulted

upper respiratory tract infection, was the most common complaint among French pilgrims to Hajj in 2007.[25] In another study, cough was reported in 83.5% and sore throat in 82% of Iranian pilgrims in 2004.[26] The isolation rate of influenza was 9.8%, parainfluenza 7.4%, rhinovirus 5.9%, adenovirus 5.4%, enterovirus 2%, and respiratory syncytial virus 1.6%.[26] Because of the proximity of the pilgrims and intense crowding, influenza virus was reported as the leading cause of upper respiratory tract infection during Hajj.[27] Another study from the United Kingdom reported rates of 13% for rhinovirus infection and 10% for influenza virus infection.[24]

Risk of the Transmission of Mycobacterium tuberculosis

Similar to the risk of other respiratory tract infections, there is a potential risk for the transmission of tuberculosis (TB) during mass gatherings in general and during the Hajj in particular. Intense congestion, living in proximity with massive crowds, and the presence of many elderly pilgrims are all factors magnifying TB risk. Moreover, many Muslims travel from countries of high TB prevalence. Air travel has been linked to the transmission of TB, especially after prolonged flights.[28] The revised WHO guidelines related to International Health Regulations (2005) are now generally applicable to transnational TB transmission.[29] This aspect is of particular importance in this era of the emergence of extremely drug-resistant TB.[29] Confined space, long journey time, recirculated air, and limited ventilation increase the risks of transmission of airborne or droplet-spread infection. Pilgrims during Hajj are encouraged to wear facemasks to reduce airborne transmission. In a small study of hospitalized patients during the 1994 Hajj season, *Mycobacterium tuberculosis* was the commonest causative organism (20%) in 46 patients who had an established diagnosis.[30] The data suggested that TB could be transmitted in the setting of overcrowding and mass gathering. This finding is further substantiated by a study from Singapore,[31] wherein the use of a QuantiFERON TB assay revealed that of the 149 Malay pilgrims who were negative before the Hajj, 15 (10%) had a significant increase in immune response to TB antigens.[31] In addition, in a nationwide community-based survey of the epidemiology of TB in Saudi Arabia, the skin reactivity to TB and annual risk of infection were 3 times higher in Saudis living in cities hosting pilgrims compared with the corresponding national average.[32] Thus, the development of strategies to reduce the transmission of TB during mass gathering is a challenge still to be addressed.

Food-Borne Diseases

Food-borne disease is a potential concern during mass gatherings, given especially that millions of meals are prepared during such gatherings. These food-borne diseases include hepatitis A, salmonella gastroenteritis, other infectious diarrheal diseases, and brucellosis. Inadequate standards of food hygiene and shortage of water could add to the possibility of outbreaks of food-borne infections. In addition, if large numbers of food handlers are asymptomatic carriers of pathogenic bacteria, the risk is intensified. The incubation period of enteropathogens may influence any outbreak. It is estimated that the incubation period for the O104:H4 is 8 days, somewhat longer than the 3 to 8 days for Shiga toxin–producing *Escherichia coli* infections. The seriousness of any potential outbreak may extend beyond the area of mass gathering. In an outbreak of shigellosis in 1988, 3175 women who attended a 5-day outdoor music festival in Michigan, USA became ill with gastroenteritis caused by *Shigella sonnei*. The peak of the outbreak was 2 days after the festival ended. Thus, patients were spread throughout the United States by the time the outbreak was recognized.[33] A similar outbreak occurred in an annual Rainbow Family Gathering, with an attack rate of 50% among 12,700 attendees. The outbreak was caused by antibiotic-resistant *S sonnei*.[34]

There are few studies on the incidence and etiology of traveler's diarrhea during the Hajj. The last study was done in 2002, and showed that diarrhea was the third most common cause (6.7%) of hospitalization during Hajj.[35] On the other hand, cholera was the cause of several outbreaks after the Hajj.[36,37] The last reported case of cholera related to Hajj was reported by the Saudi Ministry of Health in 1989.[38] The elimination of cholera outbreaks is related to the significant improvement in water supply and sewage treatment. Although cholera is under control in many developed countries, there is a real risk of having an outbreak in mass gatherings where people come from different parts of the world and where eating habits may be different. In banquet attendees in China, an outbreak of cholera was confirmed in 7% of 337 of the attendees.[39] It was suggested that a uniform instruction and checklist be used for sanitary preparation by sanitary inspectors to ensure adequate sanitation at these gatherings.[40]

Sexually Transmitted Infections and Blood-Borne Pathogens

Sexually transmitted infections (STIs) are feared consequences of mass gatherings, especially when attendees of these gatherings are engaged in the use of alcohol and/or recreational drugs. However, there are no published data on the spread of STIs during mass gatherings and the available publications talk about the theoretical risk of STI during such gatherings.[41,42] It was speculated that an increase in the number of commercial sex workers at the World Cup in Germany might result in an increase in STIs. However, this speculation was not proved.[43]

The risk of blood-borne viruses in mass gatherings is limited in most events by the nature of contact. The relatively short duration of events in comparison with the long incubation period of these infections makes identification difficult. In festivals where participants are intravenous drug users, blood-borne viruses such as hepatitis B, hepatitis C, and human immunodeficiency virus may be transmitted if preventive approaches are not instituted. During the Hajj, men terminate their religious ritual by shaving their heads (**Fig. 3**), through which the risk of acquiring blood-borne viruses was suggested.[44,45] However, hepatitis B infection is preventable through pretravel vaccination, and the risk from shaving using the same blades can be minimized or eliminated by implementing current Saudi guidelines. These regulations call for the elimination of unlicensed barbers from operating during the Hajj. Licensed and approved barbershops/government-related head-shaving areas are stationed along the Hajj routes where the rites terminate. Nevertheless, enforcing this restriction continues to be a problem in crowds more than 3 million.

Endemic Infectious Diseases of Local Importance

The location of the mass gathering and the associated climate and weather provides information regarding social and political stability. Thus, endemic disease or ongoing

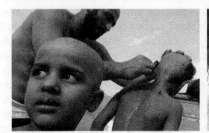
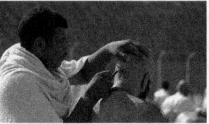

Fig. 3. Illegal unlicensed barbers operating at the Hajj.

outbreaks in mass gathering should be kept in mind as a possible risk for the people gathering at that locality. The proximity of cattle, the massive slaughter of beasts, and the intense congestion of the Hajj period makes zoonotic disease a major consideration. At the completion of the Hajj, animals continue to be predominantly slaughtered by laypersons caught up in the joy of ending their Hajj successfully. Thus, the risks of brucellosis, Rift Valley fever, Crimean-Congo hemorrhagic fever, and Orf virus are significant. However, no brucellosis outbreaks were reported during Hajj despite brucellosis being a common zoonotic disease in Saudi Arabia. In 1995, a new flavivirus was isolated in 1995 from 6 patients from south of Jeddah,[46] who presented with dengue-like viral hemorrhagic fever (VHF). The pathogen was identified as Alkhurma virus. During the 2001 Hajj season 4 cases of classic Alkhurma VHF were diagnosed in Makkah.[46]

VACCINE-PREVENTABLE DISEASES AND VACCINATION

Mass gathering is a unique situation facilitating the transmission of communicable diseases such as meningococcal infection, influenza, and measles. The spread of infectious diseases is enhanced by the presence of a large number of people coming from different countries and gathering in a small, crowded space. Thus, vaccination serves as an important preventive strategy to minimize the risk of occurrence and spread of diseases within the host community or internationally.

Meningococcal Disease

Neisseria meningitidis, a gram-negative, oxidase-positive, aerobic diplococcus organism, is the causative agent of meningococcal meningitis. Of particular importance are encapsulated strains, as they are the cause of the great majority of cases of invasive disease. Of the 13 serogroups that are described, 6 are currently recognized as the most common cause of disease (A, B, C, W135, X, and Y).[47] In relation to mass gathering, 2 major outbreaks of meningococcal disease occurred in association with the annual Hajj pilgrimage.[48–50] In 1987, the first international outbreak of meningococcal disease in association with the Hajj was caused by N meningitidis serogroup A.[51] As a result, the government of Saudi Arabia implemented mandatory bivalent meningococcal polysaccharide vaccine (A & C) for Hajj pilgrims. Although an increasing number of cases of N meningitidis serogroup A were detected in Saudi Arabia in 1992, this was not associated with further spread of the disease.[49] It was not until the 2000 Hajj season that the second international outbreak occurred, when more than 400 cases of serogroup W-135 meningococcal disease occurred in pilgrims and their close contacts reported from 16 countries.[50,52–54]

Meningococcal ACW135Y vaccination became obligatory for pilgrims to Saudi Arabia. This recommendation was made after the 2000 and 2001 outbreaks of meningococcal W135 strains. That outbreak was associated with a high mortality rate and showed the potential for rapid international spread.[55] Visitors arriving for Hajj are required to produce a certificate of vaccination with the quadrivalent vaccine (ACYW135) issued not more than 3 years previously and not less than 10 days before arrival in Saudi Arabia. The responsible authorities in the visitor's country of origin should ensure that adults and children older than 2 years are given 1 dose of the ACYW135 vaccine. The compliance with this recommendation was 96% to 98% from 2006 to 2010 (**Fig. 4**). In addition, visitors arriving from countries in the African meningitis belt, namely Benin, Burkina Faso, Cameroon, Chad, Central African Republic, Côte d'Ivoire, Eritrea, Ethiopia, Gambia, Guinea, Guinea-Bissau, Mali, Niger, Nigeria, Senegal, and Sudan, receive ciprofloxacin tablets (500 mg) chemoprophylaxis

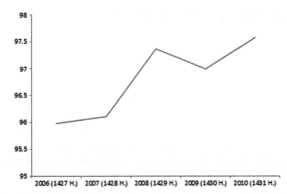

Fig. 4. Pilgrims vaccinated with the recommended meningococcal polysaccharide vaccine in their countries.

at port of entry to lower the rate of meningococcal carriage. It is estimated that about 400,000 to 460,000 pilgrims receive the recommended doses at the port of entry in Saudi Arabia (**Fig. 5**). Concerns with the lack of efficacy of meningococcal polysaccharide vaccine in children younger than 5 years, the lack of efficacy of the polysaccharide vaccine in eliminating nasopharyngeal carriage, and the need for repeat dosing every 3 to 5 years have led to greater interest in investigating the role of the newly licensed conjugated quadrivalent meningococcal vaccine during future Hajj seasons. Conjugated meningococcal vaccine is purported to address all the shortcomings of the polysaccharide vaccine.

Measles

Measles is a highly infectious disease and tends to affect all age groups, with a particular risk in those younger than 5 years and those aged 15 to 29 years. Measles is endemic in many developing countries, and outbreaks occur in multiple countries. These factors create potential for the emergence of an epidemic in the event of a mass gathering. During 2011, many European countries witnessed measles outbreaks. In addition, 13 primary measles cases occurred among unvaccinated individuals (aged 9 and 32 years) in 11 districts in Germany following the attendance of meetings in Taize, France.[56] This occurrence highlights the potential of larger outbreaks to occur in mass gatherings and delay any efforts to eradicate measles

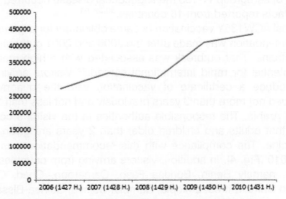

Fig. 5. Number of pilgrims given chemoprophylaxis at port of entry.

by 2015. Thus, in plans it is important to address on a global level the lapse in measles immunity and rate of measles vaccination. Measles vaccines provide 99% protection in those who receive 2 doses of the vaccine. The presence of an unvaccinated and under-vaccinated population in any locality, and especially in a mass gathering plays a major role in the spread of the disease. Thus, measles may be reintroduced by returning travelers from mass gatherings after becoming infected with the measles virus. Whether measles vaccination should be a requirement for individuals attending mass gatherings is a question that should be considered at policy-making levels, taking into consideration the pros and cons of such policies. The European Centers for Disease Control (ECDC) strongly stress the importance for European citizens to be vaccinated against measles, especially if they are planning to attend a mass gathering.[57] Moreover, it was shown that restricting community activities does not control a measles outbreak. Thus, the mainstay for the prevention of a measles outbreak is immunization and personal hygiene.

Pertussis

Pertussis, a respiratory-tract pathogen, is of particular concern during mass gatherings in general and during the Hajj in particular, because pertussis is a highly communicable but vaccine-preventable respiratory disease. In a study from Saudi Arabia, paired pre- and post-Hajj samples from 358 pilgrims showed that a greater than 4-fold increase in the level of immunoglobulin G was detected in 1.4% of pilgrims.[58] Except for influenza, this rate is higher than that of most other vaccine-preventable travel-related diseases.[59] There are no universal recommendations for pertussis vaccination for adult travelers. However, given the relatively high rate of acquisition of pertussis during mass gatherings, especially Hajj, it is reasonable to ensure that adults are vaccinated against pertussis. The availability of acellular pertussis vaccine makes it easier to achieve vaccination of adults.

Poliomyelitis

Poliomyelitis is now considered prevalent only in certain countries. The presence of visitors from these countries among people attending mass gatherings may pose a health risk for other attendees. Saudi Arabia requires that all visitors younger than 15 years traveling to Saudi Arabia from countries reinfected with poliomyelitis receive oral polio vaccine (OPV) 6 weeks before the application for an entry visa. In addition, all such visitors arriving in Saudi Arabia will receive a dose of OPV at border points.[60] Irrespective of previous immunization history, all visitors younger than 15 years arriving in Saudi Arabia will also receive a dose of OPV at border points (**Fig. 6**).

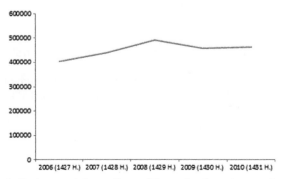

Fig. 6. Number of pilgrims receiving poliomyelitis vaccination at port of entry.

Influenza

As stated, mass gatherings pose a risk for outbreaks of influenza and other respiratory infectious diseases. The 2009 Hajj season coincided with the pandemic H1N1 infection, and at the same time the WHO declared that there were more than 300,000 laboratory-confirmed cases of pandemic influenza H1N1 and 3917 deaths in 191 countries.[61] Giving the fear of pandemic H1N1 infection in 2009-2010 the government of Saudi Arabia, while not prohibiting anyone from making Hajj, did advise other countries to follow age restrictions and vaccinations to prevent the spread of H1N1 infection.

In an attempt to reduce the risk of respiratory tract infections during the Hajj, the Saudi Ministry of Health encourages all pilgrims to wear a surgical facemask when visiting crowded places. In addition, it is recommended that all pilgrims be vaccinated against seasonal influenza before arrival in Saudi Arabia. Seasonal influenza vaccine is recommended for all health care workers working in Hajj premises.[60]

INFECTION CONTROL IN MASS GATHERINGS

Mass gatherings are associated with a large influx of patients seeking medical care. Review of recorded medical care during the 1984 Olympic Games in Los Angeles showed that the number of people seeking medical care was 5516 out of 3,447,807 visitors (0.16%).[62] In the 1996 Olympic Games in Atlanta, the frequency of use of medical services by participants was moderately higher (22.9 visits per 10,000) compared with Los Angeles (16 per 10,000).[63] Thus, increased numbers of people seeking medical care during a mass gathering may result in breakdowns in infection-control procedures. Moreover, places where mass gathering is taking place should consider the need for large-scale isolation of patients in the event of an outbreak of infectious disease.

GENERAL RECOMMENDATIONS

It is advisable to know the geography and the social activity being undertaken at any particular mass gathering, which then dictate adherence to standard and specific health requirements for vaccination. It is advisable to have up-to-date immunization against infections likely to be encountered during mass gatherings, such as influenza, measles, pertussis, hepatitis A and B, polio, and meningococcal disease. Measures to prevent infections at mass gatherings should include sufficient surveillance, proper respiratory hygiene, and an effective vaccination program. In addition, prompt diagnosis, isolation, and treatment of infectious cases would be essential in certain infectious diseases such as TB.

REFERENCES

1. WHO/CDS/EPR. Communicable disease alert and response for mass gatherings. 2008. Available at: http://www.who.int/csr/Mass_gatherings2.pdf. Accessed June 10, 2011.
2. Grange JT, Green SM, Downs W. Concert medicine: spectrum of medical problems encountered at 405 major concerts. Acad Emerg Med 1999;6:202–7.
3. Memish ZA, Alrabeeah AA. Jeddah declaration on mass gatherings health. Lancet Infect Dis 2011;11:342–3.
4. McConnell J, Memish Z. The Lancet conference on mass gatherings medicine. Lancet Infect Dis 2010;10:818–9.
5. Rashid H, Haworth E, Shafi S, et al. Pandemic influenza: mass gatherings and mass infection. Lancet Infect Dis 2008;8:526–7.

6. Farid MA. Implications of the Mecca pilgrimage for a regional malaria eradication programme. Bull World Health Organ 1956;15:828–33.

7. Baharoon S, Al-Jahdali H, Al Hashmi J, et al. Severe sepsis and septic shock at the Hajj: etiologies and outcomes. Travel Med Infect Dis 2009;7:247–52.

8. New South Wales Government. Available at: http://www.secure.nsw.gov.au/mass-gatherings/. Accessed June 1, 2011.

9. Mass gatherings and public health: the experience of the Athens 2004 Olympic Games. Available at: http://www.euro.who.int/__data/assets/pdf_file/0009/98415/E90712.pdf. Accessed June 1, 2011.

10. Khan K, Freifeld CC, Wang J, et al. Preparing for infectious disease threats at mass gatherings: the case of the Vancouver 2010 Olympic Winter Games. CMAJ 2010;182:579–83.

11. Health conditions for travellers to Saudi Arabia for the pilgrimage to Mecca (Hajj). Wkly Epidemiol Rec 2011;86(39):425–8.

12. Memish ZA, Al Rabeeah AA. Health conditions for travellers to Saudi Arabia for the pilgrimage to Mecca (Hajj) 1432 (2011). J Infect Public Health 2011;4: 105–7.

13. Centers for Disease Control and Prevention (CDC). Surveillance for early detection of disease outbreaks at an outdoor mass gathering—Virginia, 2005. MMWR Morb Mortal Wkly Rep 2006;55:71–4.

14. Centers for Disease Control and Prevention (CDC). Update: outbreak of acute febrile illness among athletes participating in Eco-Challenge-Sabah 2000—Borneo, Malaysia, 2000. MMWR Morb Mortal Wkly Rep 2001;50:21–4.

15. Sejvar J, Bancroft E, Winthrop K, et al. Leptospirosis in "Eco-Challenge" athletes, Malaysian Borneo, 2000. Emerg Infect Dis 2003;9:702–7.

16. Balkhy HH, Memish ZA, Bafaqeer S, et al. Influenza a common viral infection among Hajj pilgrims: time for routine surveillance and vaccination. J Travel Med 2004;11:82–6.

17. El Bashir H, Haworth E, Zambon M, et al. Influenza among U.K. pilgrims to Hajj, 2003. Emerg Infect Dis 2004;10:1882–3.

18. Gundlapalli AV, Rubin MA, Samore MH, et al. Influenza, Winter Olympiad, 2002. Emerg Infect Dis 2006;12:144–6.

19. Shi P, Keskinocak P, Swann JL, et al. The impact of mass gatherings and holiday traveling on the course of an influenza pandemic: a computational model. BMC Public Health 2010;10:778.

20. Khan K, Memish ZA, Chabbra A, et al. Global public health implications of a mass gathering in Mecca, Saudi Arabia during the midst of an influenza pandemic. J Travel Med 2010;17:75–81.

21. El-Sheikh SM, El-Assouli SM, Mohammed KA, et al. Bacteria and viruses that cause respiratory tract infections during the pilgrimage (Hajj) season in Makkah, Saudi Arabia. Trop Med Int Health 1998;3:205.

22. Kholeidi AN, Baksh MF, Al Hamad NA, et al. Seropositivity in clinical influenza cases among pilgrims during Hajj, 1421 H (2001). Saudi Epidemiol Bull 2001; 8:27–8.

23. Al Saleh E, Al Mazroua M, Choudhary AJ, et al. Serotypes of influenza during Hajj season, 1424H (2004). Saudi Epidemiol Bull 2005;12:1–2.

24. Rashid H, Shafi S, Haworth E, et al. Viral respiratory infections at the Hajj: comparison between UK and Saudi pilgrims. Clin Microbiol Infect 2008;14:569–74.

25. Gautret P, Soula G, Delmont J, et al. Common health hazards in French pilgrims during the Hajj of 2007: a prospective cohort study. J Travel Med 2009;16: 377–81.

26. Alborzi A, Aelami MH, Ziyaeyan M, et al. Viral etiology of acute respiratory infections among Iranian Hajj pilgrims, 2006. J Travel Med 2009;16:239–42.
27. Alzeer AH. Respiratory tract infection during Hajj. Ann Thorac Med 2009;4:50–3.
28. Kornylo-Duong K, Kim C, Cramer EH, et al. Three air travel-related contact investigations associated with infectious tuberculosis, 2007-2008. Travel Med Infect Dis 2010;8:120–8.
29. Plotkin BJ, Hardiman MC. The international health regulations (2005), tuberculosis and air travel. Travel Med Infect Dis 2010;8:90–5.
30. Alzeer A, Mashlah A, Fakim N, et al. Tuberculosis is the commonest cause of pneumonia requiring hospitalization during Hajj (pilgrimage to Makkah). J Infect 1998;36:303–6.
31. Wilder-Smith A, Foo W, Earnest A, et al. High risk of Mycobacterium tuberculosis infection during the Hajj pilgrimage. Trop Med Int Health 2005;10:336–9.
32. al-Kassimi FA, Abdullah AK, al-Hajjaj MS, et al. Nationwide community survey of tuberculosis epidemiology in Saudi Arabia. Tuber Lung Dis 1993;74:254–60.
33. Lee LA, Ostroff SM, McGee HB, et al. An outbreak of shigellosis at an outdoor music festival. Am J Epidemiol 1991;133:608–15.
34. Wharton M, Spiegel RA, Horan JM, et al. A large outbreak of antibiotic-resistant shigellosis at a mass gathering. J Infect Dis 1990;162:1324–8.
35. Al-Ghamdi SM, Akbar HO, Qari YA, et al. Pattern of admission to hospitals during muslim pilgrimage (Hajj). Saudi Med J 2003;24:1073–6.
36. Onishchenko GG, Lomov IuM, Moskvitina EA. Cholera in the Republic of Dagestan. Zh Mikrobiol Epidemiol Immunobiol 1995;(Suppl 2):3–8 [in Russian].
37. Onishchenko GG, Lomov IuM, Moskvitina EA, et al. The epidemiological characteristics of cholera in the Republic of Dagestan. An assessment of the epidemic-control measures. Zh Mikrobiol Epidemiol Immunobiol 1995;(Suppl 2):9–22 [in Russian].
38. Memish ZA. The Hajj: communicable and non-communicable health hazards and current guidance for pilgrims. Euro Surveill 2010;15:19671.
39. Tang XF, Liu LG, Ma HL, et al. Outbreak of cholera associated with consumption of soft-shelled turtles, Sichuan province, China, 2009. Zhonghua Liu Xing Bing Xue Za Zhi 2010;31:1050–2 [in Chinese].
40. Zieliński A, Gładysz K. Structured sanitary preparation to mass gatherings. Przegl Epidemiol 2010;64:9–13.
41. Richter M, Massawe D. Serious soccer, sex (work) and HIV—will South Africa be too hot to handle during the 2010 World Cup? S Afr Med J 2010;100:222–3.
42. Baleta A. South Africa prepares for the football World Cup. Lancet Infect Dis 2010;10:373–4.
43. Loewenberg S. Fears of World Cup sex trafficking boom unfounded. Lancet 2006;368:105–6.
44. Gatrad AR, Sheikh A. Hajj and risk of blood borne infections. Arch Dis Child 2001; 84:375.
45. Rafiq SM, Rashid H, Haworth E, et al. Hazards of hepatitis at the Hajj. Travel Med Infect Dis 2009;7:239–46.
46. Memish ZA, Charrel RN, Zaki AM, et al. Alkhurma haemorrhagic fever—a viral haemorrhagic disease unique to the Arabian Peninsula. Int J Antimicrob Agents 2010;36(Suppl 1):S53–7.
47. Stephens DS. Conquering the meningococcus. FEMS Microbiol Rev 2007;31: 3–14.
48. Dull PM, Abdelwahab J, Sacchi CT, et al. Neisseria meningitidis serogroup W-135 carriage among US travelers to the 2001 Hajj. J Infect Dis 2005;191:33–9.

49. al-Gahtani YM, el Bushra HE, al-Qarawi SM, et al. Epidemiological investigation of an outbreak of meningococcal meningitis in Makkah (Mecca), Saudi Arabia, 1992. Epidemiol Infect 1995;115:399–409.

50. Aguilera JF, Perrocheau A, Meffre C, et al. Outbreak of serogroup W135 meningococcal disease after the Hajj pilgrimage, Europe, 2000. Emerg Infect Dis 2002;8:761–7.

51. Moore PS, Harrison LH, Telzak EE, et al. Group A meningococcal carriage in travelers returning from Saudi Arabia. JAMA 1988;260:2686–9.

52. Mayer LW, Reeves MW, Al-Hamdan N, et al. Outbreak of W135 meningococcal disease in 2000: not emergence of a new W135 strain but clonal expansion within the electrophoretic type-37 complex. J Infect Dis 2002;185:1596–605.

53. Issack MI, Ragavoodoo C. Hajj-related *Neisseria meningitidis* serogroup W135 in Mauritius. Emerg Infect Dis 2002;8:332–4.

54. Fonkoua MC, Taha MK, Nicolas P, et al. Recent increase in meningitis caused by *Neisseria meningitidis* serogroups A and W135, Yaounde, Cameroon. Emerg Infect Dis 2002;8:327–9.

55. Shafi S, Booy R, Haworth E, et al. Hajj: health lessons for mass gatherings. J Infect Public Health 2008;1:27–32.

56. Pfaff G, Lohr D, Santibanez S, et al. Spotlight on measles 2010: measles outbreak among travellers returning from a mass gathering, Germany, September to October 2010. Euro Surveill 2010;15. pii: 19750.

57. Measles in the European Union and a reminder for EU citizens attending mass gatherings. Available at: http://ecdc.europa.eu/en/healthtopics/measles/Documents/2011_06_17_measles_update_mass%20gatherings.pdf. Accessed October 20, 2011.

58. Wilder-Smith A, Earnest A, Ravindran S, et al. High incidence of pertussis among Hajj pilgrims. Clin Infect Dis 2003;37:1270–2.

59. Steffen R, Rickenbach M, Willhelm U, et al. Health problems after travel to developing countries. J Infect Dis 1987;156:84–91.

60. Memish ZA. Health conditions for travelers to Saudi Arabia for (Hajj) for the year 1431H/2010. J Infect Public Health 2010;3:92–4.

61. World Health Organization. Global alert and response. Pandemic H1N1 (2009) update—67. Available at: http://www.who.int/csr/don/2009_09_25/en/index.html. Accessed June 20, 2011.

62. Baker WM, Simone BM, Niemann JT, et al. Special event medical care: the 1984 Los Angeles Summer Olympics experience. Ann Emerg Med 1986;15:185–90.

63. Wetterhall SE, Coulombier DM, Herndon JM, et al. Medical care delivery at the 1996 Olympic Games. JAMA 1998;279:1463–8.

Rabies

Relevance, Prevention, and Management in Travel Medicine

Christoph F.R. Hatz, MD, DTM&H[a,b,c,]*, Esther Kuenzli, MD, MSc[d],
Maia Funk, MD[c]

KEYWORDS

- Rabies • Travel • Epidemiology • Exposure • Vaccination

KEY POINTS

- Terrestrial or bat rabies is present in almost all countries of the world.
- Travelers are at risk in enzoonotic regions of being bitten; the rabies infection risk for the individual traveler and the indication for preexposure prophylaxis has to be assessed on an individual basis.
- Preexposure prophylaxis consists of one intramuscular or one intradermal injection on days 0, 7 and 21 (or 28) each.
- Postexposure prophylaxis has to be applied as quickly as possible (within 24-48 hours) after contact with a potentially rabid animal.
- In many regions of the world, antirabies immunoglobulin is not readily available. 2/3 of all travelers do not receive correct postexposure treatment.

CAUSE

Rabies is a zoonotic viral disease, transmitted only in mammals, mostly in the Orders *Carnivora* and *Chiroptera*. Terrestrial rabies (genotype 1), predominantly transmitted by dogs, is the most important rabies cycle threatening humans. The causative neurotropic virus is a negative-stranded RNA virus of the family *Rhabdoviridae*, genus

This work was supported by the employers and did not receive any contributions from third parties, including industry. Christoph Hatz has received unconditional educational grants for courses from Novartis, Sanofi-Pasteur, GSK, and Crucell.

[a] Swiss Tropical and Public Health Institute, PO Box, CH-4002, Basel, Switzerland; [b] University of Basel, Petersplatz, CH-4051 Basel, Switzerland; [c] Division of Communicable Diseases, Institute of Social and Preventive Medicine, University of Zurich, Hirschengraben 84, CH-8001, Zurich, Switzerland; [d] Division of Infectious Diseases and Hospital Epidemiology, University Hospital of Basel, Petersgraben 4, CH-4031 Basel, Switzerland
* Corresponding author. Swiss Tropical and Public Health Institute, University of Basel, Socinstrasse 57, PO Box, CH-4002, Basel, Switzerland.
E-mail address: christoph.hatz@unibas.ch

Infect Dis Clin N Am 26 (2012) 739–753
http://dx.doi.org/10.1016/j.idc.2012.05.001
0891-5520/12/$ – see front matter © 2012 Elsevier Inc. All rights reserved.

id.theclinics.com

Lyssavirus.[1–4] This genus contains several rabies-related viruses (**Table 1**).[5–8] All variants are known or suspected to cause rabies-like diseases.

Transmission occurs by the virus entering through the skin or the mucosa after bites, scratches, or preexisting injuries contaminated by the saliva of an infected mammal.

Only 51 human rabies cases that have not been transmitted by animal bites have been described. Eighteen were caused by improperly inactivated vaccine in Brazil, 15 by transplants (8 cornea, 3 kidney, 1 each for kidney-pancreas, liver, iliac artery, lung).[10–12] Eight seem to have occurred by contamination of impaired skin, 2 by aerosols in laboratory staff, and 2 have potentially originated from a stay in bat-infested caves.[13] Six cases were human-to-human transmissions and included 3 human bites. Ingesting raw meat has not been shown to be responsible for human cases.

EPIDEMIOLOGY

Rabies (terrestrial and bat transmitted) is present in more than 150 countries on all continents (**Fig. 1**). More than 95% of all human deaths are observed in Asia and Africa, mostly in rural areas. An estimated 55,000 to 70,000 persons[14,15] die from rabies every year. Severe underreporting is assumed, and 40% of all cases are children less than 15 years of age.[16,17] Forty-two deaths of imported rabies cases were reported in Europe, the United States, and Japan between 1990 and 2010.[18] Terrestrial rabies is not present in Oceania, Japan, and some Central and Western European countries. No cases have been verified in Antarctica or in New Zealand. The rabies-free status can suddenly change by (re)introduction of the disease, as documented among animals in Northeastern Italy in 2008. All but 1 country report animal rabies to the World Organization for Animal Health (Office Of Epizootics [OIE]) but only a few report to Rabnet.[19]

An area free of rabies is defined[20] as an area that (1) has no case of autochthonous infection by any Lyssavirus confirmed either in humans or in any animal species,

Genotype	Virus	Phylogroup	Identified In	Main Host
Table 1 **Rabies and rabies-related viruses**				
1	Rabies virus	I	Worldwide	Canine, bat
2	Lagos	II	Africa, Middle East	Bat
3	Mokola	II	West Africa (Nigeria)	Bat
4	Duvenhage	I	Africa	Bat
5	EBLV-1	I	Europe	Bat
6	EBLV-2	I	Europe	Bat
7	Australian bat	I	Australia	Bat
8	Aravan	I	Kyrgyzstan	Bat
9	Khujand	I	Tajikistan	Bat
10	Irkut	I	Asia	Bat
11	West Caucasian bat virus	?	Eastern Europe	Bat
	Shimoni bat virus[a]	II	Kenya	Bat
	Bokeloh bat virus[a]	I	Germany	Bat
	Ikoma virus	?	Tanzania	African civet cat[9]

Abbreviation: EBLV, European lyssa bat virus.
[a] Not definitively classified.

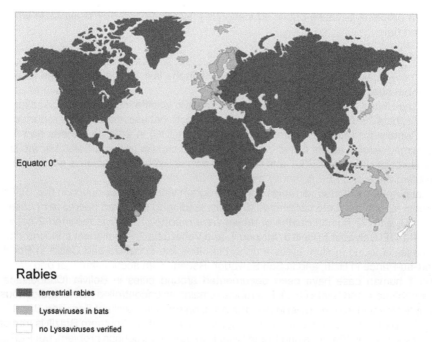

Rabies

▓ terrestrial rabies

░ Lyssaviruses in bats

☐ no Lyssaviruses verified

Fig. 1. Rabies and rabies-related diseases. (*Courtesy of* M. Funk, and Astral/SA, Tropimed; with permission.)

including bats, at any time during 2 consecutive years; (2) provides an adequate surveillance system; and (3) has an effectively controlled import policy.

More than 99% of human deaths are caused by dog bites.[21] In South America, the saliva of bats is the most important source of infection.[22] Rodents are known to be poor transmitters, and monkeys do not play an important role in transmission to humans: no confirmed transmissions to humans have been described.

Fifteen million people per year receive some form of postexposure prophylaxis (PEP), most of them in India and China. An estimated 327,000 rabies deaths annually are thus averted.[14]

Europe

The introduction of the wildlife vaccination program[19] with vaccine baits has led to the elimination of canine/fox rabies in some European countries.[23] Only bat rabies is present there,[24,25] and spillovers are rare (there are no vampire bats in Europe). Countries free of terrestrial rabies are Great Britain, Switzerland, Spain (excluding Melilla and Ceuta on the African continent), Portugal, France, Germany, Belgium, the Netherlands, Sweden, Finland, Norway (continental), Denmark, Austria, and, until 2008, Italy.[26,27] Since 2008, Italy[28] has reported new rabies cases among foxes in the northeast (Friuli-Venezia, Giulia, Veneto), entering from the northeastern neighbouring country Slovenia. From 2008 to February 2011, 287 mostly fox rabies cases were found, most in the Veneto (216), but also in Friuli (58), Trento (8), and Bolzano 85).[29–31] Fox vaccination programs were intensified[32] and cases are declining.

Eastern Europe is still reporting human cases of terrestrial rabies.[33,34] Most wildlife cases in 2005 occurred in the Russian Federation, Ukraine, Lithuania, Belarus, Croatia, and Estonia. However, human rabies in Eastern Europe is not a major public health problem, because public education is maintained and PEP is available within a short time.

Americas

Dog rabies cases have been reduced by 90% in the last 10 years. All rabies strains, even bat strains, are of genotype 1.[35]

In the United States, 6154 animal cases (most in wildlife: raccoons 36.5%, skunks 23.5%, bats 23.3%) and 2 human rabies cases, both bat associated, were reported to the Centers for Disease Control and Prevention (CDC) in 2010.[36] Canada had 123 confirmed wildlife rabies cases in 2010, mostly in skunks (60) and bats (48); the last human case dates from 2007 and originated from a bat bite.[37] Rabies is not a serious problem there and PEP is readily available.

Latin America started its rabies control program with dog vaccination in the 1980s. Almost 42 Mio dogs are vaccinated annually, leading to a marked decrease of cases. In 2003, only 27 human deaths of rabies were reported[35]: Bolivia reported 2 cases, Brazil 14, El Salvador 5, Haiti 3, Mexico 1, and Venezuela 2. The highest concentration of cases is found in slum areas around big cities like Fortaleza and Ceará in Brazil, Port-au-Prince in Haiti, and in San Salvador. Recently, an accumulation of dog cases and 1 human case have been documented around cities in Bolivia (Chuquisaca, Cochabamba, and Santa Cruz). Bat rabies remains an uncontrolled risk for indigenous people sleeping in open dwellings in the Amazon regions mainly of Peru and Brazil.[22]

A big part of the South (Chile, Uruguay, most of Argentina, Southern Brazil) is free of dog rabies, as are Panama and Costa Rica. Rabies is not a serious problem, but PEP is not available in remote areas.

Asia

More than half of all reported human rabies cases originate in the Far East and in South Asia (>30,000). Data are limited,[38,39] with substantial underreporting. Death rates in humans may be substantially higher than officially reported.[14]

Since 1995, human rabies cases in Thailand have steadily declined, also because of extensive vaccination of dogs. In 2006, most human deaths were reported in India (20,000), China (3209), Pakistan, Bangladesh, and Myanmar.[40] Malaysia is only marginally affected at the northern border areas of the mainland.

Availability of immunologicals (including rabies immunoglobulin [RIG]) against rabies is unreliable in tourist areas and big cities, and poor in rural areas.

Africa

The dimension of the rabies problem in Africa is unknown in many areas. Considerable underreporting is likely.[14] It is assumed that more than 20,000 people die of the disease every year. Most cases are acquired in rural areas. RIG is not readily available and access to active vaccines is limited.

Australia

Only Australian bat virus has been reported. Immunologicals are readily available.

RESERVOIR

All mammals are susceptible to rabies virus infection but only a few are important reservoirs. The wild reservoir is primarily maintained in *Carnivora* (dog, fox, wolf, coyote, jackal, mongoose) but also in *Omnivora* like raccoons, skunks and in *Chiroptera* (bats).

In North America, the main reservoirs are raccoons, skunks, and bats; in Latin America it is bats. In Western Europe the main wildlife reservoir is the red fox, in Eastern Europe the red fox (50%), and, increasingly, the raccoon dog (18%),[34] especially in Belarus and the Baltic states.

PATHOLOGY

The virus is transmitted by saliva of rabid animals through the skin and mucosa or into the muscle of the victim. The average incubation period is between 1 and 3 months. It ranges from a few days if the head or highly innervated body parts are affected (hands, arms), to more than 1 year.[41,42] The pathogenesis is not fully understood.[43] In the beginning, the virus does not enter the cells and may be removed by washing the wound with alkaline soap. Local replication in muscle cells is possible and was documented in animals.[44] The virus then enters the axon of peripheral nerves and moves toward the central nervous system (CNS) at a speed of 1 to 40 cm per day, leading to an acute and almost always fatal encephalomyelitis. The rabies virus attaches specifically and unspecifically to neuronal cell membranes. Specific receptor bindings may contribute to the pathogenicity only in mammals, but not in birds.[45,46] Once inside the neuronal cells, it replicates, moves transsynaptically, and eventually along somatic and autonomic nerves back to the skin, various organs, tissues, the salivary glands, and also to nerve tissue around hair follicles. Final massive replication in the salivary glands leads to the high infectiousness of saliva. Deadly functional damage is done to the hypothalamus and brain stem, thus influencing cardiac and respiratory control. No antibodies appear during the incubation period.[47]

CLINICAL SIGNS AND SYMPTOMS

Clinical signs and symptoms show a broad variety, even in patients infected with a Lyssavirus of the same genotype.[48,49] This adds to the frequent misdiagnosis of the disease and confusion with other CNS diseases and infections.

Human rabies infections other than by genotype 1 are rare. Therefore, only symptoms of this type are described here. Once symptoms of the disease develop, human rabies is nearly always fatal within 2 to 12 days.

Two forms of the genotype 1 disease are known: furious rabies and paralytic rabies. The latter form is present in 30% of human cases as well as in dog rabies, and it is often misdiagnosed.

Furious rabies starts with unspecific symptoms such as headache, malaise, fever, disconcertment, local sensations (tingling, burning, itching, anesthesia) at the bite or entry site, followed by excitability, confusion, hypersalivation, priapism, aerophobia, and eventually hydrophobia and convulsions.

Paralytic cases seem less severe and present with loss of sensation, weakness, and pain. The muscles are progressively paralyzed, starting at the virus entry site. A slow development of coma precedes death.

DIAGNOSIS

Before onset of clinical disease, there is no test to confirm rabies infection. Presumptive diagnosis from the patient's history of a potential rabies contact in any unclear acute neurologic illness is vital, even months or years after a potential exposure. Classic signs with hypersalivation and aerophobia or hydrophobia are not always present. Symptoms develop within 2 to 10 days to the full illness and death. Laboratory diagnosis in the first week of illness is rarely achieved.

Laboratory Diagnosis

Serology is not applicable for testing individuals for rabies at an early stage of infection. Seroconversion occurs late in clinical disease. A single test result is not sufficient, and should be repeated within 3 to 7 days. Tests of skin and saliva samples may be positive at day 4 to 5 of the disease. Antibodies are present in the serum on days 5 to 8, and later in the cerebrospinal fluid (CSF). New, more sensitive molecular methods are in development.[50]

For ante mortem diagnosis, all samples have to be considered infectious and should be securely sealed before transportation. A deep neck skin biopsy containing a minimum of 10 hair follicles should be at least 5 mm in diameter and taken from the neck hairline, deep enough to contain the skin nerves of the hair follicle. Lyssavirus antigen is found by direct fluorescent antibody (DFA) test or reverse-transcriptase polymerase chain reaction (RT-PCR). The DFA is the gold standard test.[49,51–53] In saliva, the detection of rabies RNA (RT-PCR) or the virus in cell culture is considered diagnostic. In serum and CSF, detection of antibodies to rabies virus in unvaccinated persons leads to the diagnosis. The tests include the indirect fluorescent antibody test (IFA), complete rabies neutralization at 1:5 dilution, or an increase in antibody levels.[49,51–53] Brain biopsy is not indicated because of lack of treatment consequences. Post mortem diagnosis is made from tissue of the brain stem,[54] cerebellum, or hippocampus and includes antigen detection by DFA . Other diagnostic tests are the direct rapid immunohistochemical test, RT-PCR,[55] enzyme-linked immunosorbent assay, Sellers stain technique (Negri bodies),[56] rabies tissue culture infection test,[57] and mouse inoculation test.[58]

MANAGEMENT

Immediate treatment is crucial in case of a possible exposition to rabies: a substantial part of the virus load can be washed out and mortality reduced by 50%.[59,60] Immediate, thorough (approximately 15 minutes) washing and flushing of all bite wounds, scratches, or injuries with alkaline soap and large amounts of water is required. Subsequent disinfection with the usual disinfectants may further reduce the risk of disease development. Apart from mandatory postexposure vaccination, antibiotic coverage according to the potential bacteriologic spectrum may be appropriate (**Table 2**).

Table 2
Categories of exposure (World Health Organization)

Cat	Category of Exposure to Animals Suspicious for Rabies	Type of PEP
I	Touching or feeding animal licks on intact skin	None
II	Nibbling of uncovered skin, minor scratches, abrasions without bleeding	Immediate vaccination, local wound cleansing. Additionally, in persons with an immunodeficiency, rabies immunoglobulin should be applied.
III	Single or multiple bites or scratches (penetration of the skin), licks on broken skin, contamination of mucous membrane with saliva from licks, bat exposure	Immediate vaccination, administration of rabies immunoglobulin, local treatment of the wound

Data from Rabies. Guide for post-exposure prophylaxis. World Health Organization, WHO; 2011. Available at: http://www.who.int/rabies/human/postexp/en/. Accessed June 20, 2012.

PEP

The type of PEP depends on the category of exposure to a suspicious animal. PEP must be applied whenever rabies exposure is suspected, and in any category II and III contact with a potentially rabid mammal. It includes application of RIG and vaccination in subjects without previous vaccination. RIG is mandatory in category III contacts in persons who have not previously been vaccinated and in category II contacts in persons with a immunodeficiency who have not previously been vaccinated.

Despite exceedingly rare failures,[41,61,62] correct and timely application of PEP in nonimmunized victims after contact with rabies virus is considered to prevent the development of disease. The rule of thumb (not evidence based) is that application of immunologicals should occur within 48 hours.

Previously vaccinated subjects need 2 vaccine doses on days 0 and 3, or 4 intradermal injections of 0.1 mL on day 0.[42] Less urgency for such boosting of memory cell function seems necessary.

Mortality in symptomatic patients is close to 100%. Only 6 patients with confirmed rabies disease have survived. All have been vaccinated after the event, and none of them had received immunoglobulin prior to the onset of the disease. Only 1 patient recovered fully, the other 5 survived with severe sequelae.[63]

Vaccination

Passive immunization Administration of human rabies immunoglobulin (HRIG), or equine rabies immunoglobulin (ERIG) in many developing countries, provides an immediate protection by virus-neutralizing antibodies to bridge the time to an active immune response. Use of HRIG (20 international units [IU]/kg) provides passive immunity that persists for a short time (half-life approximately 21 days).[64,65] ERIG or F(ab')2 products of ERIG are less effective and have a shorter half-life. Therefore, ERIG requires a higher dose (40 IU/kg). Various products of HRIG are available (eg, HyperRab S/D [Talecris Biotherapeutics], Imogam Rabies-HT [Sanofi Pasteur], Berirab [Bering]). The World Health Organization (WHO) does not recommend the use of immunoglobulin later than 7 days after the initiation of postexposure vaccination. As much as possible of the RIG should be injected into or around the wound site. If necessary, RIG can be diluted if several sites are present. The remaining immunoglobulin is applied intramuscularly at a distant site. For PEP in a category III exposure or in a category II exposure in a person with an immunodeficiency, except for persons previously vaccinated, RIG should always be administered concurrently with the first dose of vaccine.

Active immunization For all vaccines, the potency should be at least the WHO-recommended minimal potency of 2.5 IU per full intramuscular vaccine dose.[66] In industrialized countries, 0.5 to 1.0 mL intramuscular (IM) doses are generally used for both preexposure and PEP regimens. In developing countries, different IM and intradermal (ID) regimens are used.

The neutralizing antibody response appears 7 to 10 days after initiation of vaccination, and detectable levels persist for years. There are no trials to document a change of efficacy if different cell cultured vaccines are used.

Intramuscular regimens
- Essen regimen (original): 1 dose on days 0, 3, 7, 14, and 28
- Zagreb regimen: 2 doses on day 0, followed by 1 dose each on day 7 and 21
- Essen regimen (shortened): an alternative regimen for people who receive wound care plus WHO-prequalified rabies vaccine plus high-quality rabies immunoglobulin and are immunocompetent is a 4-dose intramuscular regimen of 1 dose on days 0, 3, 7, and 14[67]

Intradermal regimens Updated Thai Red Cross regimen: 2 intradermal doses on days 0, 3, 7, and 28, injected (eg, at the dorsal side of the forearm).

For IM and ID regimens, a fifth dose after at least 3 months may be administered to convey an immunologic memory, but studies confirming this protection are lacking. Thus a booster schedule (1 dose each on days 0 and 3) is necessary after every potential rabies contact (**Table 3**).

Adverse effects The need for rabies PEP after a potential contact outweighs the risks of the vaccination. Thus, hypersensitivity to components of the vaccine is a only relative contraindication. Precautions, contraindications, and adverse effects related to rabies vaccination are summarized on the following Web page: http://www.cdc.gov/rabies/specific_groups/doctors/vaccination_precautions.html.

Pregnancy
PEP is not contraindicated in pregnancy or during breast feeding.

Immunosuppression
Immune-compromising agents and treatments (corticosteroids, cancer therapy, irradiation, immune modulators, immunosuppressive medication), diseases (eg, HIV), or conditions (eg, solid organ and hematopoietic stem cell transplant recipients) may interfere with immune response and vaccination targets.[69–72] For PEP, the original Essen regimen with 5 IM doses on days 0, 3, 7, 14, and 28, plus RIG (in category II and category III exposures) and rapid fluorescent focus inhibition test (RFFIT) confirmation of adequate antibody response on day 21 should be strictly adhered to.[42]

TREATMENT OF RABIES DISEASE
Acute Treatment Measures

Life can be prolonged only for a short time. Analgesics and heavy sedation are necessary. The role of antivirals (Ribavirine), interferon-α, and ketamine is unclear. The only treatment option is palliation and supportive care.[73,74]

PREVENTION

There are 2 main prevention strategies: (1) avoid contact with unfamiliar and wild living animals, and (2) get a preexposure vaccination in case of professional risk and other exposures, as listed in **Table 4**.

Table 3
Rabies vaccines worldwide

Brand	Distribution	Culture Media
Imovax Rabies Vaccine	Sanofi Pasteur	Human diploid cell
Imovax Rabies Vero	Aventis Pasteur	Purified vero cells rabies vaccine
RabAvert	Chiron	Purified chicken embryo cell
Rabivac	Chiron	Human diploid cell
Rabipur	Novartis	Purified chicken embryo cells
Vaccin Rabique Mérieux	Sanofi Pasteur	Human diploid cell
TRC Verorab	Sanofi-Aventis	Purified vero cells rabies vaccine
Verorab	Sanofi Pasteur	Purified vero cells rabies vaccine
Rabies Vaccine Absorbed	Bioport GSK, United States (not available at this time)	Diploid fetal rhesus lung cells Rhesus cell rabies vaccine
Vaxirab (Lyssavax-N)[68]	Licensed in India (Berna Biotech)	Purified duck embryo cells

Table 4
Rabies risk groups

Risk Category	Risk Groups/Profession	Preexposure Regimens
Continuous	Rabies research, rabies biologics work	Primary course. Testing after 6 mo and booster dose if titer is <0.5 IU/mL (RFFIT)
Frequent or episodic	Rabies diagnostic workers, animal handlers, veterinarians and staff in enzootic areas, working with wild animals in enzootic areas, bat handling, caving	Primary course. Testing after 2 y and booster dose if titer is <0.5 IU/mL (RFFIT)
Infrequent	Veterinarians and staff in nonenzootic areas, work with wild animals in nonenzootic areas, travelers in regions with rabies and no access to immediate appropriate medical care (limited access to vaccine and HRIG)	Primary course
	Travelers with extensive outdoor exposure in rural high-risk areas where immediate access to appropriate medical care may be limited, regardless of duration of stay	No testing, no booster vaccination
Rare	Worldwide, if good access to medical care (biologics available)	None

Abbreviation: HRIG, human rabies immunoglobulin.
Data from Manning SE, Rupprecht CE, Fishbein D, et al. Human rabies prevention–United States, 2008: recommendations of the Advisory Committee on Immunization Practices. MMWR Recomm Rep 2008;57(RR-3):1–28.

Although vaccinating dogs is the most cost-effective public health strategy for preventing rabies in humans, the preexposure prophylaxis (PrEP) of human individuals remains a crucial option for practical reasons. Risk groups should be vaccinated before possible exposure.[75]

PrEP

At least 3 doses are necessary. In industrialized countries, a 3-dose IM regimen with human diploid cell vaccine (HDCV) or purified chicken embryo cell vaccine (PCECV) with one ampoule on days 0, 7, and 21 (or 28) injected into the deltoid area in adults or in the antelateral area of the thigh in children less than 2 years old is recommended.

Intradermal regimens with the same intervals are used in developing countries because supply of vaccine is limited. One intradermal dose consists of 0.1 mL. The Asian Rabies Expert Bureau recommends that one intradermal dose should contain ≥0.50 IU, irrespective of the vaccine used.[76]

Healthy persons tested 2 to 4 weeks after complete and correct PrEP with cell cultured vaccines showed adequate antibody response (RFFIT). Testing in immune-competent persons who do not work with potentially rabid material is not necessary.[78,79] Cross-protection to groups other than phylogroup I depends on how far the genetics differ.[77,80] Protection against the Eurasian bat virus strains Aravan (ARAV), Khujand (KHUV), and Irkut (IRKV) is not reliable.[81] Protection against West Caucasian bat virus (WCBV) is questionable.

The gold standard to measure the immune response after active vaccination is the RFFIT.[82] According to the WHO, the minimal titer showing an adequate immune response is 0,5 IU/mL 14 days after the final vaccination.[83–85]

PREVENTION OF RABIES IN TRAVELERS

The risk of rabies disease among travelers is low, but the number of potential rabies exposures is considerably higher than generally anticipated.

Twenty-two cases of rabies in travelers have been reported in the last 10 years. The highest risk was observed in migrants and visiting friends and relatives (VFRs). Most victims were men. Children have not been found to be at a higher risk among travelers in studies, but vaccination should still be recommended because children may not report an exposure to their parents and may miss PEP, and because they are more often injured on the head, because of smaller body size.[86]

Two-thirds of travelers did not receive correct PEP after a suspicious contact.[87,88]

The incidence of being licked or bitten by a potentially rabid animal (mostly dogs) was estimated at 3.6% and 0.7% respectively in a study among backpackers in southeast Asia.[89] The incidence of being injured by a potentially rabid animal varies between 2 to 32 per 1000 travelers per year according to different studies.[90,91] However, routine vaccination against rabies for all travelers to every region of the world with an increased risk of rabies is neither feasible nor sensible.

The WHO recommendations state that people "with extensive outdoor exposure in rural high-risk areas, regardless of duration of stay"[42] should be vaccinated. However, a study done in Nepal showed that trekking was not associated with an increased risk for potential rabies exposure.[90] Another study described more exposures in cities than in rural areas.[92] Length of stay cannot indiscriminately be used as an indicator for the risk of being exposed to a potentially rabid animal either. Diverging results from different studies looking at the time point of exposure among foreign backpackers in Thailand showed that 54% of all contacts happened within the first 10 days after arrival,[89] whereas the exposure occurred after a median of 5 weeks among Israeli travelers.[91]

Other contradictory results exist concerning the risk for travelers to different geographic regions. Although some countries report more cases of potential rabies exposure in travelers returning from South and Southeast Asia,[93] others report more cases from North Africa.[94] These ratios depend on the absolute number of tourists to these destinations. Furthermore, different results are reported with regard to different age groups[93,95] or sex.[96,97]

The presumed risk factor of outdoor exposure in rural high-risk areas[42] does not seem to be based on much evidence and neither travel destination nor age, sex, or length of stay are universally applicable risk factors. An alternative basis for recommendations of PrEP may be the timely availability of adequate PEP at the destination. This approach depends on several factors: (1) first and foremost, travelers must be aware of the risk of rabies at the travel destination and of the modes of transmission; (2) travelers immunized with 3 preexposure doses will be more relaxed than nonvaccinated travelers by buying some time and reducing hassle before getting postexposure treatment in case of an exposure, especially in areas where RIG is not readily available; (3) travelers need to know where correct treatment is available; (4) the required biologicals do not only have to be available within a limited amount of time but their correct application must be assured; (5) planned repeated trips to endemic areas in the future (cumulative risk) may also influence the decision for PrEP.

Even if vaccine and immunoglobulin were available in certain destinations, PrEP might be indicated for ethical reasons: every traveler who requires postexposure treatment in the developing world further depletes the already meager stocks of vaccine, possibly depriving someone else of a life-saving treatment.

The difficulty of estimating the risk for the international traveler is probably best assessed and discussed at individual level, based on travel style (eg, backpacker,

VFR), length of stay, age, and destination. Most of all, every traveler must be made aware of the risk and know what to do in case of an exposure.

REFERENCES

1. Dietzschold B, Li J, Faber M, et al. Concepts in the pathogenesis of rabies. Future Virol 2008;3(5):481–90.
2. Dietzschold B, Schnell M, Koprowski H. Pathogenesis of rabies. Curr Top Microbiol Immunol 2005;292:45–56.
3. Jackson AC. Rabies: new insights into pathogenesis and treatment. Curr Opin Neurol 2006;19(3):267–70.
4. Jackson AC. Rabies pathogenesis. J Neurovirol 2002;8(4):267–9.
5. Gould AR, Hyatt AD, Lunt R, et al. Characterisation of a novel Lyssavirus isolated from pteropid bats in Australia. Virus Res 1998;54(2):165–87.
6. Freuling CM, Beer M, Conraths FJ, et al. Novel Lyssavirus in Natterer's bat, Germany. Emerg Infect Dis 2011;17(8):1519–22.
7. Kuzmin IV, Mayer AE, Niezgoda M, et al. Shimoni bat virus, a new representative of the Lyssavirus genus. Virus Res 2010;149(2):197–210.
8. Constantine DG. Bat rabies and other Lyssavirus infections. Reston (VA): US Department of the Interior; 2009.
9. Denise AM, Daniel LH, Chanasa N, et al. Ikoma Lyssavirus, highly divergent novel lyssavirus in an African civet. Emerging Infectious Diseases 2012;18(4):664–7.
10. Hellenbrand W, Meyer C, Rasch G, et al. Cases of rabies in Germany following organ transplantation. Euro Surveill 2005;10(2):E050224–6.
11. Bronnert J, Wilde H, Tepsumethanon V, et al. Organ transplantations and rabies transmission. J Travel Med 2007;14(3):177–80.
12. Dietzschold B, Koprowski H. Rabies transmission from organ transplants in the USA. Lancet 2004;364(9435):648–9.
13. Gibbons RV. Cryptogenic rabies, bats, and the question of aerosol transmission. Ann Emerg Med 2002;39(5):528–36.
14. Knobel DL, Cleaveland S, Coleman PG, et al. Re-evaluating the burden of rabies in Africa and Asia. Bull World Health Organ 2005;83(5):360–8.
15. The Global Alliance for Rabies Control. Annual number of deaths from rabies hits 70,000 worldwide. Economic burden of disease hits US$ 4 billion. OIE, Global Conference on Eliminating Rabies. Geneva (Glasgow), September 28, 2011.
16. World Health Organization. Rabies. Immunization, vaccines and biologicals. 2010. Available at: http://www.who.int/immunization/topics/rabies/en/index.html. Accessed March 22, 2011.
17. Robertson K, Recuenco S, Niezgoda M, et al. Seroconversion following incomplete human rabies postexposure prophylaxis. Vaccine 2010;28(39):6523–6.
18. Malerczyk C, De Tora L, Gniel D. Imported human rabies cases in Europe, the United States, and Japan, 1990 to 2010. J Travel Med 2011;18(6):402–7.
19. Wandeler AI. The rabies situation in Western Europe. In: Dodet B, Fooks AR, Müller T, Tordo N, and the Scientific & Technical Department of the OIE, editors. OIE/WHO/EU International conference: towards the elimination of rabies in Eurasia, vol. 131. Basel: Karger; 2008. p. 19–25.
20. World Health Organization. WHO Expert consultation on rabies. First report. Geneva (Switzerland): World Health Organization; 2004.
21. World Health Organization. World survey of rabies. Geneva (Switzerland): World Health Organization; 1998.

22. Schneider MC, Romijn PC, Uieda W, et al. Rabies transmitted by vampire bats to humans: an emerging zoonotic disease in Latin America? Rev Panam Salud Publica 2009;25(3):260–9.

23. Poetzsch CJ, Mueller T, Kramer M. Summarizing the rabies situation in Europe. Rabies Bulletin Europe 2002;26:11–6.

24. Crowcroft N. Rabies-like infection in Scotland. Eurosurveillance Weekly 2002; 6(50):pii-1984.

25. Friedrich-Loeffler-Institut F. Bat rabies in Europe. Facts and figures Available at: http://rbe-new.fli.bund.de/About_Rabies/Bats/Facts_Figures.aspx. Accessed October 4, 2011.

26. Towards the elimination of rabies in Eurasia. Proceedings of a joint OIE/WHO/EU international conference. May 27-30, 2007. Paris, France. Dev Biol (Basel) 2008; 131:XIII–XXIV, 3–584.

27. Blancou J. The control of rabies in Eurasia: overview, history and background. Dev Biol (Basel) 2008;131:3–15.

28. De Benedictis P, Gallo T, Iob A, et al. Emergence of fox rabies in north-eastern Italy. Euro Surveill 2008;13(45):19033.

29. Istituto zooprofilattico Sperimentale delle Venezie I. Rabbia. Situazione epidemi-logica. 2011. Available at: http://www.izsvenezie.it/index.php?option=com_content&view=article&id=405&Itemid=403. Accessed October 3, 2011.

30. Ministero della Salute I. Rabbia silvestre in Italia. 2010. Available at: http://www.salute.gov.it/dettaglio/principaleFocusNuovo.jsp?id=17&area=rabbiasilvestre. Accessed October 3, 2011.

31. Istituto zooprofilattico Sperimentale delle Venezie I. Rabbia, dinamica di una malattia. 2010 [in Italian].

32. Mulatti P, Ferre N, Patregnani T, et al. Geographical information systems in the management of the 2009-2010 emergency oral anti-rabies vaccination of foxes in north-eastern Italy. Geospat Health 2011;5(2):217–26.

33. Bourhy H, Dacheux L, Strady C, et al. Rabies in Europe in 2005. Euro Surveill 2005;10(11):213–6.

34. Matouch O. The rabies situation in eastern Europe. In: Dodet B, Fooks AR, Müller T, Tordo N, and the Scientific & Technical Department of the OIE, editors. OIE/WHO/EU International conference: towards the elimination of rabies in Eura-sia, vol. 131. Paris: Karger; 2008. p. 27–35.

35. Schneider MC, Belotto A, Ade MP, et al. Current status of human rabies trans-mitted by dogs in Latin America. Cad Saude Publica 2007;23(9):2049–63.

36. Blanton JD, Palmer D, Dyer J, et al. Rabies surveillance in the United States during 2010. J Am Vet Med Assoc 2011;239(6):773–83.

37. Canadia Food Inspection Agency. Positive rabies in Canada. Animal rabies 2011. Available at: http://www.inspection.gc.ca/english/anima/disemala/rabrag/statse. shtml. Accessed October 3, 2011.

38. Gruzdev KN. The rabies situation in central Asia. In: Dodet B, Fooks AR, Müller T, Tordo N, and the Scientific & Technical Department of the OIE, editors. OIE/WHO/EU International conference: towards the elimination of rabies in Eurasia, vol. 131. Paris: Karger; 2008. p. 37–42.

39. Seimenis A. The rabies situation in the Middle East. In: Dodet B, Fooks AR, Müller T, Tordo N, and the Scientific & Technical Department of the OIE, editors. OIE/WHO/EU International conference: towards the elimination of rabies in Eura-sia, vol. 131. Paris: Karger; 2008. p. 43–53.

40. Fu ZF. The rabies situation in Far East Asia. In: Dodet B, Fooks AR, Müller T, Tordo N, and the Scientific & Technical Department of the OIE, editors.

OIE/WHO/EU International conference: towards the elimination of rabies in Eurasia, vol. 131. Paris: Karger; 2008. p. 27–35.

41. Wilde H. Failures of post-exposure rabies prophylaxis. Vaccine 2007;25(44):7605–9.
42. World Health Organization. Rabies vaccines: WHO position paper. Wkly Epidemiol Rec 2010;32(85):309–20.
43. Plotkin SA. Rabies. Clin Infect Dis 2000;30(1):4–12.
44. Charlton KM, Nadin-Davis S, Casey GA, et al. The long incubation period in rabies: delayed progression of infection in muscle at the site of exposure. Acta Neuropathol 1997;94(1):73–7.
45. Jackson AC, Park H. Experimental rabies virus infection of p75 neurotrophin receptor-deficient mice. Acta Neuropathol 1999;98(6):641–4.
46. Christine T, Klaus S, Christelle L, et al. The rabies virus glycoprotein receptor p75NTR is not essential for rabies virus infection. Journal of virology 2007; 81(24):13622–30.
47. Johnson N, Cunningham AF, Fooks AR. The immune response to rabies virus infection and vaccination. Vaccine 2010;28(23):3896–901.
48. Hemachudha T, Wacharapluesadee S, Laothamatas J, et al. Rabies. Curr Neurol Neurosci Rep 2006;6(6):460–8.
49. Hemachudha T, Laothamatas J, Rupprecht CE. Human rabies: a disease of complex neuropathogenetic mechanisms and diagnostic challenges. Lancet Neurol 2002;1(2):101–9.
50. Fooks AR, Johnson N, Freuling CM, et al. Emerging technologies for the detection of rabies virus: challenges and hopes in the 21st century. PLoS Negl Trop Dis 2009;3(9):e530.
51. Hemachudha T, Wacharapluesadee S. Antemortem diagnosis of human rabies. Clin Infect Dis 2004;39(7):1085–6.
52. Dacheux L, Reynes JM, Buchy P, et al. A reliable diagnosis of human rabies based on analysis of skin biopsy specimens. Clin Infect Dis 2008;47(11):1410–7.
53. Rabies, human. 2011 Case definition. 2011. Available at: http://www.cdc.gov/osels/ph_surveillance/nndss/casedef/rabies_human_current.htm. Accessed October 20, 2011.
54. Dean DJ, Abelseth MK. Laboratory techniques in rabies: the fluorescent antibody test. Monogr Ser World Health Organ 1973;(23):73–84.
55. Centers of Disease Control. Rabies. Diagnosis in animals and humans. 2011. Available at: http://www.cdc.gov/rabies/diagnosis/animals-humans.html. Accessed September 20, 2011.
56. Tierkel ES, Atanasiu P. Rapid microscopic examination for Negri bodies and preparation of specimens for biological tests. In: WHO, editor. Laboratory techniques in rabies. 4th edition. Geneva (Switzerland): WHO; 1996. p. 55–65.
57. Sureau P. Les techniques rapides de diagnostic de laboratoire de la rage. Arch Inst Pasteur Tunis 1986;63:183–97.
58. Webster LT, Dawson JR. Early diagnosis of rabies by mouse inoculation. Measurement of humoral immunity to rabies by mouse protection test. Proc Soc Exp Biol Med 1935;32:570–3.
59. Kaplan MM, Cohen D, Koprowski H, et al. Studies on the local treatment of wounds for the prevention of rabies. Bull World Health Organ 1962;26:765–75.
60. Warrell MJ. The challenge to provide affordable rabies post-exposure treatment. Vaccine 2003;21(7–8):706–9.
61. Shantavasinkul P, Tantawichien T, Wacharapluesadee S, et al. Failure of rabies postexposure prophylaxis in patients presenting with unusual manifestations. Clin Infect Dis 2010;50(1):77–9.

62. Hemachudha T, Mitrabhakdi E, Wilde H, et al. Additional reports of failure to respond to treatment after rabies exposure in Thailand. Clin Infect Dis 1999; 28(1):143–4.
63. Centers for Disease Control and Prevention (CDC). Recovery of a patient from clinical rabies–Wisconsin, 2004. MMWR Morb Mortal Wkly Rep 2004;53(50): 1171–3.
64. Cabasso VJ. Properties of rabies immune globulin of human origin. J Biol Stand 1974;2(1):43–50.
65. Cabasso VJ, Loofbourow JC, Roby RE, et al. Rabies immune globulin of human origin: preparation and dosage determination in non-exposed volunteer subjects. Bull World Health Organ 1971;45(3):303–15.
66. WHO Expert Committee on Rabies. World Health Organ Tech Rep Ser 1992;824: 1–84.
67. Rupprecht CE, Briggs D, Brown CM, et al. Use of a reduced (4-dose) vaccine schedule for postexposure prophylaxis to prevent human rabies: recommendations of the advisory committee on immunization practices. MMWR Recomm Rep 2010;59(RR-2):1–9.
68. Sudarshan MK, Madhusudana SN, Mahendra BJ, et al. Assessing the burden of human rabies in India: results of a national multi-center epidemiological survey. Int J Infect Dis 2007;11(1):29–35.
69. Pancharoen C, Thisyakorn U, Tantawichien T, et al. Failure of pre- and postexposure rabies vaccinations in a child infected with HIV. Scand J Infect Dis 2001; 33(5):390–1.
70. Thisyakorn U, Pancharoen C, Wilde H. Immunologic and virologic evaluation of HIV-1-infected children after rabies vaccination. Vaccine 2001;19(11–12):1534–7.
71. Tantawichien T, Jaijaroensup W, Khawplod P, et al. Failure of multiple-site intradermal postexposure rabies vaccination in patients with human immunodeficiency virus with low CD4+ T lymphocyte counts. Clin Infect Dis 2001;33(10): E122–4.
72. Kotton CN. Vaccination and immunization against travel-related diseases in immunocompromised hosts. Expert Rev Vaccines 2008;7(5):663–72.
73. Jackson AC, Warrell MJ, Rupprecht CE, et al. Management of rabies in humans. Clin Infect Dis 2003;36(1):60–3.
74. van Thiel PP, de Bie RM, Eftimov F, et al. Fatal human rabies due to Duvenhage virus from a bat in Kenya: failure of treatment with coma-induction, ketamine, and antiviral drugs. PLoS Negl Trop Dis 2009;3(7):e428.
75. Manning SE, Rupprecht CE, Fishbein D, et al. Human rabies prevention–United States, 2008: recommendations of the Advisory Committee on immunization practices. MMWR Recomm Rep 2008;57(RR-3):1–28.
76. Dodet B. Antigen content versus volume of rabies vaccines administered. Biologicals 2011;39:444–5.
77. Meslin F-X, Kaplan MM, Koprowski H, editors. Laboratory techniques in rabies. 4th edition. Geneva: World Health Organization; 1996.
78. Sehgal S, Bhattacharya D, Bhardwaj M. Ten year longitudinal study of efficacy and safety of purified chick embryo cell vaccine for pre- and postexposure prophylaxis of rabies in Indian population. J Commun Dis 1995; 27(1):36–43.
79. Wilde H, Glueck R, Khawplod P, et al. Efficacy study of a new albumin-free human diploid cell rabies vaccine (Lyssavac-HDC, Berna) in 100 severely rabies-exposed Thai patients. Vaccine 1995;13(6):593–6.

80. Brookes SM, Parsons G, Johnson N, et al. Rabies human diploid cell vaccine elicits cross-neutralising and cross-protecting immune responses against European and Australian bat lyssaviruses. Vaccine 2005;23(32):4101–9.

81. Hanlon CA, Kuzmin IV, Blanton JD, et al. Efficacy of rabies biologics against new lyssaviruses from Eurasia. Virus Res 2005;111(1):44–54.

82. Smith JS, Yager PA, Baer GM. A rapid reproducible test for determining rabies neutralizing antibody. Bull World Health Organ 1973;48(5):535–41.

83. Rupprecht CE, Hemachudha T. Rabies. In: Scheld WM, Whitley RJ, Marra CM, editors. Infections of the central nervous system. Philadelphia: Lippincott Williams & Wilkins; 2004. p. 243–59.

84. World Health Organization. Requirements for rabies vaccine for human use. Geneva (Switzerland): World Health Organization; 1981. p. 658.

85. Briggs DJ. The immunological basis for immunization series: module 17: rabies. Geneva (Switzerland): World Health Organization; 2011.

86. Meslin FX. Rabies as a traveler's risk, especially in high-endemicity areas. J Travel Med 2005;12(Suppl 1):S30–40.

87. Hatz CF, Bidaux JM, Eichenberger K, et al. Circumstances and management of 72 animal bites among long-term residents in the tropics. Vaccine 1995;13(9): 811–5.

88. Gautret P, Shaw M, Gazin P, et al. Rabies postexposure prophylaxis in returned injured travelers from France, Australia, and New Zealand: a retrospective study. J Travel Med 2008;15(1):25–30.

89. Piyaphanee W, Shantavasinkul P, Phumratanaprapin W, et al. Rabies exposure risk among foreign backpackers in Southeast Asia. Am J Trop Med Hyg 2010; 82(6):1168–71.

90. Pandey P, Shlim DR, Cave W, et al. Risk of possible exposure to rabies among tourists and foreign residents in Nepal. J Travel Med 2002;9(3):127–31.

91. Menachem M, Grupper M, Paz A, et al. Assessment of rabies exposure risk among Israeli travelers. Travel Med Infect Dis 2008;6(1–2):12–6.

92. Phanuphak P, Ubolyam S, Sirivichayakul S. Should travellers in rabies endemic areas receive pre-exposure rabies immunization? Ann Med Interne (Paris) 1994;145(6):409–11.

93. Shaw MT, O'Brien B, Leggat PA. Rabies postexposure management of travelers presenting to travel health clinics in Auckland and Hamilton, New Zealand. J Travel Med 2009;16(1):13–7.

94. Gautret P, Adehossi E, Soula G, et al. Rabies exposure in international travelers: do we miss the target? Int J Infect Dis 2010;14(3):e243–6.

95. Peigue-Lafeuille H, Bourhy H, Abiteboul D, et al. La rage humaine en France en 2004: état des lieux et prise en charge. Médecine et maladies infectieuse 2004; 34:551–60 [in French].

96. Gautret P, Schwartz E, Shaw M, et al. Animal-associated injuries and related diseases among returned travellers: a review of the GeoSentinel Surveillance Network. Vaccine 2007;25(14):2656–63.

97. Johnson N, Brookes SM, Fooks AR, et al. Review of human rabies cases in the UK and in Germany. Vet Rec 2005;157(22):715.

Parasitic Liver Disease in Travelers

Wilson W. Chan, MD[a,b], Adrienne Showler, MD[c], Andrea K. Boggild, MSc, MD[d,e],*

KEYWORDS

- Liver disease • Parasitic liver disease • Disease in travelers • Jaundice

KEY POINTS

- Parasitic infections are common in tropical and subtropical regions worldwide.
- Many protozoal and helminthic infections can lead to both acute and chronic liver disease, with jaundice being one of the most well recognized associated symptoms.
- The pathophysiology of parasitic causes of liver disease is varied, and can include mechanisms such as hemolysis, direct hepatocellular dysfunction, upregulation of inflammatory cytokines, intrahepatic cholestasis, and extrahepatic obstruction.

Liver disease is an important source of morbidity among ill returning travelers. A recent GeoSentinel study of returning travelers presenting to medical attention showed that hepatitis was responsible for 115 cases per 1000 patients presenting with nondiarrheal gastrointestinal illness, and thus 9.4 cases per 1000 patients overall.[1] Jaundice is one of the most common and obvious symptoms of liver disease, although by no means the only one. Its differential diagnosis is extensive, especially in travelers, and encompasses many causes, both infectious and noninfectious (**Table 1**).[2] Viral hepatitis, particularly hepatitis A and B, is the most common cause of jaundice in the returning traveler.[1]

Parasitic causes constitute a significant burden of liver disease in tropical and subtropical nations. Schistosomiasis, for example, affects more than 200 million people worldwide, the vast majority of whom live in tropical regions.[3] Travelers to endemic areas are not spared: a study of patients presenting to a tropical medicine clinic in Canada over a 6-year period revealed numerous cases of parasitic infections capable of causing liver disease, including malaria, schistosomiasis, amebiasis, echinococcosis, and clonorchiasis.[4] The parasites that can cause jaundice and liver dysfunction are taxonomically and biologically varied (**Table 2**). Hepatic

Funding sources: None.
Conflict of interests: None.
[a] Calgary Laboratory Services, 9, 3535 Research Road Northwest, Calgary, Alberta T2L 2K8, Canada; [b] Department of Pathology and Laboratory Medicine, University of Calgary, Calgary, Alberta T2L 2K8, Canada; [c] Division of Infectious Diseases, Department of Medicine, University of Toronto, 200 Elizabeth Street, 13EN-218, Toronto, Ontario M5G 2C4, Canada; [d] Tropical Disease Unit, UHN-Toronto General Hospital, 200 Elizabeth Street, 13EN-218, Toronto, Ontario M5G 2C4, Canada; [e] Division of Infectious Diseases, Department of Medicine, University of Toronto, 200 Elizabeth Street, 13EN-218, Toronto, Ontario M5G 2C4, Canada
* Corresponding author.
E-mail address: Andrea.boggild@utoronto.ca

Infect Dis Clin N Am 26 (2012) 755–780
http://dx.doi.org/10.1016/j.idc.2012.05.006
0891-5520/12/$ – see front matter © 2012 Elsevier Inc. All rights reserved.

id.theclinics.com

Table 1
Causes of jaundice in adults

Noninfectious	Infectious
Prehepatic	**Bacterial**
• Red blood cell destruction	• Severe sepsis
○ Intravascular hemolysis	○ Toxic shock syndrome: *Staphylococcus aureus*, *Streptococcus pyogenes*
■ Microangiopathic hemolytic anemia	○ Clostridial myonecrosis: *Clostridium perfringens*
■ Red blood cell shearing (eg, mechanical heart valve)	• Pyogenic bacteria
■ Paroxysmal nocturnal hemoglobinuria	○ Liver abscess: Enterobacteriaceae, *Streptococcus milleri*, anaerobes
○ Extravascular hemolysis	○ Typhoid fever (*Salmonella typhi*)
■ Autoimmune hemolysis (warm and cold agglutinins)	○ Shigellosis
■ Red blood cell membrane defects (eg, hereditary spherocytosis)	• Fastidious gram-negatives: brucellosis, legionellosis, Q fever
■ Enzyme deficiencies (eg, glucose-6-phosphate dehydrogenase deficiency)	• Mycobacteria: tuberculosis
■ Hemoglobinopathies: sickle cell disease, thalassemia	• Spirochetes: syphilis (secondary and tertiary), leptospirosis
■ Hypersplenism	• Rickettsiae: Rocky Mountain Spotted Fever, epidemic typhus, murine typhus, scrub typhus
■ Drug-induced (eg, dapsone, nitrites)	**Viral**
• Impaired biliary conjugation	• Picornaviridae: hepatitis A, enterovirus
○ eg, Gilbert syndrome, Dubin-Johnson syndrome, Crigler-Najjar syndrome	• Hepadnaviridae: hepatitis B
Hepatic	• Flaviviridae: hepatitis C, dengue, yellow fever
• Hepatocellular injury	• Deltaviridae: hepatitis D
○ Drugs: acetaminophen, isoniazid, rifampin, pyrazinamide, minocycline, nitrofurantoin, phenytoin, sulfasalazine, etretinate, ketoconazole, terbinafine, thiazolidinediones, monoamine oxidase inhibitors, selective serotonin reuptake inhibitors, and nonsteroidal anti-inflammatory drugs	• Hepevirus: hepatitis E
○ Toxins: alcohol, *Amanita phylloides* (poisonous mushrooms), cocaine, phencyclidine ("angel dust"), 3,4-methylenedioxymethamphetamine ("ecstasy")	• Herpesviridae: varicella zoster virus, Epstein-Barr virus, human cytomegalovirus
○ Autoimmune hepatitis	
○ Shock liver/hypoperfusion	
○ Nonalcoholic steatohepatitis	

  o Hepatic congestion, secondary to right-sided heart failure
  o Herbal supplements (eg, ma huang, jin bu huan, germander, chaparral, pennyroyal, skullcap, kava, Hydroxycut, Herbalife)
  o Wilson disease
  o Decompensated cirrhosis of any cause
- Intrahepatic cholestasis
  o Primary biliary cirrhosis
  o Drugs: oral contraceptives, anabolic steroids, total parenteral nutrition, trimethoprim/sulfamethoxazole
  o Cholestasis of pregnancy
  o Graft versus host disease
- Other
  o Budd-Chiari syndrome
  o Veno-occlusive disease
  o Infiltrative conditions (eg, amyloidosis, sarcoidosis)

Posthepatic
- Extrahepatic cholestasis
  o Intrinsic obstruction
    ■ Choledocholithiasis
    ■ Biliary stricture
    ■ Primary sclerosing cholangitis
    ■ Cholangiocarcinoma
    ■ Choledochal cyst
    ■ Sphincter of Oddi dysfunction
  o Extrinsic compression
    ■ Pancreatitis (acute and chronic)
    ■ Extrahepatic malignancy (eg, pancreatic cancer, lymphoma)

Fungal
- Candidiasis
- Histoplasmosis
Parasitic
- Please refer to Table 2

Data from Refs. [124–126]

Table 2
Summary of parasitic causes of jaundice

Name	Etiology	Transmission	Geographic Distribution	Clinical Manifestations	Diagnosis	Management	Prevention
Malaria	*Plasmodium* spp • *P falciparum* • *P vivax* • *P ovale* • *P malariae* • *P knowlesi*	Mosquito bite (*Anopheles*)	Africa: sub-Saharan Asia: Southeast, India Central & South America Middle East	Mild-moderate • Fever Severe • Cerebral malaria • Acute renal failure • ARDS • Hepatopathy	• Microscopy (blood) • RDT (ICT) • PCR	Mild-moderate (oral) • Atovaquone + proguanil • Quin + doxy Severe (parenteral) • ACT • Quin + doxy	• Insect precautions prophylaxis • Atovaquone + proguanil • Doxycycline • Mefloquine • Chloroquine in areas with susceptible Pf
Babesiosis	*Babesia* spp • *B microti* • *B divergens*	Tick bite (*Ixodes*)	USA: NE states Europe: France	Mild-moderate • Fever Severe • Hemolytic anemia • Jaundice • Multi-system organ failure	• Microscopy (blood) • Serology • PCR	Mild-moderate • Azithromycin + atovaquone Severe • Clindamycin + quinine	• Tick precautions • Long pants, tucked socks • Tick checks
Amebic liver abscess	*Entamoeba histolytica*	Ingestion (fecal-oral)	Central & South America Asia Africa	Liver abscess • Fever • RUQ pain • Leukocytosis	• Imaging (US, CT, MRI) • Serology • PCR	• Metronidazole Luminal agent • Iodoquinol • Paromomycin	Food precautions
Visceral leishmaniasis	*Leishmania* • *L donovani* • *L chagasi-infantum*	Sandfly bite (*Phlebotomus, Lutzomyia*)	Africa: Sudan, Ethiopia Asia: Indian subcontinent Central & South America: Brazil	Visceral leishmaniasis • Fever • HSM • Pancytopenia • Weight loss	• Microscopy (BM) • Serology • PCR	• Liposomal amphoB	Insect precautions

Disease	Organism	Transmission	Geography	Clinical features	Diagnosis	Treatment	Prevention
Schistosomiasis	Schistosoma • S mansoni • S japonicum • S haematobium • S mekongi • S intercalatum	Skin penetration (contaminated freshwater)	Africa: northern Asia: east, SE South America: Amazon	Acute • Fever • Eosinophilia • Cough, dyspnea • Lymphadenopathy Chronic • Portal hypertension • Ascites, varices	• Microscopy (stool) • Serology	Praziquantel	Freshwater avoidance
Fascioliasis	Fasciola • F hepatica • F gigantic	Ingestion of metacercariae (aquatic vegetables)	South America: Peru, Bolivia Middle East Europe: France	Acute • Fever • Eosinophilia • RUQ pain • Hepatomegaly Chronic • Obstructive jaundice • Cholangitis • Pancreatitis	Acute • Serology • Imaging (CT) Chronic • Microscopy (stool) • ERCP	Triclabendazole	Cooking of aquatic vegetables Treating livestock
Clonorchiasis/opisthorchiasis	Clonorchis • C sinensis Opisthorchis • O viverrini • O felineus	Ingestion of metacercariae (uncooked fish)	Clonorchis Asia: East, SE O viverrini Asia: SE O felineus Europe: eastern, USSR	• Obstruction • Recurrent pyogenic cholangitis • Cholangiocarcinoma	• Microscopy (stool) • Imaging (US, CT) • ERCP	Praziquantel	Cooking of fish

(continued on next page)

Table 2
(continued)

Name	Etiology	Transmission	Geographic Distribution	Clinical Manifestations	Diagnosis	Management	Prevention

Echinococcosis	*Echinococcus*
	• *E granulosus*
	• *E multilocularis*
		Ingestion of eggs
		(contaminated
		soil, dog fur)
			E granulosus:
			South America,
			Middle East,
			East Africa,
			Asia, Russia
			E multilocularis:
			Europe: East
			Asia: Russia, China
			North America:
			Canada, Alaska
				Cystic echinococcosis
				• RUQ pain
				• Hepatomegaly
				• Cyst rupture
				Alveolar echinococcosis
				• Hepatomegaly
				• Portal hypertension
				• Obstructive jaundice
					• Imaging
					  (US, CT)
					• Serology
					• Microscopy
					  (cyst fluid)
						Albendazole ±
						  praziquantel;
						  mebendazole
						PAIR
						surgery
							Interrupt
							  transmission
							  via disposal
							  of ruminant
							  viscera rather
							  than feeding
							  to local canids

Ascariasis	*Ascaris*
	• *A lumbricoides*
		Ingestion of egg
		(contaminated
		soil)
			Africa	Biliary ascariasis
				• Biliary colic
				• Cholangitis
				• Cholecystitis
				• Pancreatitis
					• Microscopy
					  (stool)
					• Imaging (US)
					• ERCP
						Mebendazole
						ERCP extraction
							Food precautions
							  (avoid fertilizing
							  with human
							  manure)

Visceral larva
migrans (VLM)
	Toxocara
	• *T canis*
	• *T cati*
		Ingestion of eggs
		(contaminated
		soil)
			Worldwide	VLM
				• Fever
				• Eosinophilia
				• Cough, wheeze
				• Hepatomegaly
					• Serology
					• Imaging
					  (CT, MRI)
						Albendazole	Pet deworming
							Avoidance of
							  geophagia/pica

Abbreviations: ACT, artemisinin-combination therapy; amphoB, amphotericin B; ARDS, acute respiratory distress syndrome; BM, bone marrow; CT, computed tomography; doxy, doxycycline; ERCP, endoscopic retrograde cholangiopancreatography; HSM, hepatosplenomegaly; ICT, immunochromatographic test; MRI, magnetic resonance imaging; PAIR, percutaneous aspiration, instillation, and reaspiration; PCR, polymerase chain reaction; Pf, *Plasmodium falciparum*; quin, quinine or quinidine; RDT, rapid diagnostic test; RUQ, right upper quadrant; US, ultrasound.

manifestations may arise through a spectrum of pathophysiologic processes, classi-fied broadly as prehepatic, hepatic, and posthepatic (**Fig. 1**). As travel to tropical and subtropical regions continues to rise, parasitic liver disease in travelers will remain an important entity to diagnose and treat.

We herein summarize the most common parasitic etiologies that may lead to jaun-dice in the returned traveler, visitor of friends and relatives (VFR), or new immigrant, and describe the etiology, epidemiology, and pathogenesis of clinical features of each.

MALARIA
Etiology and Epidemiology

Malaria is caused *Plasmodium* spp, a genus of sporozoan protozoa. Five species have been described to affect humans: *Plasmodium falciparum*, the agent of the most severe disease; *Plasmodium vivax*, *Plasmodium ovale*, *Plasmodium malariae*, and *Plasmodium knowlesi*,[5] all of which use the *Anopheles* mosquito as a vector. Severe disease is usually caused by *P falciparum*, although severe malaria caused by *P vivax* is well-documented.[6] *P knowlesi* has been recently described in southeast Asia, and it too has been implicated in severe disease.[7]

Malaria is endemic to more than 100 tropical and subtropical countries of the world, including Central and South America, Asia, the Middle East, and with the highest inten-sity of infection in sub-Saharan Africa.[8] Travelers to these regions are prone to infec-tion: malaria is consistently the most common diagnosis in returning travelers presenting with fever (20%–30%).[9–19] Another study showed that it was one of the most common parasitic infections in returned ill Canadian travelers, second only to nonhistolytica amebiasis.[4]

Clinical Features

After a variable incubation period, ranging from 5 to 10 days for *P falciparum*, to weeks to months for non-falciparum species,[20] malaria can exhibit a broad spectrum of severity. The cardinal symptom of malaria is fever, often intermittent, classically in species-specific patterns that are seldom elicited on patient history.[21] Mild and moderate malaria most often presents with fever, which may be accompanied by

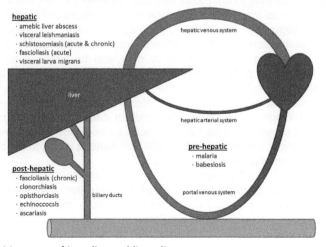

Fig. 1. Parasitic causes of jaundice and liver disease.

nonspecific, constitutional symptoms such as headache, malaise, nausea, and vomiting, and arthralgias.[20]

Severe malaria, in contrast, is a systemic, life-threatening condition that affects multiple organ systems including the brain, kidneys, and liver. Key events in the pathogenesis of P falciparum malaria include sequestration of parasitized erythrocytes (PEs) within the microvasculature of vital organs; dysregulated inflammatory responses to infection, contributing to immune-mediated tissue injury and upregulation of sequestration receptors; and uncontrolled parasite replication resulting in high parasite burdens that further enhance sequestration and host-mediated inflammatory injury.[22] Manifestations of severe disease include cerebral malaria, hyperparasitemia, severe anemia,[5] acute renal failure, and acute respiratory distress syndrome with pulmonary edema.[20] Notably, clinical jaundice (and/or icterus) is considered one of the defining criteria of severe malaria by the World Health Organization,[23] often correlating with hyperbilirubinemia of 3 mg/dL, or 50 μmol/L.[24]

Jaundice varies in incidence in studies of malaria, occurring from as rarely as 2.6% to as often as 62.0%,[25] possibly increasing in recent years.[26] Jaundice can result from hemolysis: as malarial schizonts mature and prepare to release merozoites, the erythrocyte membrane is lysed in a protease-dependent process.[27] In severe disease, disseminated intravascular coagulation with microangiopathic hemolysis may exacerbate the anemia.[28] The accumulation of the unconjugated bilirubin released during widespread hemolysis can be significant enough to cause visible jaundice.[25]

Malaria can also directly cause hepatocellular dysfunction, often referred to as malarial hepatopathy. This usually occurs only in severe disease with P falciparum, although it has been noted with severe P. vivax as well.[6] The etiology of hepatopathy is multifactorial. A major mechanism is microvascular obstruction, similar to that occurring in other organ systems affected by severe falciparum malaria, such as the brain and kidney. This is mediated by PfEMP1, a membrane protein expressed by PEs that mediates interaction with and adherence to endothelial receptors, including intercellular adhesion molecule-1, CD36, and CSA.[29] They also adhere to uninfected erythrocytes, forming rosettes.[29] Thus, PEs not only sequester in the microvasculature and avoid splenic clearance, but also form intravascular deposits that impede blood flow and cause tissue ischemia.[30]

Additionally, apoptosis is increasingly recognized as a contributor to malarial hepatopathy. An increase in apoptosis has been observed in the livers of malaria-infected mice, as was increased expression of the proapoptotic protein Bax and a decrease in antiapoptotic Bcl-2.[31] It is hypothesized that this mechanism is driven by trophozoite production of hydroxyl radicals, and resultant oxidative stress, in the hepatocytes.[31] The host cytokine response may also be instrumental in hepatic dysfunction. A study of patients infected with P. vivax suggested an association between significantly higher levels of the cytokines interleukin (IL)-1, IL-4, IL-6, IL-10, tumor necrosis factor (TNF), and interferon-gamma (IFN-γ) and hepatic dysfunction.[32] A murine model using Plasmodium chabaudi also suggested TNF was an important cytokine involved in hepatocellular necrosis.[33] Other mechanisms of hepatocellular injury may include intrahepatic cholestasis owing to impaired biliary flow, and obstruction of portal venules by PEs.[30]

Together, these pathways of hepatic injury lead to pathologic changes of necrosis, without a marked inflammatory response. A series of autopsies of liver tissues in cases of fatal malaria found widespread Kupffer cell hyperplasia and retention of malarial hemozoin pigment. Significant hepatocellular necrosis was seen in 41%; these were notable for a paucity of inflammation infiltrates, compared with those seen in viral hepatitis.[28] Clinically, this pathophysiology may manifest as jaundice, hepatomegaly, and biochemical derangement of liver function tests.[30,34] Transaminases are elevated, although the increase may be modest (2–3 times the upper limit of normal).[26] Jaundice may arise from a combination of hemolysis, and hepatocellular dysfunction and destruction, as described previously. The presence of jaundice itself is a marker associated with more severe disease and higher mortality.[26] In severe cases, the degree of hepatic dysfunction may be critical enough to mimic fulminant hepatic failure.[30] Even in these situations, however, malaria hepatopathy has a better prognosis than other causes of fulminant hepatic failure (24% vs 76% mortality without transplantation).[34] The diagnostic picture may be complicated by adverse effects of drugs. In particular, hepatotoxicity has been reported with certain antimalarial drugs, such as mefloquine and sulfadoxine-pyrimethamine,[30] and in particular, fulminant hepatic failure requiring transplantation secondary to amodiaquine use has been reported.[35]

In sum, jaundice in malaria can arise as a result of a number of pathophysiologic mechanisms mediated by both host and parasite, and is often, although not exclusively, a marker of more severe clinical disease. Jaundice in a traveler with malaria, particularly one who is nonimmune, warrants close inpatient observation, and likely parenteral therapy.

BABESIOSIS
Etiology and Epidemiology

Babesiosis is caused by protozoan members of the genus *Babesia*. *Babesia microti* is the most common species in North America, whereas most European cases are caused by *Babesia divergens*.[36] Although these 2 species were thought to cause virtually all babesiosis, a growing body of evidence has implicated other *Babesia* species, such as *Babesia duncani* (formerly known as species WA1), as agents in human disease.[37]

Humans are intermediate hosts; other mammals, especially rodents for *B microti* and cows for *B divergens*, are important reservoirs. Organisms are transmitted by the bite of a tick, in most cases *Ixodes* spp. In particular, *Ixodes scapularis* is the main vector for *B microti*. Aside from tick bites, blood transfusions are a well-documented source of human infections.[37–39]

B microti is endemic in the United States, with most disease occurring in the northeastern coast, including Connecticut, Rhode Island, New York, and New Jersey,[40] and as far west as Wisconsin and Minnesota.[41] Cases of *B duncani* infection have been reported in California and Washington State, whereas most *B divergens* cases have been reported from Europe, primarily France and England.[37] Travelers to endemic areas are at risk of contracting babesiosis; one recent case report describes a patient from Ohio with travel to Connecticut who contracted severe babesiosis, complicated by cardiac arrhythmias and pancytopenia, despite lack of documented tick exposure.[42]

Clinical Features

Infection with *B microti* in immunocompetent hosts is commonly asymptomatic; even when there are symptoms, it often causes mild to moderate disease. Fever is the main presenting complaint, often accompanied by nonspecific symptoms, such as headache, malaise, and myalgia. Other symptoms, including cough, nausea and vomiting, and abdominal pain, may be present. Anemia, and less commonly jaundice from the released bilirubin, may be present,[40] secondary to hemolysis during the parasite's replication, with merozoite egress. *Babesia* spp have been observed to produce superoxide anions through lipid peroxidation in vitro; the subsequent oxidative damage may contribute to anemia.[43] Overall, if untreated, the symptoms may last for weeks to months.[36]

Severe babesiosis is most common in immunocompromised patients, with multisystem organ failure and death occurring in 5% to 8% of patients with *B microti*, and more than 40% of patients with *B divergens*.[41] Asplenia is the most significant risk factor for severe babesiosis, and for *B divergens* in particular,[36] highlighting the importance of the spleen in clearance of *Babesia*-infected erythrocytes. Human immunodeficiency virus (HIV), immunosuppressive medications, malignancy, and older age (>50) are other known risk factors.[40] In severe babesiosis, much higher levels of parasitemia (80% or more) may be seen, which can result in a severe hemolytic anemia and jaundice.[37] Disseminated intravascular coagulation, acute respiratory distress syndrome (ARDS), and congestive heart failure may be complications of severe disease.[36] Hepatic failure, evidenced by rising transaminases and decreased hepatic synthetic function (including rising international normalized ratio), may occur.[39] The pathogenesis of severe babesiosis is not fully elucidated. It has been shown that a CD4+ immune response, and in particular IFN-γ, is critical for control and clearance of the infection.[40] However, proinflammatory cytokines may simultaneously contribute to complications of *B duncani* infection: TNF and IFN-γ levels were elevated in pulmonary tissues of mice infected with *B duncani* that developed ARDS, but were normal in *B microti*–infected animals.[44] In addition, *Babesia* spp have been shown to be capable of cytoadherence by means of VESA1, a secreted membrane protein similar to *P falciparum*'s PfEMP-1, which can lead to microvasculature obstruction and downstream hypoxia. This has not been observed in *B microti* or *B divergens*, however, the 2 most common human pathogens.[40]

Babesiosis is an important tick-associated illness, and should be included on the differential diagnosis for febrile patients with an appropriate epidemiologic history. Although mild babesiosis is the norm in those with unimpaired immune systems, severe disease may occur in immunocompromised hosts, with complications that include jaundice and hepatic dysfunction.

AMEBIC LIVER ABSCESS
Etiology and Epidemiology

Amebic liver abscess (ALA) is the most common extraintestinal complication of infection with *Entamoeba histolytica*, an entero-invasive, amebic protozoan endemic to Central and South America, Africa, and the Indian subcontinent. Although ALA develops in fewer than 1% of *E histolytica* infections,[45] it represents a substantial burden of disease, given the high worldwide prevalence of amebiasis. *E histolytica* thrives in urban and peri-urban regions of developing countries, where poor sanitation practices facilitate fecal-oral transmission of infective cysts through contaminated food and water. In adults, 90% of those who develop abscesses are men,[46] most commonly in the 20 to 40 age group.[47]

Clinical Presentation

Trophozoites penetrating large bowel mucosa may cause bloody diarrhea, abdominal pain, and in severe cases, fulminant colitis. Entering the portal circulation, trophozoites travel to the liver, obstruct intrahepatic portal venules, and digest hepatocytes with proteolytic enzymes.[47,48] Focal collections of necrotic hepatocytes and acellular debris coalesce to form a larger amebic abscess cavity containing a thick reddish-brown homogeneous fluid that classically resembles "anchovy paste." Abscesses are commonly solitary right hepatic lobe lesions,[49] but in one major study, 35% of patients had isolated left lobe involvement and 16% had multiple bilateral lesions.[50]

Liver abscesses typically present within 2 to 5 months of travel or residence in an endemic area,[48] although symptoms occasionally manifest years after potential exposure.[51] Concurrent amebic colitis is usually absent, with diarrhea occurring in only 18% to 33% at the time of abscess diagnosis.[52] Between 85% and 90% of patients present with the combination of fever and right upper quadrant pain,[52,53] typically of fewer than 10 days' duration. Abdominal pain is frequently the earliest symptom, described as a heavy sensation in the right hypochondria, subcostal area or epigastrium, and which may evolve into a sharp pain that radiates to the shoulder, neck, or back.[54] Subacute presentations with nonspecific symptoms, such as nausea, anorexia, and low-grade fever, may also occur.[48,49] Hepatomegaly is present in 30% to 50%,[52] and may be visible as an epigastric mass or manifest as dyspnea owing to upward extension and diaphragmatic compression.[54] Most patients with ALA have elevation of the right hemidiaphragm on chest x-ray owing to right lobe hepatic abscesses,[49] and 10% to 30% complain of cough.[52] Leukocytosis without eosinophilia and mild transaminitis are common. The classic ultrasound appearance is that of a round, homogeneous, hypoechoic lesion with well-defined borders located near the liver surface.[46]

Jaundice occurs in a minority of 8% to 22% of cases, and is associated with acute onset of symptoms, male sex, and history of alcohol abuse.[46,53,55] Clinical jaundice is also a marker of more advanced disease: patients with multiple abscesses and with larger lesions are more likely to have jaundice, and several studies report significantly higher mortality rates in jaundiced patients owing to increased risk of abscess rupture.[54,55] Multiple mechanisms for jaundice have been implicated. Pressure on hepatic ducts caused by the abscess itself may result in obstructive jaundice, particularly in those with large abscesses immediately below the liver surface near the porta hepatis.[53,55] Hepatocyte necrosis may lead to biliovascular fistula formation, as endoscopic retrograde cholangiopancreaticography performed in a small series of patients with ALA demonstrated communication between the abscess cavity and biliary system with concurrent contrast extravasation into hepatic veins.[56] Other postulated mechanisms include intrahepatic cholestasis and widespread destruction of liver parenchymal cells.[55]

Mortality is less than 1% with early treatment,[57] but ranges from 2% to 18% depending on the clinical context.[58] Complications occur primarily because of abscess rupture. Rupture into the peritoneum occurs in 2% to 7% of patients and presents with acute onset peritonitis followed by shock.[48,57] Abscess rupture through the diaphragm results in pleuropulmonary amebiasis in 10% to 20%,[46] and may be further complicated by empyema and hepatobronchial fistulization. Rupture into the pericardium is uncommon, but may occur with left-sided abscesses, and is associated with pericarditis, tamponade, and a 30% mortality rate.[48] Hematogenous spread to distal sites, including skin and brain, is rare.

Amebic liver abscess is an infrequent complication of *E histolytica* infection that presents with fever and right upper quadrant abdominal pain within months of travel to an endemic area. Jaundice is associated with larger abscesses, increased risk of abscess rupture, and higher mortality rates.

VISCERAL LEISHMANIASIS
Etiology and Epidemiology

Leishmaniasis is a vector-borne illness caused by protozoan members of *Leishmania*. There are more than 30 different species that cause disease in humans, many possessing different geographic distributions and disease tropisms. These include cutaneous (CL), mucocutaneous (MCL), and visceral leishmaniasis (VL). Notably, VL is principally caused by the *Leishmania donovani* complex, including *L. donovani* and *Leishmania chagasi-infantum*, although rarely, *Leishmania tropica* has been implicated as an etiologic agent.[59,60] In addition, species such as *Leishmania viannia braziliensis*, which are primary agents of cutaneous and mucosal disease, are known to visceralize in hosts with immune compromise owing to HIV or solid organ transplantation.

Leishmania parasites are transmitted by the bite of sandflies belonging to the genus *Phlebotomus* in the Old World and *Lutzomyia* in the New World.[61] More than 90% of VL cases occur in India, Nepal, Bangladesh, Sudan, Ethiopia, and Brazil.[62] There has been an increased concern of widening locales of endemicity, such as Europe[63] and the southern United States[64]; still, these autochthonous cases have been mainly cutaneous forms of the disease. However, both CL and VL have been increasingly well-documented in travelers to endemic areas.[61]

Clinical Features

VL is a multisystem disease that is invariably fatal unless treated.[62] Shortly after inoculation by the sandfly bite, *Leishmania* promastigotes are phagocytosed by macrophages wherein they transform into amastigotes. The immunobiological interactions of *Leishmania* are complex, and a detailed discussion is beyond the scope of this review, but in brief, host clearance of amastigotes relies on a strong T-helper cell type 1 (Th1) response to upregulate cell-mediated immunity and to activate macrophages, using cytokines such as TNF, IFN-γ, and IL-12.[65] However, *Leishmania* itself can modulate the immune system toward a less effective Th2 response, which renders the host more vulnerable to intracellular infection. In particular, the expression of IL-10 has been found to be particularly important to increase host susceptibility and the virulence of VL.[66] Once intracellular infection has been established, amastigotes can spread throughout the reticuloendothelial system. The exact mechanism of hepatic injury is unclear, but histopathologic changes on liver biopsy include inflammation with lymphocytes and macrophages, ballooning degeneration of hepatocytes, and hypertrophy and hyperplasia of Kupffer cells.[67]

The incubation period may last from 2 to 6 months, after which symptoms reflect the systemic nature of the disease. Cardinal symptoms include fever and hepatosplenomegaly. Nonspecific symptoms may include fatigue, lymphadenopathy, anorexia, and weight loss. By late disease, this may progress to cachexia, along with edema and ascites. Blood work often shows pancytopenia, especially thrombocytopenia, and hypergammaglobulinemia.[68] Although spleen enlargement tends to be predominant, almost all patients present with some degree of hepatosplenomegaly.[61] In one recent series of 114 patients with VL prospectively followed for liver derangement, a small minority (13%) presented with jaundice. Hepatic dysfunction was associated with poor outcome: of the 11 patients who died, 9 showed markedly elevated liver markers.[69] Liver injury was demonstrably reversible in survivors: by the end of their course of treatment, aspartate aminotransferase and alanine aminotransferase normalized in 87% and 92% of patients, respectively.[69] Pediatric VL leading to fulminant hepatic failure has been reported, and in a review of 12 such patients, 6 died despite therapy.[70] Rarely, VL has been reported to present as chronic liver disease, with portal hypertension, ascites, and esophageal varices.[69,71] Although death can be caused by hepatic failure, patients more commonly die of bacterial superinfection or of bleeding.[61]

VL is a disease affecting the entire reticuloendothelial system, including the liver, and hepatosplenomegaly is common. Jaundice in VL is an infrequent entity, but its presence is an ominous finding, and should induce physicians to treat promptly.

SCHISTOSOMIASIS
Etiology and Epidemiology

Schistosomiasis is caused by trematodes or flukes of the genus *Schistosoma*, which infect humans through freshwater exposure. Cercariae, the infective stage, are released by freshwater snails that penetrate intact human skin and travel to venous plexi where they mature into adult flukes. *Schistosoma* spp migrate to specific venous plexi: *Schistosoma japonicum* and *Schistosoma mekongi* to the superior mesenteric venules, *Schistosoma mansoni* to the inferior mesenteric venules, and *Schistosoma haematobium* to the veins supplying the bladder. The lifespan of an adult fluke is 3 to 7 years on average, but can exceed 3 decades.[72]

S mansoni, *S japonicum,* and *S haematobium* cause most of the disease in more than 200 million people in 76 countries.[73] *S mansoni* is found in the Middle East, Africa, parts of South America, and the Caribbean, whereas *S japonicum* is endemic to China, the Philippines, Thailand, and Indonesia.[74] *S haematobium* is endemic to Africa and the Middle East. *Schistosoma mekongi* and *Schistosoma intercalatum* are also pathogenic in humans, but cause disease in limited regions: *S mekongi* inhabits the Mekong River Valley in Cambodia and Laos, and *S intercalatum* is found only in pockets of sub-Saharan Africa. Transmission occurs primarily in rural areas.[72] Thus, schistosomiasis is a risk to travelers with freshwater exposure in many parts of the developing world. Next to cutaneous larva migrans, schistosomiasis was the most common helminthic infection diagnosed among ill returned travelers presenting for care post travel or immigration in Canada.[4]

Clinical Presentation

More than one-third of *Schistosoma*-infected travelers are asymptomatic at diagnosis, likely because of low fluke burden.[75] Travelers frequently present with acute schistosomiasis, or Katayama fever, which is caused by an acute hypersensitivity reaction to schistosomal antigens.[75] Katayama fever occurs 2 to 8 weeks after exposure, mainly in patients with their first infection, but occasionally in those with chronic schistosomiasis.[76] Patients present with acute onset of fever, myalgia, and lethargy.[77] Nonproductive cough, wheezing, and dyspnea occur in up to 70%, often accompanied by patchy pulmonary infiltrates.[78] Eosinophilia may be marked, and is present in 80% of cases.[79] Lymphadenopathy and hepatomegaly are common, and splenomegaly is found in a third of patients.[74,77] Nonbloody diarrhea and abdominal pain may also occur. Acute transverse myelitis is a rare complication.[78] Full recovery from Katayama fever usually occurs with supportive treatment, without chronic hepatic sequelae.

Chronic symptoms of schistosomiasis arise from prolonged granulomatous inflammatory responses to schistosome eggs trapped in various host tissues. Chronic hepatic involvement is a feature of *S mansoni*, *S japonicum*, and *S mekongi* infection. Hepatic manifestations occur in 2 distinct forms: early inflammatory hepatic schistosomiasis and late fibrotic disease. The early inflammatory variety affects adolescents and up to 80% of infected children.[72] Schistosome eggs in the liver generate presinusoidal and periportal granulomatous inflammation, resulting in mild to severe hepatosplenomegaly. Abdominal ultrasonography reveals diffuse mild fibrosis, although liver function typically remains normal.

Late fibrotic liver disease develops in 4% to 8% of young and middle-aged adults with heavy chronic infection.[74] Periportal inflammation stimulates collagen deposition that ultimately results in pathognomonic "Symmer pipestem fibrosis" and noncirrhotic portal hypertension. Symptoms develop insidiously over 5 to 15 years in *S mansoni* infection,[72] whereas *S japonicum* is associated with more severe and quickly evolving disease. Complications of late fibrotic schistosomiasis are mainly portal hypertension related, and include bleeding esophageal and gastric varices, splenomegaly, and pancytopenia because of hypersplenism. Ascites occurs in decompensated cases, whereas other stigmata of chronic liver disease are typically absent on physical examination.[80] Hepatocyte function is usually preserved, and therefore hepatic encephalopathy, jaundice, and coagulopathies do not occur except in very advanced decompensated disease.[80] When hepatocyte dysfunction is present, it is often associated with superimposed viral hepatitis or alcoholic liver disease.[72,74] Although esophageal and gastric variceal bleeding are common, mortality is relatively low compared with similar bleeding events in patients with cirrhosis. Variceal bleeding from schistosomal liver disease is more likely to spontaneously resolve, given the absence of coexisting coagulopathy. Unlike cirrhosis, variceal bleeding in schistosomiasis rarely precipitates hepatic encephalopathy, as the liver is able to process the gut ammonia load produced by gastrointestinal bleeding.[80]

Travelers infected with schistosomiasis through freshwater exposure are commonly asymptomatic or may present with acute Katayama syndrome, which includes fever, pulmonary complaints, and hepatosplenomegaly. Jaundice occurs in the setting of advanced fibrotic liver disease and noncirrhotic portal hypertension, which affects only long-term residents of endemic areas with heavy chronic fluke burden. Jaundice owing to schistosomiasis is therefore a complication seen in long-term residents of the developing world, although is extremely unlikely in a typical returned traveler.

FASCIOLIASIS
Etiology and Epidemiology

Fascioliasis is caused by *Fasciola*, a genus of hepatobiliary trematodes. *Fasciola hepatica* and *Fasciola gigantica* are the 2 species that affect humans; they are separate in their epidemiology but morphologically and clinically similar. Infection is typically acquired by ingestion of metacercarial cysts attached to aquatic vegetation, such as watercress, although transmission by drinking contaminated water or consumption of inadequately cooked animal liver has been reported.[81] Once within the gastrointestinal tract, metacercariae excyst, penetrate the intestinal wall into the peritoneal space, and migrate to the liver and ultimately the biliary tree. There, the flukes finish their maturation process and spend their adulthood, where they can live an estimated 9 to 13 years.[82]

Fasciola infection is distributed worldwide in domestic livestock, especially sheep, and is an important veterinary disease. Human infection is more geographically localized, with the most intense foci in South America (Peru and Bolivia), as well as Egypt, Iran, Cuba, and western Europe (France).[83] Sporadic cases are described widely, including the United States[84] and southeast Asia.[85] Although seldom seen in returning in travelers, a case of travel-acquired acute fascioliasis has been reported in a patient from New Zealand with travel to India, Pakistan, and China.[85]

Clinical Features

Fasciola infection usually presents in 2 distinct, sequential phases, related to the parasite's life cycle. The acute phase can be seen as early as 6 weeks after ingestion and lasts for up to 4 months.[83] The fluke larvae create hemorrhagic tracts as they translocate through the liver; these progress to necrotic lesions and generate a substantial eosinophilic response.[86] The evolving lesions can also be visualized by computed tomography (CT).[87] Symptoms are related to tissue damage as the larvae migrate,[83] and include right-upper quadrant abdominal pain, fever, hepatomegaly, and eosinophilia.[88] Other nonspecific symptoms may include nausea, vomiting, anorexia, and urticaria. Jaundice is rare during this stage, but extrahepatic migration to the eye, brain, subcutaneous tissues, pancreas, and stomach have been described.[88] The diaphragm may become inflamed during the larvae's peritoneal migration, and results in cough or other respiratory symptoms.[82] This phase is self-limited: as the fluke larvae reach the biliary ducts, the necrotic lesions in their wake are repaired by fibroblasts, undergoing hepatic regeneration.[86] Systemic eosinophilia also declines as the acute phase passes.

The chronic phase of fascioliasis follows, and can last for more than 10 years. This stage is often asymptomatic, as the fluke matures to adulthood, growing and reproducing in the biliary tract; however, direct blockage of the common bile and pancreatic ducts by worms can occur, resulting in cholestasis, jaundice, and pruritus.[89] Further complications include cholecystitis, cholangitis, and pancreatitis.[90] Aside from physical obstruction, *Fasciola* spp are known to induce biliary duct hypertrophy and hyperplasia in host tissues, possibly mediated by the secretion of high levels of proline,[91] as well as direct irritation.[92] Rarely, fibrosis of the biliary tracts may follow, progressing to periportal fibrosis, portal hypertension, and cirrhosis.[81] Chronic *Fasciola* infection, and even dead flukes, may also predispose patients to cholelithiasis and bacterobilia.[83]

Fascioliasis may be acquired by travelers ingesting contaminated food or water, although this is rare. Acute disease results in hepatic injury as larvae migrate through the liver parenchyma, whereas jaundice in the chronic phase is caused by biliary obstruction and fibrosis. Severity of symptoms correlates with higher fluke burdens; severe chronic fascioliasis may necessitate endoscopic removal of the worms.

CLONORCHIASIS/OPISTHORCHIASIS
Etiology and Epidemiology

Clonorchis sinensis and *Opisthorchis* spp are hepatobiliary flukes that reside in the human bile ducts and gallbladder. These flat, 8-mm to 15-mm long,[87] leaf-shaped trematodes all have similar life cycles and disease pathogenesis, but differ in geographic distribution. *Clonorchis sinensis*, also known as the "Chinese liver fluke," is found primarily in northeast China, Korea, Taiwan, and Vietnam. *Opisthorchis viverrini* is endemic to Laos and Thailand, whereas *Opisthorchis felineus* inhabits parts of Eastern Europe, Southeast Asia, the former Soviet Union, and Siberia.[87] Immigrants from endemic areas commonly harbor chronic infection; one study detected fluke ova in stool in 26% of Asian immigrants to New York City.[93] Infection of short-term travelers to endemic areas has been documented: of 24 cases of clonorchiasis diagnosed in returned Canadian travelers and immigrants, 10 occurred in immigrants, 5 in VFRs (those traveling for the purpose of "visiting friends and relatives"), 7 in tourists, and 2 in business travelers.[4]

Humans become infected by ingesting undercooked, smoked, dried, and pickled freshwater fish containing *Clonorchis* or *Opisthorchis* larvae (metacercariae). Metacercariae excyst in the duodenum and migrate via the ampulla of Vater into the bile ducts, where they mature into adult worms.[87] Unlike fascioliasis, where migration of larvae lead to direct tissue penetration and destruction, clonorchiasis and opisthorchiasis infections are established by retrograde migration of larvae within the biliary system.

Clinical Manifestations

Clonorchis and *Opisthorchis* adult worms reside in the medium and small intrahepatic bile ducts, and occasionally in the extrahepatic ducts, gallbladder, and pancreatic ducts. Chronic presence of adult worms results in bile duct obstruction, inflammation, epithelial cell adenomatous hyperplasia, progressive periductal fibrosis, and biliary duct wall thickening.[87,94] Adult worms can live for 20 to 30 years,[95] and cause a variety of symptoms largely depending on infection duration and worm burden. Most chronic infections are asymptomatic, particularly with "light" infections of fewer than 100 flukes.[95] Higher worm burdens are associated with increasing symptoms of flatulence, dyspepsia, and right upper quadrant pain, as well as nausea, diarrhea, and anorexia.[96]

Heavy infections consisting of 1000 to 20,000 adult worms affect older individuals living in endemic areas who are persistently reexposed.[95] Those with substantial fluke burden are more likely to present with acute complications. Acute biliary obstruction can occur when flukes block the narrowed fibrosed bile ducts, or in the setting of intrahepatic pigment stone formation associated with fluke infection. *Clonorchis* and *Opisthorchis* are implicated in the syndrome of recurrent pyogenic cholangitis, as it is hypothesized that stones, parasite material, and biliary stasis create a nidus for bacterial infection.[97] Pigment stones form within the intrahepatic and extrahepatic bile ducts rather than in the gallbladder, and stones are present in 50% to 70% of individuals with this syndrome, including those who have undergone cholecystectomy.[97] Patients with recurrent pyogenic cholangitis typically present with multiple acute episodes of fever, nausea, right upper quadrant pain, and jaundice.[98] Clinical jaundice occurs in approximately 77% of patients with the syndrome, which is more likely to affect adults of low socioeconomic status between the ages of 20 and 40.[97] Acute pancreatitis may also occur because of pancreatic duct obstruction by liver flukes.

Long-term hepatobiliary fluke infection results in chronic biliary inflammation that may cause biliary strictures, and has also been linked to cholangiocarcinoma. The incidence of cholangiocarcinoma is significantly higher in biliary fluke endemic areas, and may present with weight loss, jaundice, and ascites. Although most symptoms are related to long duration of infection and high disease burden, an acute serum sickness–like reaction has also been described, mainly with *Opisthorchis viverrini* infection. Fever, abdominal pain, urticaria, myalgia, arthralgia, lymphadenopathy, hepatomegaly, and high eosinophilia[99] may develop within 10 to 26 days of contaminated fish consumption, and lasts for 2 to 4 weeks.

In summary, *Clonorchis* and *Opisthorchis* infections occur sporadically in short-term travelers who consume undercooked freshwater fish, but are common in Asian immigrants to North America. Chronic heavy infections in endemic populations cause intrahepatic bile duct fibrosis, which has been linked to obstructive jaundice, pyogenic cholangitis, and cholangiocarcinoma.

ECHINOCOCCOSIS
Etiology and Epidemiology

Echinococcosis is a zoonotic infection caused by the larval stage of *Echinococcus granulosus* ("cystic echinococcus") and *Echinococcus multilocularis* ("alveolar echinococcus"). Polycystic echinococcal infections with the less prevalent *Echinococcus vogeli* and *Echinococcus oligarthrus* infrequently cause human disease.

Cystic echinococcosis (CE) is endemic to sheep-raising areas worldwide, but predominantly affects southern South America, the Mediterranean littoral, Eastern Europe, parts of the Middle East, east Africa, central Asia, China, and Russia.[100] CE is reemerging in Western European pastoral communities, notably in Spain, Italy, and Wales, owing to collapse of local control programs.[101] Dogs and other canids are the definitive hosts, harboring adult worms in the small intestine and shedding eggs in feces. Humans typically become accidental intermediate hosts through close contact with sheep-dogs and subsequent fecal-oral transmission of eggs present on dog fur. Eggs hatch in the intermediate host small bowel, penetrate the intestinal mucosa, travel via hematogenous or lymphatic routes to other organs, and develop into cysts. Again, infection of short-term travelers is rare, and most cases of CE observed in nonendemic areas occur in immigrants from the aforementioned regions. In a study of parasitic infections among returned Canadian travelers and immigrants, cases of CE in immigrants and VFRs outnumbered cases in tourists by 3:1.[4]

Alveolar echinococcosis (AE) is less prevalent, and limited to northern areas, including parts of Central and Eastern Europe, Russia, China, northern Japan, the Near East, northwestern Canada, and Alaska.[100] Foxes, wolves, coyotes, and occasionally domestic dogs and cats act as definitive hosts in a cycle involving infected rodents as intermediate hosts. Hunting, trapping, and contact with dogs in endemic areas are major risk factors for human exposure.[102]

Clinical Presentation

Clinical presentation varies depending on the location, growth rate, and size of the resulting cysts or liver infiltrates; symptoms typically develop as a result of compression of adjacent structures or cyst rupture.

CE primarily affects the liver and lung, causing hepatic and pulmonary involvement in 65% and 25% of patients, respectively.[102] In rare cases, cysts form in other organs, including the kidney, spleen, muscle, bone, and brain.[102] Approximately 80% of patients present with disease limited to a single organ.[100] Although most primary echinococcal infections occur in childhood, most patients present in adulthood because of relatively slow cyst growth. Cysts may persist for years without any change in dimension, and may also involute, regress, or form characteristic internal "daughter cysts" without external expansion.[100] Echinococcal cyst growth rates are highly variable, ranging from 1 to 50 mm per year.[100] When hepatic cysts become large enough to cause symptoms, patients often develop right upper quadrant pain, nausea, vomiting, and hepatic enlargement. A palpable right upper quadrant mass may also be observed.

Echinococcal cysts frequently compress small adjacent segments of the biliary tree, but clinical jaundice is unusual. Obstructive jaundice occasionally results from extrinsic common bile duct compression by a large liver cyst or one located near the pancreatic head. Occult rupture of cyst contents into the biliary system occurs in 10% to 37% of patients, but is typically asymptomatic.[103] Rarely, frank cyst rupture into the bile ducts leads to intrinsic blockage and stasis, which presents as obstructive jaundice associated with complications, including acute cholangitis, pancreatitis, liver abscess, and septicemia.[103] Lung cysts may rupture directly into bronchi, where they are either expelled through coughing or partially retained, creating a nidus for superimposed bacterial or fungal infection.[102] Direct cyst rupture through both endocyst and pericyst layers is potentially fatal, as cyst contents released into the pleura, peritoneum, or blood stream provoke an allergic response ranging from mild hypersensitivity to anaphylactic shock.

AE is a chronic infection primarily involving the liver. *E multilocularis* growth resembles that of a malignancy, as larvae expand in the liver through external budding without cyst formation, and directly infiltrate adjacent organs or metastasize hematogenously. AE typically presents late in the disease course, following a prolonged asymptomatic period ranging from 5 to 15 years.[104] In contrast with CE, an estimated 34% of patients with AE have already progressed to multiorgan involvement at the time of presentation.[105] Early symptoms are often vague, including nonspecific right upper quadrant and epigastric pain in one-third of patients.[100] An additional 25% to 44% present with cholestatic jaundice resulting from extrinsic biliary compression.[106] The remaining one-third of AE infections are found incidentally during investigation of nonspecific symptoms including fever, weight loss, and anemia.[100] Presenting symptoms are highly correlated with mass location within the liver, as patients with hilar liver masses are more likely to have compressive jaundice, whereas patients with posterior segment involvement alone are more often asymptomatic.[106] The natural disease course involves progression to hepatomegaly, symptoms of portal hypertension, severe hepatic dysfunction, and worsening cholestatic jaundice.[107] Rare complications include invasion of the hepatic veins or inferior vena cava, transdiaphragmatic fistulization between liver and lung, and cutaneous abdominal lesions resulting from larval penetration of the abdominal wall.[106]

In summary, CE primarily affects immigrants from sheep-raising communities worldwide. Cyst rupture is the major feared complication and contained rupture into the bilary tree causes obstructive jaundice leading to cholangitis.

ASCARIASIS
Etiology and Epidemiology

The most common helminthic infection, ascariasis caused by *Ascaris lumbricoides* is estimated to infect as many as 1.4 billion people worldwide, with prevalence of infections as high as 90% in highly endemic areas.[108] Infection is acquired when embryonated eggs in the soil are ingested, either directly or from contamination of food and water supplies. The eggs hatch, releasing larvae that penetrate the intestinal wall, following which a migratory lung phase takes place. Final localization to the gastrointestinal tract via a cough-swallow mechanism occurs, where they complete development into adults.[109] Adults are roundworms that can grow to a length of 50 cm; females can produce up to 200,000 eggs daily. These are excreted in the stool, where they are not immediately infective; they require weeks to embryonate outside of the body before the eggs are ready to hatch on ingestion.

Widely distributed throughout the tropics, ascariasis occurs principally in Central and South America, sub-Saharan Africa, and Asia, with more than 50% of cases originating from China.[110] Domestically acquired infection has been reported in Europe. It is a frequent infection found on screening immigrants from endemic areas,[109] and cases of travel-related acquisition are well documented.[111] Ascariasis was the third most common enteric helminth infection, next to strongyloidiasis and intestinal tapeworm infection, diagnosed in a series of parasitic infections in returned Canadian travelers and immigrants.[4]

Clinical Features

As with acute strongyloidiasis and hookworm infection, the migratory larval lung phase of acute ascariasis may lead to a "pulmonary infiltrates with eosinophilia" syndrome, or Loeffler syndrome, although this is atypical. If symptoms occur, diagnosis of acute ascariasis is clinical and requires a high degree of suspicion, as confirmatory laboratory tests, such as identification of eggs in stool, are absent. Chronic ascariasis is most often asymptomatic, especially when worm burden is light; however, heavier infestations, where the worms may entangle or aggregate in larger clumps, may result in intestinal obstruction, which may resolve or be complicated further by volvulus, intussusception, or perforation, all of which are most commonly seen in children living in endemic areas.[108] Appendicular ascariasis is another manifestation, where appendicitis can be caused by *Ascaris* exploration and obstruction of the appendicular orifice.[109] Similarly, exploration and occlusion can occur in the common bile duct, and gives rise to biliary ascariasis.[87]

Biliary ascariasis is uncommon, but may constitute almost 20% of admissions for ascariasis in endemic regions.[81] Patients with a dilated sphincter of Oddi have a higher risk of *Ascaris* intrusion into their biliary tract. Thirty percent of affected patients had previously undergone cholecystectomy, which led to a dilated common bile duct, increased cholecystokinin secretion, and relaxation of the sphincter.[112] Prior sphincterotomy is also a risk factor, as is pregnancy, during which time the sphincter relaxation is attributed to high levels of progesterone.[81]

Most obstructions are transient if the worms are alive, and the worms typically can move in and out of the common bile duct,[81,109] thus presenting as biliary colic.[113] The obstruction can become persistent if the *Ascaris* adult becomes coiled,[114] if the sphincter of Oddi undergoes spasm in response to secretion of worm antigens,[81] or if the worms die in situ.[113] Clinical presentations depend on the ducts involved. Cholecystitis and cholangitis are relatively common, especially as the worms aid translocation of bacterial flora into the common bile duct.[114] Gallstones, usually pigment stones, can use live and dead worms as a nidus.[110] These are more common after an episode of cholangitis, where the precipitation of bilirubin glucuronide may result from its deconjugation by bacterial β-glucuronidase.[97] Recurrent pyogenic cholangitis, discussed in the *Clonorchis* section, has also been attributed to *Ascaris*.[97] The inflammatory response arising from the bodies of dead worms can give rise to biliary strictures, which can cause chronic biliary obstruction.[114] Jaundice may arise either acutely or chronically, principally as a result of biliary obstruction either by the worm, stones, or strictures. Pancreatitis is a less common complication (4%–36% of biliary ascariasis), but may occur when *Ascaris* worms obstruct either the pancreatic duct or the common bile duct, with consequent inflammation of the pancreas from reflux of pancreatic secretions or bile respectively.[112] Recurrent pancreatitis has been reported, possibly caused by the transience of *Ascaris* in the biliary ducts.[115] Hepatic abscess is a rare but serious complication,[116] resulting from heavy parasite load with migration of ascarid worms upstream to the parenchyma of the liver, where they cause local inflammation, necrosis, and finally, abscess formation.[112]

Ascariasis is a common infection in travelers to tropical and subtropical regions, and the proclivity of *Ascaris* to explore orifices may lead to a wide range of hepatobiliary manifestations. Obstruction of the biliary tracts or ampulla of Vater are often transient and may lead to jaundice; if the obstruction fails to resolve, endoscopic or surgical removal of worms may be necessary.

VISCERAL LARVA MIGRANS/TOXOCARIASIS
Etiology and Epidemiology

Visceral larva migrans (VLM) is a clinical syndrome most commonly caused by ingestion of the eggs of *Toxocara* spp, the most common of which are *Toxocara canis* and *Toxocara cati*. The definitive hosts are domestic pets (dogs and cats, respectively), which pass the helminth's eggs in their stool; egg embryonation occurs in the environment. Infection in humans is typically acquired by ingestion of embryonated *Toxocara* eggs, which can be present in contaminated sand and soil.[117,118] Humans are incidental hosts, however, as the larvae are unable to mature to adulthood in the human body. Instead, they remain in larval form and migrate to various organs, where they generate an inflammatory response, especially on death.[117]

Because of the popularity of domestic dogs and cats throughout the world, toxocariasis is considered to be a cosmopolitan disease with global distribution. Thus, travel-related acquisition of disease in short-term travelers is difficult to document owing to probable past competing exposures. Seroprevalences vary from country to country but healthy seropositive individuals exist throughout the world.[119] Children are particularly predisposed to acquisition of infection because of exposure to dog and cat feces while playing in sandboxes and playgrounds.[120]

Clinical Features

There are 2 major manifestations of toxocariasis: VLM and ocular larva migrans (OLM). The latter describes the syndrome where *Toxocara* larvae migrate only to the eye, where they can cause retinal granuloma formation and optical symptoms, including loss of vision. VLM is a broader term describing *Toxocara* involvement of any other organ, the most common being the liver and lungs.[120] Larvae shed and secrete antigens, collectively referred to as *T canis* excretory secretory antigens (TEX); these generate a strong inflammatory response, which is thought to be responsible for hepatomegaly.[121] Organ pathology is further propagated on larval death, with triggering of immediate and delayed-type hypersensitivity reactions.[117] Inflammation results in the formation of eosinophilic granulomas,[121] which can be observed histologically on liver biopsy. Irregular, focal areas of necrosis, surrounded by granulomas consisting of multinucleated giant cells, epithelioid cells, with eosinophils and mononuclear cells on the periphery may be seen.[119]

Fever and eosinophilia are considered hallmarks of the syndrome, the latter reaching levels as high as 70%,[117] although its absence does not exclude the disease.[122] Lung involvement can present as chronic cough and wheeze, and possibly reactive airways; pulmonary infiltrates or nodules may be observed on chest radiograph.[120] Liver involvement manifests most often as hepatomegaly, which affects as many as 87% of patients.[123] Elevated transaminases are less common, and jaundice is infrequent. There are infrequent reports of severe hepatic disease. One case of severe, granulomatous hepatitis, followed by irreversible portal fibrosis leading to chronic cholestasis has been described.[122] Rarely, eosinophilic cholecystitis has been reported.[119] Less common complications of VLM include myocarditis, arthritis, and nephritic syndrome.[119] Toxocariasis affecting the central nervous system may cause eosinophilic meningitis and seizures,[123] as well as rarer manifestations, including encephalitis, myelitis, optic neuritis, and cerebral vasculitis.[119]

VLM is a cosmopolitan infection whose incidence in travelers is difficult to ascertain. It can cause hepatic injury resulting from inflammation associated with both living and dead larval worms, and although disease is often mild and self-limited, severe manifestations of hepatic dysfunction may result.

SUMMARY

The etiologic agents of parasitic liver disease are diverse, and remain important as health issues for travelers as international travel continues to increase. Pathogenic mechanisms leading to jaundice in these infections are equally diverse. Practitioners may find it prudent to consider these agents in their differential diagnosis when travelers return from endemic areas of disease, especially when they present with stigmata of liver disease, such as jaundice or with elevated liver transaminases.

REFERENCES

1. Freedman DO, Weld LH, Kozarsky PE, et al. Spectrum of disease and relation to place of exposure among ill returned travelers. N Engl J Med 2006;354(2): 119–30.
2. Wall E, Cooke G. Jaundice in the traveller. Medicine (Abingdon) 2010;38(1): 14–7.
3. Feasey N, Wansbrough-Jones M, Mabey DC, et al. Neglected tropical diseases. Br Med Bull 2010;93(1):179–200.

4. Boggild AK, Yohanna S, Keystone JS, et al. Prospective analysis of parasitic infections in Canadian travelers and immigrants. J Travel Med 2006;13(3): 138–44.

5. Greenwood BM, Bojang K, Whitty CJ, et al. Malaria. Lancet 2005;365(9769): 1487–98.

6. Alexandre MA, Ferreira CO, Siqueira AM, et al. Severe *Plasmodium vivax* malaria, Brazilian Amazon. Emerg Infect Dis 2010;16(10):1611–4.

7. Cox-Singh J, Davis TM, Lee KS, et al. *Plasmodium knowlesi* malaria in humans is widely distributed and potentially life threatening. Clin Infect Dis 2008;46(2): 165–71.

8. Hay SI, Guerra CA, Tatem AJ, et al. The global distribution and population at risk of malaria: past, present, and future. Lancet Infect Dis 2004;4:327–36.

9. Wilson ME, Weld LH, Boggild AK, et al. Fever in returned travelers: results from the GeoSentinel Surveillance Network. Clin Infect Dis 2007;44:1560–8.

10. Antinori S, Galimberti L, Gianelli E, et al. Prospective observational study of fever in hospitalized returning travelers and migrants from tropical areas, 1997-2001. J Travel Med 2004;11(3):135–42.

11. Bottieau E, Clerinx J, Schrooten W, et al. Etiology and outcome of fever after a stay in the tropics. Arch Intern Med 2006;166(15):1642–8.

12. Doherty JF, Grant AD, Bryceson AD. Fever as the presenting complaint of travellers returning from the tropics. QJM 1995;88(4):277–81.

13. Hagmann S, Neugebauer R, Schwartz E, et al. Illness in children after international travel: analysis from the GeoSentinel Surveillance Network. Pediatrics 2010;125(5):e1072–80.

14. Hill DR. Health problems in a large cohort of Americans traveling to developing countries. J Travel Med 2000;7(5):259–66.

15. Klein JL, Millman GC. Prospective, hospital based study of fever in children in the United Kingdom who had recently spent time in the tropics. BMJ 1998; 316(7142):1425–6.

16. O'Brien D, Tobin S, Brown GV, et al. Fever in returned travelers: review of hospital admissions for a 3-year period. Clin Infect Dis 2001;33(5):603–9.

17. Parola P, Soula G, Gazin P, et al. Fever in travelers returning from tropical areas: prospective observational study of 613 cases hospitalised in Marseilles, France, 1999-2003. Travel Med Infect Dis 2006;4(2):61–70.

18. Steffen R, Rickenbach M, Wilhelm U, et al. Health problems after travel to developing countries. J Infect Dis 1987;156(1):84–91.

19. West NS, Riordan FAI. Fever in returned travellers: a prospective review of hospital admissions for a 2(1/2) year period. Arch Dis Child 2003;88(5): 432–4.

20. Trampuz A, Jereb M, Muzlovic I, et al. Clinical review: severe malaria. Crit Care 2003;7(4):315–23.

21. Tuteja R. Malaria—an overview. FEBS J 2007;274(18):4670–9.

22. Idro R, Jenkins NE, Newton CR. Pathogenesis, clinical features, and neurological outcome of cerebral malaria. Lancet Neurol 2005;4(12):827–40.

23. Public Health Agency of Canada. Canadian recommendations for the prevention and treatment of malaria among international travellers. Can Commun Dis Rep 2009;35(S1):1–90.

24. World Health Organization. Severe falciparum malaria. Trans R Soc Trop Med Hyg 2000;94(Suppl 1):S1–90.

25. Anand AC, Puri P. Jaundice in malaria. J Gastroenterol Hepatol 2005;20(9): 1322–32.

26. Ahsan T, Ali H, Bkaht SF, et al. Jaundice in falciparum malaria; changing trends in clinical presentation—a need for awareness. J Pak Med Assoc 2008;58(11): 616–21.

27. Bannister LH. Looking for the exit: how do malaria parasites escape from red blood cells? Proc Natl Acad Sci U S A 2001;98(2):383–4.

28. Rupani AB, Amarapurkar AD. Hepatic changes in fatal malaria: an emerging problem. Ann Trop Med Parasitol 2009;103(2):119–27.

29. Pasternak ND, Dzikowski R. PfEMP1: an antigen that plays a key role in the pathogenicity and immune evasion of the malaria parasite Plasmodium falciparum. Int J Biochem Cell Biol 2009;41(7):1463–6.

30. Bhalla A, Suri V, Singh V. Malarial hepatopathy. J Postgrad Med 2006;52(4): 315–20.

31. Guha M, Kumar S, Choubey V, et al. Apoptosis in liver during malaria: role of oxidative stress and implication of mitochondrial pathway. FASEB J 2006; 20(8):1224–6.

32. Yeom JS, Park SH, Ryu SH, et al. Serum cytokine profiles in patients with Plasmodium vivax malaria: a comparison between those who presented with and without hepatic dysfunction. Trans R Soc Trop Med Hyg 2003;97(6):687–91.

33. Seixas E, Oliveira P, Moura Nunes JF, et al. An experimental model for fatal malaria due to TNF-alpha-dependent hepatic damage. Parasitology 2008;135(6):683–90.

34. Devarbhavi H, Alvares JF, Kumar KS. Severe falciparum malaria simulating fulminant hepatic failure. Mayo Clin Proc 2005;80(3):355–8.

35. Markham LN, Giostra E, Hadengue A, et al. Emergency liver transplantation in amodiaquine-induced fulminant hepatitis. Am J Trop Med Hyg 2007;77(1):14–5.

36. Homer MJ, Aguilar-Delfin I, Telford SRI, et al. Babesiosis. Clin Microbiol Rev 2000;13(3):451–69.

37. Leiby DA. Tranfusion-transmitted Babesia spp.: bull's-eye on Babesia microti. Clin Microbiol Rev 2011;24(1):14–28.

38. Fox LM, Wingerter S, Ahmed A, et al. Neonatal babesiosis: case report and review of the literature. Pediatr Infect Dis J 2006;25(2):169–73.

39. Babu RV, Sharma GA. 57-year-old man with abdominal pain, jaundice, and a history of blood transfusion. Chest 2007;132(1):347–50.

40. Vannier E, Gewurz BE, Krause PJ. Human babesiosis. Infect Dis Clin North Am 2008;22(3):469–88.

41. Kreuziger LM, Tafur AJ, Thompson RJ. 79-year-old man with fever, malaise, and jaundice. Mayo Clin Proc 2009;84(3):281–4.

42. Chiang E, Haller N. Babesiosis: an emerging infectious disease that can affect those who travel to the northeastern United States. Travel Med Infect Dis 2011; 9(5):238–42.

43. Otsuka Y, Yamasaki M, Yamato O, et al. Increased generation of superoxide in erythrocytes infected with Babesia gibsoni. J Vet Med Sci 2001;63(10):1077–81.

44. Hemmer RM, Ferrick DA, Conrad PA. Up-regulation of tumor necrosis factor-alpha and interferon-gamma expression in the spleen and lungs of mice infected with the human Babesia isolate WA1. Parasitol Res 2000;86(2):121–8.

45. Haque R, Huston CD, Hughes M, et al. Amebiasis. N Engl J Med 2003;348(16): 1565–73.

46. Wells CD, Arguedas M. Amebic liver abscess. South Med J 2004;97(7):673–82.

47. Chavez-Tapia N, Hernandez-Calleros J, Tellez-Avila FI, et al. Image-guided percutaneous procedure plus metronidazole versus metronidazole alone for uncomplicated amoebic liver abscess. Cochrane Database Syst Rev 2009;(1):CD004886.

48. Stanley SL. Amoebiasis. Lancet 2003;361(9362):1025–34.

49. Petri WA, Singh U. Enteric amebiasis. In: Guerrant R, Walker DH, Weller PF, editors. Tropical infectious diseases: principles, pathogens, and practice. 2nd edition. Philadelphia: Elsevier; 2006. p. 967–83.
50. Sharma MP, Ahuja V. Amebiasis; correspondence. N Engl J Med 2003;349: 307–8.
51. Knobloch J, Mannweiler E. Development and persistence of antibodies to *Entamoeba histolytica* in patients with amebic liver abscess: analysis of 216 cases. Am J Trop Med Hyg 1983;32(4):727–32.
52. Petri WA, Chadee K. Recent advances in amebiasis. Crit Rev Clin Lab Sci 1996; 33(1):1–37.
53. Sharma N, Sharma A, Varma S, et al. Amoebic liver abscess in the medical emergency at a North Indian hospital. BMC Res Notes 2010;3(21):1–4.
54. Salles JM, Moraes LA, Salles MC. Hepatic amebiasis. Braz J Infect Dis 2003; 7(2):96–110.
55. Sarda AK, Kannan R, Gupta A, et al. Amebic liver abscess with jaundice. Surg Today 1998;28(3):305–7.
56. Singh V, Bhalla A, Sharma N, et al. Pathophysiology of jaundice in amoebic liver abscess. Am J Trop Med Hyg 2008;78(4):556–9.
57. Ravdin JI. Amebiasis. Clin Infect Dis 1995;20(6):1453–64.
58. Sharma MP, Dasarathy S, Verma N, et al. Prognostic markers in amoebic liver abscess: a prospective study. Am J Gastroenterol 1996;91(12):2584–8.
59. Sacks DL, Kenney RT, Neva FA, et al. Indian kala-azar caused by *Leishmania tropica*. Lancet 1995;345(8955):959–61.
60. Alborzi A, Rasouli M, Shamsizadeh A. *Leishmania tropica*-isolated patient with visceral leishmaniasis in southern Iran. Am J Trop Med Hyg 2006;74(2):306–7.
61. Pavli A, Maltezou HC. Leishmaniasis, an emerging infection in travelers. Int J Infect Dis 2010;14(12):e1032–9.
62. Chappuis F, Sundar S, Asrat H, et al. Visceral leishmaniasis: what are the needs for diagnosis, treatment and control? Nat Rev Microbiol 2007;5(11):873–82.
63. Ready PD. Leishmaniasis emergence in Europe. Euro Surveill 2010;15(10): 19505.
64. Wright NA, Davis LE, Aftergut KS, et al. Cutaneous leishmaniasis in Texas: a northern spread of endemic areas. J Am Acad Dermatol 2010;58(4):650–2.
65. Murray HW, Berman JD, Davies CR, et al. Advances in leishmaniasis. Lancet 2005;366(9496):1561–77.
66. Nylén S, Sacks D. Interleukin-10 and the pathogenesis of human visceral leishmaniasis. Trends Immunol 2007;28(9):378–84.
67. el Hag IA, Hashim FA, el Toum IA, et al. Liver morphology and function in visceral leishmaniasis (Kala-azar). J Clin Pathol 1994;47(6):547–51.
68. Wilson ME, Streit JA. Visceral leishmaniasis. Gastroenterol Clin North Am 1996; 25(3):535–51.
69. Mathur P, Samantaray JC, Samanta P. High prevalence of functional liver derangement in visceral leishmaniasis at an Indian tertiary care center. Clin Gastroenterol Hepatol 2008;6(10):1170–2.
70. Baranwal AK, Mandal RN, Singh R. Fulminant hepatic failure complicating visceral leishmaniasis in an apparently immunocompetent child. Indian J Pediatr 2007;74(5):489–91.
71. Prakash A, Singh NP, Sridhara G, et al. Visceral leishmaniasis masquerading as chronic liver disease. J Assoc Physicians India 2006;54:893–4.
72. Gryseels B, Polman K, Clerinx J, et al. Human schistosomiasis. Lancet 2006; 368(9541):1106–18.

73. Steinmann P, Keiser J, Bos R, et al. Schistosomiasis and water resources development: systematic review, meta-analysis, and estimates of people at risk. Lancet Infect Dis 2006;6(7):411–25.

74. Ross AG, Bartley PB, Sleigh AC, et al. Schistosomiasis. N Engl J Med 2002; 346(16):1212–9.

75. Nicolls DJ, Weld LH, Schwartz E, et al. Characteristics of schistosomiasis in travelers reported to the GeoSentinel Surveillance Network 1997-2008. Am J Trop Med Hyg 2008;79(5):729–34.

76. Ross AG, Sleigh AC, Li Y, et al. Schistosomiasis in the People's Republic of China: prospects and challenges for the 21st century. Clin Microbiol Rev 2001;14(2):270–95.

77. Doherty JF, Moody AH, Wright SG. Katayama fever: an acute manifestation of schistosomiasis. BMJ 1996;313(7064):1071–2.

78. Bethlem EP, Schettino Gde P, Carvalho CR. Pulmonary schistosomiasis. Curr Opin Pulm Med 1997;3(5):361–5.

79. Gray DJ, Ross AG, Li YS, et al. Diagnosis and management of schistosomiasis. BMJ 2011;342:d2651.

80. Rebouças G. Clinical aspects of hepatosplenic schistosomiasis: a contrast with cirrhosis. Yale J Biol Med 1975;48(5):369–76.

81. Rana SS, Bhasin DK, Nanda M, et al. Parasitic infestations of the biliary tract. Curr Gastroenterol Rep 2007;9:156–64.

82. Keiser J, Utzinger J. Food-borne tremodiases. Clin Microbiol Rev 2009;22(3): 466–83.

83. Mas-Coma S, Bargues MD, Valero MA. Plant-borne trematode zoonoses: fascioliasis and fasciolopsiasis. In: Murrell KD, Fried B, editors. Food-borne parasitic zoonoses: fish and plant-borne parasites (World Class Parasites), vol. 11. New York: Springer; 2007. p. 293–334.

84. Fried B, Abruzzi A. Food-borne trematode infections of humans in the United States of America. Parasitol Res 2010;106(6):1263–80.

85. Kang ML, Teo CH, Wansaicheong GK, et al. *Fasciola hepatica* in a New Zealander traveler. J Travel Med 2008;15(3):196–9.

86. Masake RA, Wescott RB, Spencer GR, et al. The pathogenesis of primary and secondary infection with *Fasciola hepatica* in mice. Vet Pathol 1978;15(6):763–9.

87. Lim JH, Kim SY, Park CM. Parasitic diseases of the biliary tract. AJR Am J Roentgenol 2007;188(6):1596–603.

88. Marcos LA, Terashima A, Gotuzzo E. Update on hepatobiliary flukes: fascioliasis, opisthorchiasis and clorchiasis. Curr Opin Infect Dis 2008;21(5):523–30.

89. Umac H, Erkek AB, Ayaslioglu E, et al. Pruritus and intermittent jaundice as clinical clues for *Fasciola hepatica* infestation. Liver Int 2006;26(6):752–3.

90. Sezgin O, Altintas E, Tombak A, et al. *Fasciola hepatica*-induced acute pancreatitis: report of two cases and review of the literature. Turk J Gastroenterol 2010; 21(2):183–7.

91. Isseroff H, Sawma JT, Reino D. Fascioliasis: role of proline in bile duct hyperplasia. Science 1977;198(4322):1157–9.

92. Dias LM, Silva R, Viana HL, et al. Biliary fascioliasis: diagnosis, treatment and follow-up by ERCP. Gastrointest Endosc 1996;43(6):616–20.

93. Schwartz DA. Cholangiocarcinoma associated with liver fluke infection: a preventable source of morbidity in Asian immigrants. Am J Gastroenterol 1986;81(1): 76–9.

94. Lai CH, Chin C, Chung HC, et al. Clonorchiasis-associated perforated eosinophilic cholecystitis. Am J Trop Med Hyg 2007;76(2):396–8.

95. Papachristou GI, Schoedel KE, Ramanathan R, et al. *Clonorchis sinensis*-associated cholangiocarcinoma: a case report and review of the literature. Dig Dis Sci 2005;50(11):2159–62.
96. Upatham ES, Viyanant V, Kurathong S, et al. Relationship between prevalence and intensity of *Opisthorchis viverrini* infection, and clinical symptoms and signs in a rural community in north-east Thailand. Bull World Health Organ 1984;62(3): 451–61.
97. Lim JH. Oriental cholangiohepatitis: pathologic, clinical, and radiologic features. AJR Am J Roentgenol 1991;157(1):1–8.
98. Hawn TR, Jong EC. Trematodes. In: Jong EC, Sanford CA, editors. The travel and tropical medicine manual. 4th edition. Philadelphia: Saunders; 2008. p. 626–36.
99. Harinasuta T, Pungpak S, Keystone JS. Trematode infections: opisthorchiasis, clonorchiasis, fascioliasis, and paragonimiasis. Infect Dis Clin North Am 1993; 7(3):699–716.
100. Brunetti E, Kern P, Vuitton DA, et al. Expert consensus for the diagnosis and treatment of cystic and alveolar echinococcosis in humans. Acta Trop 2010; 114(1):1–16.
101. Rojo-Vazquez FA, Pardo-Lledias J, Francos-von Hunefeld M, et al. Cystic echinococcosis in Spain: current situation and relevance for other endemic areas in Europe. PLoS Negl Trop Dis 2011;5(1):e893.
102. Moro P, Schantz PM. Echinococcosis: a review. Int J Infect Dis 2009;13(2): 125–33.
103. Spârchez Z, Osian G, Onica A, et al. Ruptured hydatid cyst of the liver with biliary obstruction: presentation of a case and review of the literature. Rom J Gastroenterol 2004;13(3):245–50.
104. Ammann RW, Eckert J. Cestodes: Echinococcus. Gastroenterol Clin North Am 1996;25(3):655–89.
105. Kern P, Bardonnet K, Renner E, et al. European echinococcosis registry: human alveolar echinococcosis, Europe, 1982-2000. Emerg Infect Dis 2003;9(3):343–9.
106. Bresson-Hadni S, Vuitton DA, Bartholomot B, et al. A twenty-year history of alveolar echinococcosis: analysis of a series of 117 patients from eastern France. Eur J Gastroenterol Hepatol 2000;12(3):327–36.
107. Kern P. Clinical features and treatment of alveolar echinococcosis. Curr Opin Infect Dis 2010;23(5):505–12.
108. Shah OJ, Zargar SA, Robbani I. Biliary ascariasis: a review. World J Surg 2006; 30:1500–6.
109. Khuroo MS. Ascariasis. Gastroenterol Clin North Am 1996;25(3):553–77.
110. Khandelwal N, Shaw J, Jain MK. Biliary parasites: diagnostic and therapeutic strategies. Curr Treat Options Gastroenterol 2008;11(2):85–95.
111. Sing A, Bogner JR. The end of wanderlust. Am J Med 2004;117(1):66–7.
112. Sanai FM, Al-Karawi MA. Biliary ascariasis: report of a complicated case and literature review. Saudi J Gastroenterol 2007;13(1):25–32.
113. Alam S, Mustafa G, Rahman S, et al. Comparative study on presentation of biliary ascariasis with dead and living worms. Saudi J Gastroenterol 2010;16(3):203–6.
114. Astudillo JA, Sporn E, Serrano B, et al. Ascariasis in the hepatobiliary system: laparoscopic management. J Am Coll Surg 2008;207(4):527–32.
115. Lee KH, Shelat VG, Low HC, et al. Recurrent pancreatitis secondary to pancreatic ascariasis. Singapore Med J 2009;50(6):e218–9.
116. Alam S, Mustafa G, Ahmad N, et al. Presentation and endoscopic management of biliary ascariasis. Southeast Asian J Trop Med Public Health 2007;38(4):631–5.

117. Despommier D. Toxocariasis: clinical aspects, epidemiology, medical ecology, and molecular aspects. Clin Microbiol Rev 2003;16(2):265–72.
118. Magnaval JF, Glickman LT, Dorchies P, et al. Highlights of human toxocariasis. Korean J Parasitol 2001;39(1):1–11.
119. Rubinsky-Elefant G, Hirata CE, Yamamoto JH, et al. Human toxocariasis: diagnosis, worldwide seroprevalences and clinical expression of the systemic and ocular forms. Ann Trop Med Parasitol 2010;104(1):3–23.
120. Hotez PJ, Wilkins PP. Toxocariasis: America's most common neglected infection of poverty and a helminthiasis of global importance? PLoS Negl Trop Dis 2009; 3(3):e400.
121. Kayes SG. Human toxocariasis and the visceral larva migrans syndrome: correlative immunopathology. Chem Immunol 1997;66:99–124.
122. Hartleb M, Januszewski K. Severe hepatic involvement in visceral larva migrans. Eur J Gastroenterol Hepatol 2001;13(10):1245–9.
123. Mok CH. Visceral larva migrans: a discussion based on review of the literature. Clin Pediatr 1968;7:565–73.
124. Friedman LS, Gee MS, Misdraji J. Case records of the Massachusetts General Hospital. Case 39-2010. A 19-year-old woman with nausea, jaundice, and pruritus. N Engl J Med 2010;363(26):2548–57.
125. Roche SP, Kobos R. Jaundice in the adult patient. Am Fam Physician 2004; 69(2):299–304.
126. Feldman M, Friedman LS, Brandt LJ, editors. Sleisenger and Fordtran's gastrointestinal and liver disease. 9th edition. Philadelphia: Saunders; 2010. p. 1343–69.

Eosinophilia in the Returning Traveler

Andrew Ustianowski, PhD(Lond), FRCP(Lond), DTM&H[a],*,
Alimuddin Zumla, MD, MSc, PhD, FRCP(Lond), FRCP(Edin), FRCPath(UK), FSB[b]

KEYWORDS

- Eosinophilia • Traveler • Helminth • Screening

KEY POINTS

- Eosinophilia is common in returning travellers and is frequently associated with helminth infection, though there are multiple potential causes.
- Some of the helminthic causes have potential future implications for the individual and public health.
- Screening algorithms for asymptomatic eosinophilia based on geographical exposure have been developed.
- A travel history, combined with accurate symptomatology, is important in determining the cause of eosinophilia in symptomatic patients.

INTRODUCTION

An elevated eosinophil count is a common, frequently underrecognized finding in travelers returning from the tropics and elsewhere. Although there are multiple causes of eosinophilia in a traveler, from infections to malignancies, it is often related to an acquired helminth infection. In some cases these infections can be benign and self-limiting, but in others it may lead to severe sequelae for the individual or others.

BIOLOGY AND FUNCTION OF EOSINOPHILS

Eosinophils are leukocytes derived from the bone marrow whose predominant subsequent location is within the tissues, although eosinophil levels are routinely assessed by counting the relatively small proportion that are located within the blood. Eosinophils are multifunctional proinflammatory cells that have pivotal roles in allergic responses and immunity against multicellular parasites, but also are involved in organ formation (eg, mammary gland development) and probably many other processes.

[a] Regional Infectious Diseases Unit, North Manchester General Hospital, Delaunays Road, Manchester, M8 5RB, UK; [b] Centre for Infectious Diseases & International Health, University College London Medical School, Royal Free Hospital, Rowland Hill Street, London, NW3 2PF, UK
* Corresponding author.
E-mail address: andrew.ustianowski@pat.nhs.uk

Infect Dis Clin N Am 26 (2012) 781–789
http://dx.doi.org/10.1016/j.idc.2012.05.004
0891-5520/12/$ – see front matter © 2012 Elsevier Inc. All rights reserved.

id.theclinics.com

Eosinophils can also be directly pathogenic. Hypereosinophilia may be associated with tissue damage secondary to the effects of released granule proteins (eg, major basic protein, eosinophilic cationic protein, eosinophil peroxidase, and eosinophil-derived neurotoxin).

DEFINITIONS AND FREQUENCIES

The upper range of normal for the eosinophil count varies with age and between laboratories. There is also marked diurnal variation in counts (with up to 40% variation coinciding with cortisol levels).[1] However, in adults it is generally agreed that a count greater than 0.45×10^9/L is elevated. Counts greater than 1.5×10^9/L are classified as moderate and greater than 5×10^9/L as severe. The term hypereosinophilia is sometimes used to classify counts greater than 1.5×10^9/L.

There are multiple causes, which may be subclassified as primary or secondary. Primary eosinophilia is caused by clonal expansion of eosinophils associated with hematological malignancies, such as leukemias and myeloid disorders. Secondary eosinophilia can be due to allergies, infections, neoplastic and autoimmune conditions, and a variety of other causes (**Box 1**).[2]

The relative frequencies of the different causes of eosinophilia vary considerably in different populations. In those that reside or have traveled to the tropics, parasitic

---

Box 1
Main causes of eosinophilia

Allergic Conditions

    Atopic dermatitis

    Asthma

    Allergic rhinitis

    Reactions to medications

Infections

    Helminth infections

    Fungal infections (allergic bronchopulmonary aspergillosis and coccidioidomycosis)

Neoplastic and Hematological Conditions

    Lymphoma (especially Hodgkin)

    Leukemia (especially acute eosinophilic leukemia)

    Multiple other malignances

    Hypereosinophilic syndromes

    Mastocytosis

Rheumatologic and Immunologic Conditions

    Vasculitides (especially Churg-Strauss)

    Idiopathic eosinophilic synovitis

    Hyper–immunoglobulin E syndrome

    Omenn syndrome

Other

    Adrenal insufficiency

    Cholesterol embolism

infections are a common cause, and these are the focus of the following sections of this article. Other infections should be borne in mind, however, including fungal infections. Certain conditions, such as human immunodeficiency virus, have been associated with eosinophilia, but it is unclear whether this is directly causal or related to other undiagnosed causes.

In those individuals with helminth infection not all will have an eosinophilia[3–5] and, in those that do, the degree of eosinophilia and the associated symptoms depend on several factors, especially whether this is the first encounter of the host with the helminth, but also the parasite burden and the time since infection. In general there are higher eosinophil counts and more associated other symptoms if the host is naïve to the parasite. Therefore, the symptoms and clinical and laboratory findings will vary for many infections between travelers (in whom the host is generally naïve to the helminth) and immigrants or people still residing in endemic areas (where chronic heavy infections are more common).[6]

RATES AND ASSOCIATIONS OF EOSINOPHILIA IN TRAVELERS AND IMMIGRANTS

New-onset eosinophilia during or after a stay in the tropics is most likely attributable to a helminth infection. In asymptomatic returning travelers eosinophilia has been detected in 8% to 10%,[7–9] and of these 14% to 64% have acquired worm infections.[8–10] However these studies, and others that failed to detect such rates,[11,12] have methodological issues such as retrospective designs, targeted or small patient groups, or short intervals between exposure and testing (see the section Prepatent Period), therefore true rates in differing patient populations are hard to establish. The GeoSentinel Surveillance Network includes large numbers of patients and has provided data on several specific helminth infections, including filariasis[13] and schistosomiasis,[14] and has associated the longer time spent in the tropics to an increased chance of developing eosinophilia.[15] In immigrants from tropical areas eosinophilia has been detected in 12% to 23%,[16,17] and a large proportion of these individuals has detectable helminth infections.

Some helminth infections may have little consequence; however it has been estimated that between 10% and 73% of returning travelers and immigrants from tropical areas with eosinophilia could have a potentially serious infection, which may have direct health consequences for the individuals themselves or their contacts.[4,8,10,16–20]

PARASITIC CAUSES

Tissue-helminth infections are often associated with eosinophilia. However, some tissue helminths become effectively separated from host immune surveillance and therefore lose their propensity to induce an eosinophilia until any barriers become breached or weakened; for example, a hydatid is often associated with eosinophilia only if there has been cyst leakage. Gut-lumen helminths are not usually associated with increased eosinophil counts, except during or soon after tissue migratory phases. Eosinophilia is generally not caused by infection with unicellular parasites such as amoebae and other protozoae (perhaps with the exception of *Isospora* infection).

The principal helminthic causes in individuals depend on their geographic and other exposures, and can be further subdivided by symptoms and clinical findings.

Geographic Exposure

Some helminth infections can be acquired in many continents (eg, *Ascaris*) whereas others can be quite focal (eg, *Loa loa*), and some are generally associated with only rural exposure whereas others may also be acquired in urban environments. A detailed

Table 1
The more common symptomatic helminth infections associated with eosinophilia after tropical exposure

Geographic Exposure	Predominant Symptom Complex	Infection	More Common Presentations/Specifics
Global	Rash	Schistosomiasis	Acute schistosomiasis may be associated with a widespread urticarial rash (part of Katayama fever)
		Strongyloides stercoralis	Larva currens
		Cutaneous larva migrans (Ancyclostoma spp)	Not usually associated with eosinophilia
	Gastrointestinal/hepatic	Hookworm Acyclostoma/Necator	Usually asymptomatic but can be associated with diarrhea, abdominal pain, and iron-deficiency anemia
		Ascaris lumbricoides	Usually asymptomatic but can be associated with diarrhea and abdominal pain or biliary obstruction
		Strongyloides stercoralis	May cause diarrhea and abdominal pain; more severe in hyperinfestation syndrome
		Fasciola hepatica	Right upper quadrant pain and fever, jaundice, biliary obstruction
		Toxocara visceral larva migrans	Abdominal pain, hepatosplenomegaly
	Respiratory	Hookworm Acyclostoma/Necator	Loeffler syndrome during pulmonary migratory phase
		Wuchereria bancrofti (filariasis)	Dry cough and wheeze (tropical pulmonary eosinophilia)
		Strongyloides stercoralis	Loeffler syndrome during pulmonary migratory phase; severe in hyperinfestation syndrome
	Other	Toxocara visceral larva migrans	Wheeze, cough, infiltrates
		Wuchereria bancrofti (filariasis)	Lymphangitis and lymphadenitis
		Trichinella	Myalgia, periorbital edema, myocarditis

Region	Category	Organism	Clinical features
Africa	Rash	Schistosomiasis	Acute schistosomiasis may be associated with widespread urticarial rash (part of Katayama fever)
		Loa loa	Calabar swelling, eye worm (West African exposure)
		Onchocerca volvulus	Pruritus, dermatitis, nodules
	Gastrointestinal/hepatic	Schistosoma mansoni	Abdominal pain, diarrhea, portal hypertension with hepatosplenomegaly
	Respiratory	Paragonimus	Chest pain, cavitatory lesions, pleural effusions, hemoptysis
	Neurologic	Schistosomiasis	Transverse myelitis
	Other	Schistosoma haematobium	Hematuria, urinary obstruction, bladder carcinoma
		Onchocerca volvulus	Blindness
America (South & Central) and Caribbean	Rash	Schistosoma mansoni	Acute schistosomiasis may be associated with widespread urticarial rash (part of Katayama fever)
		Gnathostoma spinigerium	Migrating subcutaneous swellings
	Gastrointestinal/hepatic	Anisakis and Pseudoterranova spp	Abdominal pain, vomiting
		Schistosoma mansoni	Abdominal pain, diarrhea, portal hypertension with hepatosplenomegaly
		Angiostrongylus costaricensis	Abdominal pain, diarrhea
	Respiratory	Paragonimus	Chest pain, cavitatory lesions, pleural effusions, hemoptysis
	Neurologic	Angiostrongylus cantonensis	Eosinophilic meningitis (mostly Caribbean exposure)
		Gnathostoma spinigerium	Meningoencephalitis, myelitis
Asia and Oceania	Rash	Gnathostoma spinigerium	Migrating subcutaneous swellings
		Schistosoma japonicum	Acute schistosomiasis may be associated with widespread urticarial rash (part of Katayama fever); rare in Caribbean
	Gastrointestinal/hepatic	Anisakis and Pseudoterranova spp	Abdominal pain, vomiting
		Clonorchis sinensis and Opisthorchis spp	Right upper quadrant pain and fever, jaundice, biliary obstruction
		Schistosoma japonicum	Abdominal pain, diarrhea, portal hypertension with hepatosplenomegaly
	Respiratory	Brugia malayi (filariasis)	Dry cough and wheeze (tropical pulmonary eosinophilia)
		Paragonimus	Chest pain, cavitatory lesions, pleural effusions, hemoptysis
	Neurologic	Angiostrongylus cantonensis	Eosinophilic meningitis
		Gnathostoma spinigerium	Meningoencephalitis, myelitis
	Other	Brugia malayi (filariasis)	Lymphangitis and lymphadenitis

travel history is therefore vital to correctly investigate and diagnose a returning traveler with eosinophilia.

Other Relevant Exposures

Helminths can be acquired via a variety of routes; therefore, a history examining particular exposures and contact with specific vectors is important. For instance, exposure to fresh water may lead to schistosomiasis, and specific food intake may hint at specific etiology (eg, the consumption of water vegetation [*Fasciola*], raw or undercooked crabs/shellfish [*Paragonimus*], fish [*Anisakis* and *Gnathostoma*], snails [*Angiostrongylus cantonensis*], frog/snake [*Gnathostoma*] or pork, bear, and crocodile [*Trichinella*]).

Syndromic Classifications

Symptoms may also aid in the establishment of a definitive diagnosis. Most helminthic infections can be grouped by syndromic clinical features, particularly those that cause rash, those associated with fever, and those that are most commonly asymptomatic.

A summary of the more common helminthic causes by geographic exposure and symptomatology is given in **Table 1**.

OTHER DIAGNOSTIC ISSUES

There are other issues specific to parasitic infections that need to be considered in the approach to a traveler with eosinophilia. Prominent among these are the prepatent period (and its relevance to the timing of investigations) and the frequency of cross-reactivity of helminth serology assays.

Prepatent Period

Many tropical diagnostics require the direct visualization of ova or the parasites themselves. Ova will only be produced by adult helminths, but early in infection symptoms and eosinophilia may be caused by larvae or immature parasites that cannot yet produce ova or larval forms. Therefore the diagnostic tests available will be negative, and the infection can remain unconfirmed until a later date when sufficient ova, or the parasites themselves, are produced. The time between exposure (and potentially clinical symptoms) and the ability to detect the infection with such assays is termed the prepatent period. Similar issues can occur with serologic tests; either there can be delayed antibody responses only detectable on convalescent samples, or the antibody responses assayed are those directed to antigens of a later developmental stage (eg, some serologic assays for schistosomiasis detect antibodies directed toward egg antigens that will only be detectable once egg production has ensued). As a result, it is common practice in those who are asymptomatic to delay performing a tropical screen until 1 to 4 months after exposure, and in those with symptoms to potentially treat on clinical grounds and attempt to confirm the diagnosis only several weeks later.

Serologic Cross-Reactivity

Although diagnostics dependent on direct visualization of a parasite, its ova or cysts can usually allow an experienced parasitologist to make a definitive diagnosis, those dependent on antibody responses can frequently lead to false-positive results attributable to cross-reactivity. Common examples are the cross-reactivity between filarial and *Strongyloides* serology, between schistosomiasis and *Fasciola*, and between cysticercosis and hydatid. Therefore a comparative determination of the specific titers, changes in titer as a result of specific treatment, and/or expert advice are often required to fully establish a helminth diagnosis by these routes.

SCREENING ALGORITHMS FOR ASYMPTOMATIC OR PAUCISYMPTOMATIC PATIENTS

Although likely diagnoses may be suggested by exposure history and clinical symptoms (if present), often a series of screening tests is performed to establish the diagnosis and exclude other infections. Some helminths can solely be acquired in specific continents, and others, though more generally distributed, are almost exclusively acquired by humans only in certain areas. Therefore, most screening algorithms are based largely on geographic exposure.[9,21] Such an algorithm is shown in **Fig. 1**.

Some screening algorithms suggest using empiric broad-spectrum antihelminthics. The most commonly used is albendazole; however, this drug is not truly broad spectrum, having inadequate efficacy against many helminths. Such empiric therapy should generally be reserved for those cases of persistent eosinophilia that have remained undiagnosed despite extensive investigation, and it is vital that such treatment leads to the permanent resolution of the eosinophilia, to ensure that continuing infection, or alternative causes (see **Box 1**), are not missed.

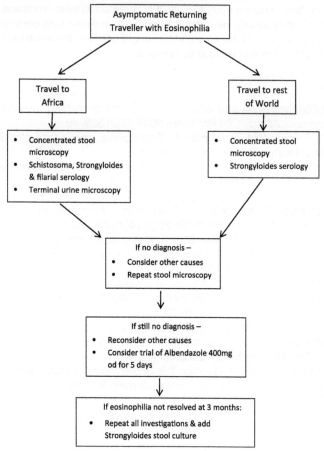

Fig. 1. Potential screening algorithm for asymptomatic eosinophilia in returning travelers.

COMMON HELMINTH INFECTIONS CAUSING EOSINOPHILIA

The more commonly encountered parasitic causes of eosinophilia in returning travelers are summarized by geographic exposure and the most common symptomatology in **Table 1**. More detailed descriptions are available from a variety of sources (eg, Checkley and colleagues[21]); however, it must also be acknowledged that there are many rarer parasitic causes (some of which have yet to have reliable diagnostics developed), so more expert advice should be sought if these initial diagnoses are excluded and/or there is no response to empiric antihelminthic therapy (eg, albendazole).

SUMMARY

The causes of eosinophilia are multiple. In a returning traveler it may well be related to an acquired helminth infection; however, other causes such as malignancies, atopy, and autoimmune conditions should also be considered. A detailed travel history determining specific geographic, environmental, and cultural exposures may help to narrow down the list of likely helminths; however, screening for several is often required, and screening algorithms have been developed. In an asymptomatic individual, delaying screening until several weeks after exposure is likely to increase the yield of the assays, and in those who are symptomatic it is common to treat on clinical suspicion, as the diagnosis may initially be difficult to confirm. In those with persisting eosinophilia or symptoms, expert advice should be sought because the available diagnostics are frequently suboptimal or difficult to interpret.

REFERENCES

1. Nutman TB. Evaluation and differential diagnosis of marked, persistent eosinophilia. Immunol Allergy Clin North Am 2007;27(3):529–49.
2. Tefferi A, Patnaik MM, Pardanani A. Eosinophilia: secondary, clonal and idiopathic. Br J Haematol 2006;133(5):468–92.
3. Fryatt RJ, Teng J, Harries AD, et al. Intestinal helminthiasis in ex-patriates returning to Britain from the tropics. A controlled study. Trop Geogr Med 1990;42(2): 119–22.
4. Schulte C, Krebs B, Jelinek T, et al. Diagnostic significance of blood eosinophilia in returning travelers. Clin Infect Dis 2002;34(3):407–11.
5. Bierman WF, Wetsteyn JC, van Gool T. Presentation and diagnosis of imported schistosomiasis: relevance of eosinophilia, microscopy for ova, and serology. J Travel Med 2005;12(1):9–13.
6. O'Brien DP, Leder K, Matchett E, et al. Illness in returned travelers and immigrants/refugees: the 6-year experience of two Australian infectious diseases units. J Travel Med 2006;13(3):145–52.
7. Whitty CJ, Carroll B, Armstrong M, et al. Utility of history, examination and laboratory tests in screening those returning to Europe from the tropics for parasitic infection. Trop Med Int Health 2000;5(11):818–23.
8. Libman MD, MacLean JD, Gyorkos TW. Screening for schistosomiasis, filariasis, and strongyloidiasis among expatriates returning from the tropics. Clin Infect Dis 1993;17(3):353–9.
9. Meltzer E, Percik R, Shatzkes J, et al. Eosinophilia among returning travelers: a practical approach. Am J Trop Med Hyg 2008;78(5):702–9.
10. Whetham J, Day JN, Armstrong M, et al. Investigation of tropical eosinophilia; assessing a strategy based on geographical area. J Infect 2003;46(3):180–5.

11. Baaten GG, Sonder GJ, van Gool T, et al. Travel-related schistosomiasis, strongy-loidiasis, filariasis, and toxocariasis: the risk of infection and the diagnostic relevance of blood eosinophilia. BMC Infect Dis 2011;11:84.
12. Boggild AK, Yohanna S, Keystone JS, et al. Prospective analysis of parasitic infections in Canadian travelers and immigrants. J Travel Med 2006;13(3): 138–44.
13. Lipner EM, Law MA, Barnett E, et al. Filariasis in travelers presenting to the Geo-Sentinel Surveillance Network. PLoS Negl Trop Dis 2007;1(3):e88.
14. Nicolls DJ, Weld LH, Schwartz E, et al. Characteristics of schistosomiasis in travelers reported to the GeoSentinel Surveillance Network 1997-2008. Am J Trop Med Hyg 2008;79(5):729–34.
15. Chen LH, Wilson ME, Davis X, et al. Illness in long-term travelers visiting GeoSentinel clinics. Emerg Infect Dis 2009;15(11):1773–82.
16. Seybolt LM, Christiansen D, Barnett ED. Diagnostic evaluation of newly arrived asymptomatic refugees with eosinophilia. Clin Infect Dis 2006;42(3):363–7.
17. Lopez-Velez R, Huerga H, Turrientes MC. Infectious diseases in immigrants from the perspective of a tropical medicine referral unit. Am J Trop Med Hyg 2003; 69(1):115–21.
18. Weller PF. Eosinophilia in travelers. Med Clin North Am 1992;76(6):1413–32.
19. Harries AD, Myers B, Bhattacharrya D. Eosinophilia in Caucasians returning from the tropics. Trans R Soc Trop Med Hyg 1986;80(2):327–8.
20. Pardo J, Carranza C, Muro A, et al. Helminth-related eosinophilia in African immigrants, Gran Canaria. Emerg Infect Dis 2006;12(10):1587–9.
21. Checkley AM, Chiodini PL, Dockrell DH, et al. Eosinophilia in returning travellers and migrants from the tropics: UK recommendations for investigation and initial management. J Infect 2010;60(1):1–20.

rends and Patterns of
ssociated Morbidity

, MB ChB, MD, FRCP(Lond)[a,b,*],
, BSc, RN[b]

ravel trends • Travel-associated morbidity
essment

e and patterns of international travel alter morbidity and mortality during

data collection can provide a more accurate picture of travel-associ-
More accurate denominator data will improve the validity of risk

n risk traveller groups and factors which contribute to ill-health will lead
and relevant interventions.

is of the largest and fastest growing economic sectors in the world,
eases so too will travel-associated morbidity and mortality. Inter-
al bodies exist to promote better health among travelers and the
ponsible and sustainable tourism. At an international level, the
nization publishes guidance for travel health providers, as do
ies including the Centers for Disease Control (CDC) in the United
alth Protection Agency and its affiliates in the United Kingdom.
nd national societies also exist to provide educational and training
el medicine. Interest in the provision of travel medicine services
ly since the specialty was formed and, despite its short history
ture on travel-associated health risks has been published across
f topics.

es to the advisory board of Sigma Tau and Norgine and has received travel
Tau.

pter provides an overview of the trends in travel and groups of travelers at
and examines patterns of morbidity during and after travel. The epidemio-
ssment depends on the type and quality of data available, which plays a crit-
n defining an individual's risk at the pretravel assessment and provides
tive on the nature of morbidity among travelers.

TRAVEL

f travel-associated morbidity inform health professionals of the likely threats
el. With international travel becoming more accessible and affordable, there
a rapid growth in overseas travel, particularly to developing countries. This
the volume of travel, destinations visited, duration, age, and activities under-
avelers all have a major bearing on patterns of illness developing during and
. Understanding change is an essential part of understanding the threats
ravelers and deciding on ways to mitigate threats and prevent illness.

vel Trends

el statistics are prepared by The World Tourism Organization (WTO), a special-
cy of the United Nations. Using questionnaire responses from overseas
ts and the travel industry, tourist arrivals are reported from frontier posts.
ast 6 decades there has been an estimated 38-fold increase in international
als, from 25 million in 1950 to 940 million in 2010, with a projection that inter-
rivals will reach nearly 1.6 billion by the year 2020. Of these worldwide arrivals
2 billion will be intraregional and 0.4 billion will be long-haul travelers **Fig. 1.**[1]
w destinations are in developing countries and the emerging and devel-
nomies receive a steadily increasing proportion of tourists, from 31% in
% in 2010.

t be predicted, destinations visited by travelers change over time: although
nains the most popular destination, with just more than 50% of all interna-
st arrivals in 2010, there has been a strong growth in travel to Asia and the
th almost 204 million international arrivals in 2010 (accounting for 21.7% of
al tourist arrivals). Major destinations within the region include China,

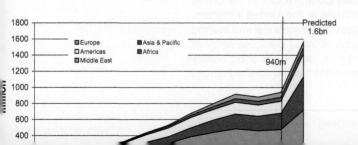

Malaysia, and Thailand. The Middle East accounted for 6.4% of all tourist arrivals and was the fastest growing region in 2010. The Americas accounted for 15.9% of international tourist arrivals in 2010, with Mexico the second leading destination in the Americas. Arrivals in South America were up by 11% with around 23 million international arrivals. Africa accounted for 5.2% of international tourist arrivals, receiving 49 million international tourists in 2010 **Fig. 2.**[1]

By 2020, the WTO projects that the top 3 receiving regions will be Europe (717 million tourists), east Asia (397 million), and the Americas (282 million), followed by Africa, the Middle East, and south Asia.[1]

UK Travel Trends

Since 1961, UK travel statistics have been collected by the Office for National Statistics as part of the International Passenger Survey (IPS). The IPS is a year-round survey of incoming and outgoing passengers' at all major ports and samples around 0.2% of all travelers for the governments' understanding of incoming and outgoing currency. The survey estimates the total annual overseas visits made by UK residents. Since, 1961 there has been a greater than 16-fold increase in UK residents' travel, from 3.3 million to 55.6 million in 2010.[2] This methodology, unique in the Western Hemisphere, provides the most accurate denominator data on travel and is used in this chapter in the discussion of travel by UK residents.

In 2010, 6.2 million visits were made by UK residents to tropical countries. The burden of morbidity in this population is significant, because a predicted 8% of travelers require medical care,[3] around 1% require hospital treatment, and 1 in 86,000 US citizens (2007) die abroad from a non-natural cause during travel.

UK travelers are making fewer visits to the traditional tourist areas of Europe (eg, Spain, Italy, Greece, and Cyprus) and increasingly visit medium-haul destinations outside the Eurozone, such as Turkey and Tunisia. Turkey has become the eighth most popular destination among UK travelers, with 1.82 million visits from the United Kingdom in 2010. Since the 1980s, when long-haul destinations became popular with UK travelers, visits to countries outside Europe and North America increased from 1.5 million in 1985 to 9.3 million in 2010. Visits to tropical countries are increasing with an average annual growth rate of 8%. Visits to Asia (1.3 million visits in 2010), the Caribbean, and South and Central American countries are making up an increasing share of the UK travel market.

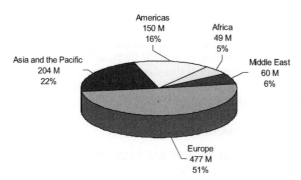

Fig. 2. International tourist arrivals (million [M]) by region visited 2010. (*Data from* World Tourism Organization. Tourism highlights 2011 edition. Available at: http://mkt.unwto.org/sites/all/files/docpdf/unwtohighlights11enhr_0.pdf. Accessed September 14, 2011.)

Purpose of Travel

The reason people travel has a bearing on their risks and patterns of morbidity. Globally in 2010, travel for leisure, recreation, and holidays accounted for slightly more than half of all international tourist arrivals worldwide (51%, or 480 million arrivals). Some 15% of international tourists reported traveling for business and professional purposes and another 27% traveled for other purposes, such as visiting friends and relatives (VFR), religious reasons and pilgrimages, and health tourism.

UK residents tend to travel primarily for holidays; however, VFR travel has grown markedly, from 2.3 million (13.2% of the total visits) in 1980 to 10.8 million (20%) in 2010, reflecting ongoing migration into the United Kingdom. The foreign-born population make up around 9% of the total UK population. VFR travel is disproportionately large, constituting more than 20% of all visits abroad annually, and, of the 2 million visits made by UK residents to Africa, 44% are VFRs. Since 2001, VFRs have been the most frequently stated reason for visiting West Africa, with the proportion of total visits increasing from 25% in 1993 to 57% in 2006. In the United States, of the total overseas travel (excluding travel to Canada and Mexico), which was 27 million in 2004, 46% (11.8 million) were VFRs.

This increased proportion of visits for the purpose of VFR is likely to continue to grow in future years.

Business travel among UK residents has increased from 3.2 million visits in 1985 to 6.6 million in 2010.[2] Business trips are of shorter duration than travel for other purposes, and half of all business visits are from 1 to 3 nights. Business travelers are predominantly men (5.4 million business trips vs 1.4 million made by women in 2010).

Length of Stay

Visits abroad by UK residents have become shorter (with a gradual decline from 16 nights in 1970 to 10.9 in 2010), although the duration of travel to longer-haul destinations has increased in some destinations.[2] VFR travel is longer (averaging 15.9 nights in 2010) and a significant proportion travel for more than 4 weeks.

A recent UK population-based survey of 548 travelers to malaria risk areas showed that most (69%) spent less than 1 month abroad, 21% stayed for between 1 and 3 months, and 9% stayed for more than 3 months. Twenty-three percent of those who stayed for longer visits were backpackers and 10% were VFRs.

Although it has been reported that longer duration of stay increases the health threat to travelers, there is little evidence to support or refute this, and given the number of travelers that stay for prolonged periods abroad, this is a question that needs closer examination.

Age

Around 75% of travel by UK residents is made by those between the ages of 25 and 54 years. However, a sizable amount of travel is now made by those older than 65 years (5.3 million visits in 2010),[2] accounting for 9.5% of all visits and an increase of 1.2 million visits from a decade earlier.

MORBIDITY DURING INTERNATIONAL TRAVEL

An accurate understanding of the type and frequency of health problems occurring during travel is fundamental when identifying preventative measures to reduce morbidity and inform policy. There are limited scientific data on the problems that are encountered and their severity. The complexity of ascertaining health events during travel has led to several proxy markers of morbidity, particularly infectious health problems reported in

Trends and Patterns of Travel-Associated Morbidity 795

eturn, but many of these are questionable as representative markers
uring travel. It is therefore important to understand the methods that
define the risk of ill health, and their validity.

etermine Risk of Morbidity

nowledge and epidemiologic data remain, because most of these
ods have inherent weaknesses. The geographic distribution of
only used as a measure of endemicity and therefore exposure,
many infectious agents globally. These data reflect diseases iden-
opulation of the country or region, their methods of ascertainment
their accuracy and contemporaneous nature often unknown
on, there is often poor regional precision, which makes advising
pular regions inaccurate. The susceptibilities to infectious risks
are likely to be different to those faced by the native population
e better protected by different living conditions and a shorter expo-
ealth problems acquired during travel by travelers rather than local
measure. However, case reports of illness in travelers gives little
obability of illness because they are without a denominator and
ntative of all travelers. Surveillance reports of travel-related illness
GeoSentinel network provides a picture of morbidity as a proportion
blems encountered by travelers, stratified by region of exposure
el.[3] However, these data are not incidences and reflect returned
the GeoSentinel surveillance sites. Expert consensus (in which
specialty, eg, malaria, decide on risks and interventions) is widely
isk because it is easy to implement but may have little or no

ness of methods used to estimate morbidity and travel-associated risk

	Strengths	Weakness
tion	Widely available	Reflects patterns in local population Historical Quality and method of collection unknown
s	Fits with traditional surveillance methods	Under reporting No denominator
es	Specific to travelers	May not reflect all groups Underreporting Denominator quality unknown No time frame
idence d time)	Specific and sensitive	Denominator difficult to obtain Time frame usually historical

Carroll

with the true risk. A further problem associated with consensus is that the
dvice, varies between different consensus bodies. In a survey of European
malaria recommendations to specific destinations there was a clear band-
commendations around geographic regions of Europe with significant
etween European experts.[4] A proxy of severe morbidity is mortality among
providing a more objective measure of severe disease during travel, but this
reliable because of reporting biases and ascertainment. Incidence based on
(infectious and noninfectious) adjusted by the denominator of travelers
over time would provide the most valuable risk indicators.[5,6] However,
tries do not collect country-specific data on numbers of travelers or nonin-
orbidity, and the data are usually historical and change over time.

Associated with Travel

avel increasing year on year, there has been no evidence of an associated
imported infections to the United Kingdom. The opposite has been noted
and hepatitis A. Few deaths result from infections acquired during travel
ose that do, the largest proportion (around 7 to 10 deaths annually in the
gdom) are from malaria.[7] There are significant changes in the global epide-
many infectious threats including malaria, human immunodeficiency virus
tidrug resistant tuberculosis, and vector-borne viruses (Chikungunya and
and policy should reflect these trends.

Deaths in Travelers When Abroad

ures for deaths during travel abroad are not available in most Western coun-
use many of the countries receiving travelers do not have centralized death
Injuries account for a high proportion of deaths, with road injuries being
ause. If available, data on deaths serve as a proxy for severe morbidity
road trauma, drowning, crime, and complications of preexisting health
particularly cardiovascular disease. Severe infections among travelers
r only a small proportion of deaths (approximately 1%–4%; **Fig. 3**).

G MORBIDITY

higher risk groups, such as older people, many of whom have significant
ties, and visits to friends and relatives is pertinent because of the problems

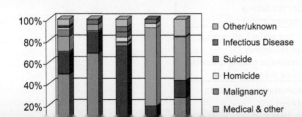

they develop during travel. In the United Kingdom, travel by residents aged 65 years and older has increased by 30% in the past decade, with 5.3 million traveling in 2010. By examining the cause of death during travel, it is obvious that preexisting medical problems such as cardiovascular disease, diabetes, respiratory diseases, and other noncommunicable diseases contribute to most medical deaths in older travelers. By proxy, most of the severe but nonfatal health problems encountered during travel are likely to be from similar causes. What remains unknown, and for which future research is vital, is whether traveling itself contributes to or exacerbates the risk of complications or relapse of existing health problems. In one comparison, cardiovascular death rates were similar in travelers to rates in nontraveling Americans.[8]

Ensuring the purchase of travel health insurance including medical evacuation cover is particularly important for travelers with preexisting illness and those planning to undertake hazardous activities. Although there is likely to be a higher purchase premium in older individuals and travelers participating in risky sports and activities, these travelers need to be persuaded of its value and relevance.

Traffic Crashes and Trauma

Between a fifth to a quarter of deaths in travelers are caused by injuries, predominantly road traffic crashes,[8-11] but, among some groups, the fatality rate caused by injury has been reported to be as high as 70%.[12] This cause of death and severe injury reflects the differences in rates of road traffic deaths between low-income/middle-income countries and high-income countries. Road traffic injury deaths are predicted to increase to the fifth leading cause of death globally by 2030. The death rates in Americans abroad is approximately 3 times that of deaths from crashes in the United States.[8]

In low-income regions of the world, road deaths are 21.5 per 100 000 population, compared with high-income countries (10.3 per 100 000).[13] More than 90% of the world's fatalities on the roads occur in low-income and middle-income countries. The 10 countries with the highest numbers of deaths are China, India, Nigeria, the United States, Pakistan, Indonesia, the Russian Federation, Brazil, Egypt, and Ethiopia.

Travelers behave differently abroad, engaging in riskier activities such as driving without seatbelts or safety helmets and consuming alcohol before driving, and they are unfamiliar with road conditions and driving practices, which places travelers at greater risk of injury even compared with local drivers. Road accident deaths in American travelers during travel are nearly double local population death rates (**Fig. 4**).

MALARIA

Malaria is an example of the changing threat and risk of a travel-associated disease. Over a 20-year period (1987–2006), the pattern of malaria species imported to the United Kingdom has changed markedly. The proportion of imported *Plasmodium vivax*

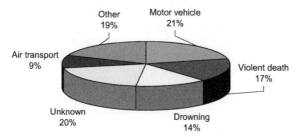

Fig. 4. Injury deaths in Americans abroad. (*Data from* Guse CE, Cortes LM, Hargarten SW et al. Fatal injuries of US citizens abroad. J Travel Med 2007;14:279–87.)

infections has decreased from 42% to 16% in these 2 decades, and *Plasmodium falciparum* now constitutes 72% of all imported species, with most cases (67%) acquired in West Africa.[7] There has also been a decline in imported malaria from West Africa in the past 10 years. Despite a 200% increase in visits by UK residents to West Africa, there has been a 60% decrease in imported *P falciparum* cases during the period. The evidence is that this reflects the change in local transmission rather than wider use of preventative measures by travelers.[6]

Outside Africa, much of the remaining imported malaria to the United Kingdom comes from Asia, 92% of which is caused by *P vivax* infection. There are also European and UK data showing a low and declining risk of malaria from many Asian and southeast Asian countries despite the 3-fold increase in tourist travel to these regions in the period 1990 to 2009 (21–62 million visits to southeast Asia and 3.2 to 10.1 million to south Asia).[5]

YELLOW FEVER

Yellow fever is endemic in many countries of sub-Saharan Africa and South America and is the only disease for which an International Certificate of Vaccination or Prophylaxis may be required for entry. An estimated 769,000 UK residents made visits to countries where there may be a risk of yellow fever infection in 2010. Yellow fever is considered as a risk despite there having been no recognized travel-associated cases of yellow fever in UK residents and only 9 cases (8 deaths) in travelers globally in the past 3 decades. The likelihood of an adverse event leading to serious injury or death associated with yellow fever immunization is around 1 event for every 200,000 naive recipients and approximately 1 in every 50,000 naive recipients more than 60 years of age, which makes the intervention rather than the disease itself an important health risk. Using Kenya as an example, Kenya receives around 1.5 million tourist arrivals annually and nearly all visit a game park during their stay (Kenyan Tourist Authority). Under new international recommendations, all these travelers would need to be protected by a yellow fever vaccination because the Kenyan game parks are within a yellow fever endemic region.[14] The threat of an adverse event is therefore higher in all travelers who are vaccine naive, and in particular older tourists, than the illness from yellow fever. Iatrogenic morbidity needs to be fully appreciated by health professionals and travelers. Prophylaxis used for low-level threats can be a noteworthy cause of travel-associated morbidity.[15]

COMMON HEALTH PROBLEMS

Health problems that are frequent in the general population occur commonly in travelers too. Headaches and malaise, viral respiratory infections, and skin infections are among the most frequent of these. Fever is a symptom of many common conditions in travelers and is often not associated with a tropical infection.

Skin problems after return have been reported in 12% of all cases presenting to a tropical disease hospital.[16] Local bacterial infection and cellulitis, and, less frequently, systemic sepsis, can follow an insect bite or skin abrasion and may require a medical consultation and antibiotic therapy.

Influenza is the most frequently occurring vaccine-preventable disease associated with travel. Two percent of Swiss travelers acquired evidence of infection after returning from traveling.[17] Other respiratory tract infections encountered include chronic sinusitis, acute otitis media, streptococcal pharyngitis, and tonsillitis.[18]

Travelers' diarrhea affects between 20% and 50% of individuals traveling to developing and/or tropical areas,[19] and 10% of affected individuals go on to develop more serious symptoms of dysentery, but few (less than 1%) require hospitalization. Around a third of those affected are unable to pursue planned activities, and this is an important consideration for most travelers.[20] The cause and pathogenesis show *Escherichia coli* as the most commonly identified organism, but invasive bacterial enteropathogens are also important.

The widely perceived vaccine-preventable infectious diseases are infrequent in returned travelers. Hepatitis A is now at least 4-fold lower than reported 3 decades ago in south-central Asia,[21] with an overall incidence by 2004 of 11 cases per 100,000 travelers. This decline is in part caused by the widespread uptake of the hepatitis A vaccine and in part by economic and hygiene improvements in the destinations. Rabies occurs rarely, although contact with animals in endemic regions is common in 1% to 3% of travelers. Hepatitis B acquisition is through sexual exposure and almost never via parenteral infection, and it is a disease identified more often in VFRs.[22] Meningococcal infection is predominantly a hazard associated with pilgrims on the Haj, and is rare in other travelers.

RISK GROUPS

Several high-risk travel groups have been identified through clinical and epidemiologic studies and are covered elsewhere in this issue by Visser and Maatelli. Three groups who pose different challenges and face a variety of risks are highlighted here.

Immunocompromised Travelers

One of the more complex group of travelers to deal with are those who are immunocompromised. A wide range of medical conditions exist that place a traveler at risk of infectious threats during travel and risk of vaccines before travel. Preexisting problems, including chronic renal and liver disease, diabetes, HIV, asplenia, and inflammatory bowel disease leave the traveler susceptible to complications and hospitalization during their journey. Treatment and medication for cancer, rheumatologic disorders, and autoimmune disease, including high-dose corticosteroids, methotrexate, azathioprine, and rituximab, and the recently introduced immunobiological agents, including etanercept, infliximab, and adalimumab predispose to infectious threats, particularly tuberculosis.

The Older Traveler

Older travelers have several factors that increase their risk of morbidity during travel. The Health Survey for England (2005) states that 66% to 78% of the UK population who are 65 years old and older report having a self-reported long-standing illness and up to 70% have mobility impairment. With such a high prevalence of preexisting morbidity, restricted mobility, and frailty, there is a high risk of health problems, falls, and injury during travel, in particular in destinations that do not have an aging population and therefore do not provide disabled access support or health care for older patients. For older travelers, purchasing travel health insurance can be problematic and many insurers decline cover to this age group. When receiving immunizations before travel, there is evidence of a diminished serologic response to hepatitis A and rabies vaccines.[23] When older individuals acquire an infection, their immunologic and physiologic responses result in more severe disease, as in hepatitis A,[24] influenza, and malaria.[25]

VFR Travelers

The term VFR generally refers to immigrants from low-income countries who now reside in high-income countries and are returning to their country of origin to visit friends and relatives. It has been estimated that VFRs make up 25% to 40% of all travelers. With increased migration globally, travel among this group of travelers will undoubtedly increase.

The lack of a standardized definition for VFR travelers makes it difficult to compare morbidity data for this group of travelers; however, there is evidence to suggest that travelers, identified as immigrants and traveling for the purpose of VFR, experience a greater proportion of serious and potentially preventable travel-related illness.[26] VFRs are at higher risk of acquiring certain infections (eg, malaria, and tuberculosis) linked to several factors including exposure (more likely to stay in family homes, rather than hotels), often in villages and remote areas, and longer stays. Many VFRs are insufficiently protected because they do not seek pretravel health advice and are less likely to use prophylaxis. There is evidence that VFRs perceive their health risks to be less serious because they are returning to their country of origin. An example of this is malaria. VFR travelers accounted for 65% of all malaria reports imported into the United Kingdom in the past 2 decades. Seventy-one percent of cases were following travel to Africa, of which two-thirds were in travelers to West Africa, with Nigeria and Ghana accounting for more than half of all imported P falciparum infections. Since 2001, VFR travel has been the predominant reason for visits to West Africa, with the proportion of visits increasing from 25% in 1993 to 57% in 2006. Seventy-six percent of all malaria cases acquired in West Africa were in VFRs and only 7% reported using a recommended chemoprophylaxis, compared with 24% of people traveling for other reasons.

The malaria cases were heavily concentrated in ethnic communities in central London, where 45% of the UK minority population reside.

VFRs are disproportionately affected by a range of other infections including hepatitis A, enteric fever, sexually transmitted diseases, and tuberculosis. Enteric fever is a disease predominantly identified in Indian, Pakistani, or Bangladeshi travelers, who have a relative risk of 3 to 8 times higher than non-VFR travelers.[27]

SUMMARY

As data collection methods have improved, a clearer picture of travel-associated health risks and at-risk travelers has emerged. The early emphasis on vaccine-preventable disease has had some impact on hepatitis A incidence but a wider examination of the causes of mortality and morbidity has highlighted behavior-related health problems such as injuries arising from road crashes and high-risk sporting activities, malaria, and sexually transmitted diseases, and has led to a change in emphasis on ways of reducing morbidly. There remain many unanswered questions that relate to the contribution of medical comorbidities on travel-associated illness, how improved communication could enhance or influence behavior change and increase the uptake of advice, and the best strategies to influence those groups of travelers at greatest risk, for instance VFRs, who do not seek pretravel advice. Enhanced data collection methods and better denominator data are necessary to provide more precise risk information and help inform policy and thereby reduce morbidity in tourists and travelers.

REFERENCES

1. Tourism highlights 2011 edition. World Tourism Organization. Available at: http://mkt.unwto.org/sites/all/files/docpdf/unwtohighlights11enhr_0.pdf. Accessed September 14, 2011.
2. National statistics. Travel trends 2010. A report on the International Passenger Survey. Available at: http://www.ons.gov.uk/ons/search/index.html?newquery=travel+trends; http://www.statistics.gov.uk/downloads/theme_transport/traveltrends2004.pdf. Accessed June 20, 2012.

3. Freedman DO, Weld LH, Kozarsky PE, et al. Spectrum of disease and relation to place of exposure among ill returned travelers. N Engl J Med 2006;354: 119–30.
4. Calleri G, Behrens RH, Bisoffi Z, et al. Variability in malaria prophylaxis prescribing across Europe: a Delphi method analysis. J Travel Med 2008;15:294–300.
5. Behrens RH, Carroll B, Hellgren U, et al. The incidence of malaria in travellers to South-East Asia: is local malaria transmission a useful risk indicator? Malar J 2010;9:266.
6. Behrens RH, Carroll B, Smith V, et al. Declining incidence of malaria imported into the UK from West Africa. Malar J 2008;7:235.
7. Smith AD, Bradley DJ, Smith V, et al. Imported malaria and high risk groups: observational study using UK surveillance data 1987-2006. BMJ 2008;337:103–6.
8. Hargarten SW, Baker TD, Guptill K. Overseas fatalities of United States citizen travelers: an analysis of deaths related to international travel. Ann Emerg Med 1991;20:622–6.
9. Paixao MA, Dewar RD, Cossar JH, et al. What do Scots die of when abroad? Scott Med J 1991;36:114–6.
10. Lunetta P. Injury deaths among Finnish residents travelling abroad. Int J Inj Contr Saf Promot 2010;17:161–8.
11. MacPherson DW, Gushulak BD, Sandhu J. Death and international travel–the Canadian experience: 1996 to 2004. J Travel Med 2007;14:77–84.
12. Hargarten SW, Baker SP. Fatalities in the Peace Corps. JAMA 1985;254:1326–9.
13. Global status report on road safety. Time for action. World Health Organization. Available at: http://www.who.int/violence_injury_prevention/road_traffic/global_status_report/en/index.html. Accessed June 20, 2012.
14. Jentes ES, Poumerol G, Gershman MD, et al. The revised global yellow fever risk map and recommendations for vaccination, 2010: consensus of the Informal WHO Working Group on Geographic Risk for Yellow Fever. Lancet Infect Dis 2011;11:622–32.
15. Behrens RH. Yellow fever recommendations for tourists to Kenya: a flawed risk assessment? J Travel Med 2008;15:285–6.
16. Herbinger KH, Siess C, Nothdurft HD, et al. Skin disorders among travellers returning from tropical and non-tropical countries consulting a travel medicine clinic. Trop Med Int Health 2011;16:1457–64.
17. Mutsch M, Tavernini M, Marx A, et al. Influenza virus infection in travelers to tropical and subtropical countries. Clin Infect Dis 2005;40:1282–7.
18. Leder K, Sundararajan V, Weld L, et al. Respiratory tract infections in travelers: a review of the GeoSentinel surveillance network. Clin Infect Dis 2003;36: 399–406.
19. von Sonnenburg F, Tornieporth NG, Waiyaki P, et al. Risk and aetiology of diarrhoea at various tourist destinations. Lancet 2000;356:133–4.
20. Steffen R. Epidemiology of traveler's diarrhea. Clin Infect Dis 2005;41(Suppl 8): S536–40.
21. Mutsch M, Spicher V, Gut C, et al. Hepatitis A virus infections in travelers, 1988-2004. Clin Infect Dis 2006;42.
22. Sonder GJ, van Rijckevorsel GG, Van Den HA. Risk of hepatitis B for travelers: is vaccination for all travelers really necessary? J Travel Med 2009;16:18–22.
23. Leder K, Weller PF, Wilson ME. Travel vaccines and elderly persons: review of vaccines available in the United States. Clin Infect Dis 2001;33:1553–66.
24. Forbes A, Williams R. Increasing age - an important adverse prognostic factor in hepatitis A virus infection. J R Coll Physicians Lond 1988;22:237–9.

25. Muhlberger N, Jelinek T, Behrens RH, et al. Age as a risk factor for severe manifestations and fatal outcome of falciparum malaria in European patients: observations from TropNetEurop and SIMPID Surveillance Data. Clin Infect Dis 2003;36: 990–5.
26. Barnett ED, MacPherson DW, Stauffer WM, et al. The visiting friends or relatives traveler in the 21st century: time for a new definition. J Travel Med 2010;17:163–70.
27. Health Protection Agency. Pilot of enhanced surveillance of enteric fever in England, Wales, and Northern Ireland, 1 May 2006 to 30 April 2007. London: Health Protection Agency; 2008. p. 1–35.

Laboratory Investigations and Diagnosis of Tropical Diseases in Travelers

Rosemarie Daly, MBBS[a], Peter L. Chiodini, MB, PhD[a,b],*

KEYWORDS

- Tropical diseases • Travel • Laboratory tests

KEY POINTS

- Type of traveler (some infections, such as malaria, are more common in migrants or those travelers visiting friends and relations).
- Geographic location visited; rural or urban; standard of accommodation; activities undertaken (work or recreational); dietary history; contact with ill patients; sexual contact; bites (animal, insect, snake); exotic foods; swimming in rivers or canals.
- Date and duration of travel; date of onset of illness and its duration.

INTRODUCTION

Illness in a traveler who returns from the tropics suffering from an illness may fall into four groups: (1) a condition that may be noninfective and possibly unrelated to travel, (2) an infectious disease that has a cosmopolitan distribution but may be more common in resource-poor settings, (3) a classical tropical disease that is endemic in a distinct geographic location,[1,2] or (4) a new or emerging disease not readily identified.[3] Consequently, evaluation of an individual traveler requires consideration of a greater range of possible diagnoses than would be entertained at home.

Detailed discussion of the clinical features and likely presentation of tropical diseases in travelers is outside the scope of this article, and the reader is referred to other sources.[1,2] In trying rapidly to identify the cause of the presenting illness in the traveler, knowledge of their natural history and a carefully taken account of the location of the trip undertaken and potential exposure to exotic infections helps narrow the range of possibilities and the amount of laboratory investigation and imaging needed to confirm a diagnosis.

PLC is supported by the UCL Hospitals Comprehensive Biomedical Research Centre Infection Theme.
[a] Hospital for Tropical Diseases, Mortimer Market, London WC1E 6JB, UK; [b] London School of Hygiene and Tropical Medicine, Keppel Street, London WC1E 7HT, UK
* Corresponding author.
E-mail address: peter.chiodini@uclh.nhs.uk

Infect Dis Clin N Am 26 (2012) 803–818
http://dx.doi.org/10.1016/j.idc.2012.06.001
id.theclinics.com

GENERAL STRATEGY FOR LABORATORY INVESTIGATION OF THE SICK TRAVELER

It is important to consider whether or not there is a risk of a viral hemorrhagic fever (VHF) at the earliest stage of investigation, because this has implications for infection control and safety of specimen handling. If suspicion exists, only essential blood tests, such as malaria, should be done whilst urgent investigations for VHF are performed.

Many of the more advanced and specialist tests may be obtainable only from national or international reference laboratories. Liaison with local microbiology networks is advisable. Because of the range and plethora of potential diagnoses, the rapidity with which the clinical situation may change, and the potential need for access to specialist treatments, it is wise to seek immediate advice and help from local infectious or tropical diseases teams.

The common presentations of illness in travelers attending tropical and infectious diseases units are fever, diarrhea, skin diseases, and eosinophilia.

Fever

The following initial investigations should be considered in all cases[2,4]:

1. Malaria thin and thick blood films and rapid malaria diagnostic test
2. Full blood count and differential count
3. Blood cultures
4. Urine analysis and culture
5. Serum biochemistry
6. Save serum for paired serology if required
7. EDTA sample for polymerase chain reaction (PCR) if arboviral or VHF infection suspected;
8. Chest radiograph and liver ultrasound (in some cases)
9. Bone marrow microscopy and culture may be required in cases of fever of unknown origin

Diarrhea

Perform stool bacterial culture; fecal viral antigen detection assays or PCR; hot stool microscopy for *Entamoeba histolytica*; stool concentration for ova, cysts, and parasites; and fecal protozoal antigen detection assays or PCR. Many components of the fever screen may be required because diarrhea may be caused by nonintestinal infection (eg, legionnaires disease and *Plasmodium falciparum* malaria).

Skin Disease

Perform bacterial culture of pus; viral PCR or culture of vesicle fluid; electron microscopy of vesicle fluid (now seldom used); microscopy and fungal culture of skin scrapings; microscopy, culture, and PCR of skin biopsy for *Leishmania* spp; skin snips for *Onchocerca* spp; microscopy of scrapings for scabies mites; and microscopy of extruded bot fly larvae or curetted jigger fleas.

Eosinophilia

Geography plays a central role in determining the strategy for investigation of eosinophilia in the returning traveler, because some helminths have well-demarcated geographic distributions. Checkley and colleagues[5] summarize a practical geography-based approach to the investigation of eosinophilia, as used at the Hospital for Tropical Diseases in London.

GENERAL LABORATORY TESTS

Investigations often start with basic hematology and biochemistry. They are never diagnostic of tropical diseases but can provide key pointers toward underlying infectious etiology.

Hematology

Various conditions point toward a diagnosis:

- Neutrophilia: high polymorphonuclear leukocyte neutrophil counts are often seen in bacterial infections, but are notable in amoebic liver abscess.
- Eosinophilia: high eosinophil counts are seen in parasitic diseases, especially helminth infections (not usually seen with protozoa except for *Toxoplasma* spp or *Isospora* spp); fungal infections; viral infections (HIV, human T-lymphotropic virus); and sometimes tuberculosis.
- Lymphopenia: low lymphocyte counts are seen in viral infections (HIV, dengue fever) and typhoid fever.
- Lymphocytosis: high mononuclear cell counts are seen in Epstein-Barr virus, cytomegalovirus (CMV), and *Toxoplasma* spp infections.
- Thrombocytopenia: malaria; viral (dengue fever, HIV); typhoid fever; and severe sepsis.

Biochemistry

In the case of raised bilirubin, consider the following: if unconjugated bilirubin, (hemolysis), malaria or babesiosis; if conjugated bilirubin, viral hepatitis, malaria, leptospirosis, septicemia, or VHF. In the case of raised transaminases, consider hepatitis or severe sepsis. If alkaline phosphatase is elevated, consider hepatitis, cholangitis, or amoebic liver abscess.

SPECIMENS USED FOR DIAGNOSIS OF TROPICAL INFECTIONS
Blood Specimens

The following blood specimens are used for diagnosis[6]:

- EDTA blood specimen: for malaria screen; *Babesia* spp screen; viral PCRs (including Lassa fever virus); reverse transcription (RT) PCR (where required); and bacterial PCRs (eg, *Ehrlichia* spp, *Anaplasma* spp [first week of illness]).
- Clotted blood for serology: viral (available for many viruses, especially the hepatitides, also VHF); some bacterial infections (eg, antistreptolysin O); some fungal infections. Serology plays a major part in the detection of parasitic infections in nonendemic areas, especially amebiasis and schistosomiasis.
- Citrate anticoagulated blood for the detection of microfilariae by filtration (midday and midnight samples).
- Blood for interferon-γ release assay for tuberculosis (requires appropriate sample tubes and liaison with laboratory).
- Blood cultures: standard or more specialized culture bottles may be available for certain bacterial, mycobacterial, and fungal cultures. It is important to provide information to the laboratory about travel history, and any infections considered reasonably likely or that need to be excluded, especially *Brucella*, typhoid, paratyphoid, and *Penicillium marneffei*. This is not just to permit the laboratory to take precautions, but to enable special culture requirements to be met. For example, *P marneffei* is thermally dimorphic. A mold-form grows at 30°C, and a yeast-form at 37°C. Identification of blood culture isolates may be made by a range of

biochemical methods, including the use of kits, such as APIs, automated biochemical systems (eg, Vitek), matrix-assisted laser desorption/ionization time of flight (MALDI-TOF) mass spectrometry, serologic and DNA-based techniques, and increasingly by combinations of these approaches.

Respiratory Samples

Respiratory samples include the following:

- Viral throat swabs for PCR and culture.
- Viral swabs (oral), where the gum-line is swabbed with a sponge. This enables virus identification by PCR or culture but also permits IgM antibodies to be detected. It is particularly useful for measles and mumps, and more practical and acceptable than blood tests in children.
- Microbiologic throat swab for bacterial or fungal culture and sensitivities.
- Pernasal swabs; these should be plated out immediately on selective media for culture for *Bordetella pertussis*, or may be sent for PCR where available.
- Saliva can be used for HIV point-of-care testing, CMV PCR, rabies RT-PCR, or virus isolation. It is likely to prove useful for the diagnosis of an increasing number of infections.
- Sputum for bacterial and fungal culture. Microscopy for parasites may reveal *Strongyloides* larvae or eggs of *Paragonimus*.
- Bronchoalveolar lavage for microscopy (which may occasionally reveal *Strongyloides*); viral culture; bacterial, mycobacterial, and fungal staining and cultures; PCR; or immunofluorescence tests for *Pneumocystis* and respiratory viruses.
- Pleural effusion aspirate for bacterial, mycobacterial and fungal microscopy and culture
- Pleural biopsy for bacterial, mycobacterial, and fungal microscopy and culture, and for histology.

Urine Samples

Urine samples include the following:

- Urinary antigen detection for *Legionella* type 1, pneumococcal antigen.
- Urine culture for bacteria and fungi.
- Microscopy of membrane-filtered urine samples for the detection of *Schistosoma haematobium* eggs (**Fig. 1**). A terminal urine sample (the last 10–20 mL of urine passed on each occasion) is required.

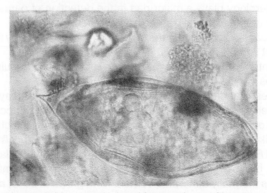

Fig. 1. *Schistosoma haematobium* egg isolated by membrane filtration of terminal urine.

- Urine nucleic acid tests for *Chamydia* and CMV. Some other viruses may be detected in urine samples, including BK virus, and adenovirus in very immunosuppressed patients.

Central Nervous System Samples

These samples include the following:

- Cerebrospinal fluid (CSF) bacterial, fungal and viral culture, or PCR (**Fig. 2**).
- Antibodies and antigen detection tests (eg, cryptococcal antigen, bacterial antigen detection tests for *Streptococcus pneumoniae* and *Neisseria meningitidis*). Culture or PCR for *Naegleria fowleri* and *Balamuthia mandrillaris*.
- CSF microscopy and serology for stage 2 human African trypanosomiasis (*Trypansoma brucei rhodesiense*).

Gastrointestinal Samples

Tests on faecal samples include the following:

- Bacterial culture, especially for *Salmonella* spp, *Shigella* spp, *Campylobacter* spp, *Vibrio cholerae*, and *Escherichia coli* O157.
- Electron microscopy for viruses (eg, *Rotavirus*) is available in some centers.
- Antigen detection enzyme-linked immunosorbent assay (ELISA) is available for a variety of pathogens (eg, *Rotavirus*, *Entamoeba histolytica* lectin).
- Fecal PCR is now widely used for the detection of viruses (eg, *Norovirus*) and now introduced in reference laboratories for intestinal protozoa, notably *E histolytica*, *Giardia intestinalis*, and *Crytosporidium* spp.
- Light microscopy for ova, cysts, and parasites. Diagnosis of amoebic dysentery requires examination of a stool specimen for trophozoites within 20 minutes of voiding (the so-called "hot stool"). A fecal concentration method must be performed on all fecal samples submitted for parasitology to permit optimal detection of fecal parasites. Fecal smears may be stained with trichrome, modified acid-fast, or other stains to enhance species identification. Fluorescent-conjugated monoclonal antibodies may be used to visualize *Cryptosporidium* spp or *G intestinalis*.
- Charcoal culture of feces enhances the detection of *Strongyloides stercoralis* larvae.

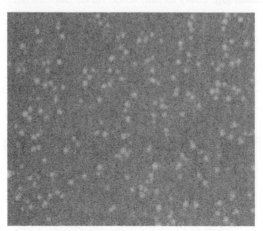

Fig. 2. India ink stain of cerebrospinal fluid showing negative stain of *Cryptococcus* spp (size range 5 to 15 μm per yeast). (*Courtesy of* Ken Aknai, East and North Herts NHS Trust.)

Duodenal and jejunal aspirates increase the sensitivity of detection for *G intestinalis trophozoites; S stercoralis larvae*; and ova of liver flukes *Fasciola hepatica*, *Clonorchis* spp, and *Opisthorcis* spp (**Fig. 3**).

Perianal adhesive tape smear taken first thing in the morning from the perianal skin and attached sticky side down to a microscope slide is the appropriate specimen for detecting *Enterobius vermicularis* ova. Although adult *Enterobius* may be present in stool samples, a negative stool result for worms and ova does not exclude the diagnosis because the ova are laid on the perianal skin.

Adult worms in stool samples (eg, roundworm *Ascaris lumbricodes*, whipworm *Trichuris trichiuria*, pinworm *E vermicularis*, segments of pork tapeworm, *Taenia solium* or beef tapeworm *Taenia saginata*) should be sent for microscopic identification. PCR is available in some centers to identify the species of *Taenia* present.

Biopsy material from rectum or sigmoid colon is valuable for the detection of *Schistosoma* spp ova by crush preparation and, if unfixed, permits assessment of their viability. If biopsies are taken, fixed material should also be sent for histology. CMV and *E histolytica* may be revealed on histology of colonic biopsies or by PCR. Rectal scrapings are examined by microscopy for *E histolytica*.

Skin Samples

Skin samples include the following:

- Skin biopsy: send for histology; bacterial culture; mycobacterial, fungal, and viral culture; and PCR. For the diagnosis of cutaneous leishmaniasis, a punch biopsy from the edge of the lesion must be sent to the laboratory in viral transport medium containing antibiotics, but not antifungals. *Leishmania* spp culture is undertaken, with subsequent PCR to identify species.
- Skin snips for demonstration of *Onchocerca volvulus* microfilariae.
- Swabs of skin lesions for viral PCR, viral culture, bacterial culture, and fungal culture.
- Pus and wound debridement samples for bacterial and fungal culture.
- Skin scrapings for fungal microscopy and culture.
- Nail clippings for fungal microscopy and culture.
- Removal of insects or arachnids from the skin or subcutaneous tissues for microscopic inspection (eg, botfly larvae, ticks, *Tunga penetrans*).

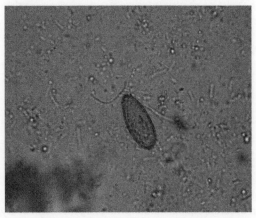

Fig. 3. Operculate ovum of *Clonorchis* spp. (*Courtesy of* Monika Manser, UKNEQAS.)

Bone Marrow Biopsy

Bone marrow biopsy includes bone marrow microscopy for *Leishmania* spp amastigotes and mycobacteria (*Mycobacterium tuberculosis* and atypical mycobacteria); and bone marrow cultures for *Mycobacterium* spp, *Salmonella typhi* (typhoid fever), and *Brucella* spp (brucellosis).

Lymph Node Aspirate or Biopsy

Lymph node aspirate and biopsy include the following:

- Microscopy after staining for trypanosomes, mycobacteria, fungi, *Toxoplasma gondii* and *Leishmania* spp.
- Culture for bacteria, mycobacteria and fungi, viruses and *Leishmania* spp.
- Histology and staining for trypanosomes, mycobacteria, fungi, *Toxoplasma gondii* and *Leishmania* spp.

Pericardial Effusion Aspirate

Pericardial effusion aspirate or biopsy for bacterial, mycobacterial, viral, and fungal culture, and histology.

Other Sample Types

Muscle biopsy specimens may be examined for *Trichinella spiralis* larvae. Deep wedge biopsy of the lesions is required in cases of Madura foot. Splenic aspirate is used for *Leishmania* spp. Xenodiagnosis is occasionally used for *Trypanosoma cruzi*. Clean, uninfected triatomine bugs are fed on the patient and then examined 3 weeks later for trypanosomes. This method will eventually be replaced by PCR.

BLOOD CULTURES FOR BACTERIA OR FUNGI

Automated blood culture systems for bacterial detection are now well established. Infections rarely seen in temperate climates, such as those caused by *Burkholderia pseudomallei*, *Brucella* spp, *S typhi* (typhoid), and *Salmonella paratyphi* (paratyphoid), may be detected in blood cultures of sick patients after tropical travel. It is important to provide the laboratory with details of area of travel and any suspected infections to enable laboratory staff to handle samples safely in category 3 or 4 conditions where necessary, or provide special growth requirements. Biochemical and serologic identification methods are applied to cultures or, where available, Matrix-Assisted Laser Desorption-Ionization Time-Of-Flight (MALDI-TOF) is deployed. In MALDI-TOF mass-spectrometry, a sample bound in a matrix undergoes desorption by an ultraviolet laser creating a hot plume which is then ionised. A Time-of-Flight mass spectrometer is used to acquire a profile spectrum of the plume which is then analysed to predict the identity of the pathogen. There are some limitations on its ability to correctly identify certain groups of related bacteria (eg, distinguishing *S pneumoniae* from *Streptococcus milleri* group). If bacterial, mycobacterial, or fungal infection is suspected but culture is unproductive, samples may be sent for 16s ribosomal DNA (for bacteria) or 18s ribosomal DNA (for fungi) or for *M tuberculosis* PCR.

Viral cultures are still used in some centers. Tissue cultures are observed for cytopathic effects, followed by confirmatory techniques, such as hemagglutination, immunofluorescence, or PCR, to determine identity. Tissue cultures may fail due to fungal or bacterial contamination, but have the advantage that novel viruses may be detected.

MICROSCOPY OF BLOOD FILMS

Blood film examination is still the method used for the primary diagnosis of malaria parasites (*Plasmodium* spp); trypanosomes (*Trypanosoma* spp); and *Babesia* spp (**Figs. 4–6**).

MICROSCOPY FOR MICROFILARIAE

Diagnosis of *O volvulus* is by microscopic examination of skin snips, but for other filariases, definitive diagnosis is usually made by demonstrating microfilariae by filtration of anticoagulated peripheral blood (citrate tube). Day blood (for *Loa loa*) should be taken between 12 noon and 2 PM local time and night blood (for *Wuchereria bancrofti*) between 12 midnight and 2 AM.

SEROLOGY

Serologic tests detect either antibodies to the pathogen or antigens of the pathogen itself. Common serologic tests used are ELISA, immunoblot, agglutination, precipitation, complement-fixation, and immunofluorescence-based microscopy. Newer techniques and formats are being developed.

Viral Serology

Given the large number of viral infections to which a traveler might be exposed, it is useful to discuss with the virologist what is relevant to symptoms and travel. Arthropod-borne viruses (arboviruses) feature strongly in the differential diagnosis in travelers from Southeast Asia. Exposure to monkeys and dogs (rabies), bats (rabies), rodents (Lassa fever), or ticks (Crimean-Congo hemorrhagic fever) is highly relevant to the differential diagnosis and selection of tests. Important viruses to consider are *Flavivirus* infections (dengue virus, West Nile virus, tick-borne encephalitis virus, yellow fever virus, St. Louis encephalitis virus, and Japanese encephalitis virus); alphaviruses including western equine encephalitis virus, Venezuelan equine encephalitis virus, eastern equine encephalitis virus, chikungunya virus, and Ross River

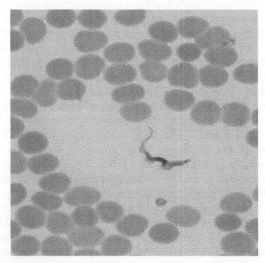

Fig. 4. *Trypanosoma brucei* spp in blood film. Giemsa stain. Original magnification ×1000 (*Courtesy of* Monika Manser.)

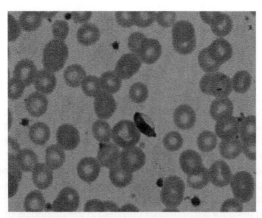

Fig. 5. *Plasmodium falciparum* gametocyte in peripheral blood film. Giemsa stain. Original magnification ×1000 (*Courtesy of* Monika Manser.)

virus; bunyaviruses, such as Crimean-Congo hemorrhagic fever and *Hantavirus*; arenaviruses (eg, Lassa fever); and filoviruses (Ebola virus and Marburg virus). For rabies, detection of neutralizing serum or CSF antibodies in an unvaccinated person is diagnostic but they are usually only detectable late in the illness.

Bacterial Serology

Many systemic bacterial infections are more readily identified by serologic methods than by culture. Serology is frequently performed to diagnose infections caused by *Bartonella* spp (bartonellosis); *Brucella* spp (brucellosis); *Leptospira* spp (leptospirosis); *Coxiella burnetii* (Q fever); *Franciscella tularensis*; *Rickettsia* spp; *Treponema pallidum* (syphilis); *Mycoplasma pneumoniae*; and *Borrelia burgdoferi* (Lyme disease). Antibodies to *B pertussis* and to *Corynebacterium diphtheriae* may be available from

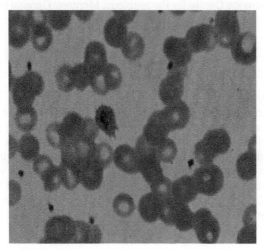

Fig. 6. *Plasmodium ovale* trophozoite in blood film. Giemsa stain. Original magnification ×1000 (*Courtesy of* Monika Manser.)

public health laboratories where monitoring is performed in conjunction with vaccination programs. Complement fixation tests, which are very laborious, have been largely superseded by ELISA but are still used to detect antibodies to some organisms (eg, *Mycoplasma* spp).

Fungal Serology

Immunodiffusion tests for histoplasmosis detect precipitins directed against M and H antigens. Antibodies against M antigen appear first in acute pulmonary histoplasmosis. Antibodies to H antigen occur later and less frequently, and are often linked to extrapulmonary dissemination.

Complement fixation tests for aspergillosis: A titer of 1:8 or greater is a strong suggestion of *Aspergillus* spp infection or allergy. However, approximately 5% of the population has circulating antibodies against *Aspergillus* spp.

Immunodiffusion tests for aspergillosis can help in the diagnosis of allergic bronchopulmonary aspergillosis and aspergilloma, the forms of aspergillosis seen in immunocompetent individuals. Precipitins can be found in more than 90% of patients with aspergilloma and in 70% of patients with allergic bronchopulmonary aspergillosis. Growth of *Aspergillus* spp in the tissues of an immunosuppressed host does not correlate with an increase in anti-*Aspergillus* spp antibody titers.

Enzyme immunoassay tests are used for coccidioidomycosis and blastomycosis. Immunodiffusion tests are used for paracoccidioidomycosis.

Parasite Serology

Although the gold standard for parasite diagnosis is to visualize the organism, serology plays a major role in clinical parasitology, especially for tissue parasites (eg, *Toxocara* spp) or where microscopy is relatively insensitive (eg, *S stercoralis*).

Parasite serology is mainly available in specialist or reference laboratories. In-house methods are often used, so the range and type of tests deployed vary between centres. The following section reflects the repertoire available in the UK. Those working in North America should consult their national reference facilities, eg, the Division of Parasitic Diseases, Centers for Disease Control and Prevention, Atlanta GA, USA; National Reference Centre for Parasitology, Montreal General Hospital, Quebec, Canada.

Babesia

Serology is not an alternative to blood film examination to detect the parasite, but can be helpful in the diagnosis of low-level *Babesia microti* infections.

Entamoeba histolytica

Antibody detection is an essential test in cases of suspected amoebic liver abscess. Such cases produce high Indirect Fluorescent Antibody Test (IFAT) titers of about 1/160 to 1/320, and the test is positive in more than 95% of cases of amoebic liver abscess by the end of the first 14 days. A negative result early in the illness should be followed with a repeat sample 7 days later. The IFAT also gives very good results in cases of amoeboma. In amoebic colitis the test is positive in about 75% of cases, so hot stool, fecal PCR, rectal scrapes, and rectal biopsy are also required if amoebic colitis is suspected.

Fascioliasis

Fasciola hepatica eggs in feces are often scanty and may not easily be found. Serology (eg, by IFAT) is the best method of diagnosis in the early stage of the infection.

Filariasis
Serology is not the best way to diagnose filariasis; demonstration of microfilariae or, in the case of *W bancrofti*, use of an antigen-detection test, is preferred. The filaria ELISA for antibody using *Brugia pahangi* as the antigen is a nonspecific screening test that is positive in many types of filariasis and in some cases of strongyloidiasis. A positive result should prompt more detailed investigation. The test is most useful in the diagnosis of tropical pulmonary eosinophilia, where high antifilarial antibody levels are required to support the diagnosis. Serology for the detection of onchocerciasis has been developed using a recombinant antigen.

Hydatid disease
Serology (ELISA or Western blot) plays a major part in diagnosis of cystic echinococcosis caused by *Echinococcus granulosus* and alveolar echinococcosis caused by *Echinococcus multilocularis*. Expert interpretation and review of imaging is essential.

Human African trypanosomiasis
Serology plays no part in the diagnosis of acute *T brucei rhodesiense* infection (East African trypanosomiasis) but is used to detect CSF antibody in suspected stage 2 infection. Early *T brucei gambiense* infection may show scanty parasitemia, so antibody detection plays an important part in case finding and individual diagnosis, in addition to its role in the evaluation of stage 2 disease.

Leishmaniasis
The direct agglutination test for leishmaniasis using formalinized promastigotes of *Leishmania donovani* stained with Coomassie blue is the standard method. An immunochromatography-based rapid diagnostic test (RDT) using K39 recombinant leishmanial antigen permits rapid field-based detection of antileishmanial antibody (**Fig. 7**). Negative serology does not exclude the diagnosis of visceral leishmaniasis in sera from HIV-positive patients. Serology is not helpful in the diagnosis of cutaneous infections.

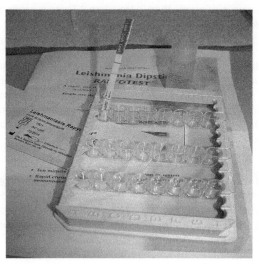

Fig. 7. Rapid rK39 immunochromatographic dipstick test for anti-leishmanial antibody. (*Courtesy of* Patricia Lowe, Hospital for Tropical Diseases, London, UK.)

Malaria

Serology is not suitable for diagnosing current infection. Urgent thick and thin blood film examination is the method of choice. Antigen may be detected by immunochromatography-based RDTs. Serology for antimalarial antibody is central to the diagnosis of hyperreactive malarial splenomegaly (tropical splenomegaly syndrome) and is sometimes used to make a retrospective diagnosis, but its main role is in blood bank screening in nonendemic areas. It is not recommended for the investigation of acute fever.

Neurocysticercosis (larval Taenia solium infection)

Neurocysticercosis, caused by the presence of the larval stage (cysticercus) of T solium in the central nervous system, is diagnosed by neuroimaging and serology by enzyme-linked immunoelectrotransfer blot (EITB). Sensitivity of the EITB is high in the presence of multiple cysts, but as low as 28% with solitary lesions. Specificity is as high as 99%, except for tests in which only a 50-kDa band is seen.[5]

Schistosomal serology

The ELISA based on soluble egg antigen of Schistosoma mansoni is reported to detect about 96% of S mansoni and 92% of S haematobium infections with 98% specificity. The test does not distinguish active from treated infections and is not helpful in post-treatment follow-up.

American trypanosomiasis (Chagas disease)

Diagnosis of acute infection is made by examining stained blood films for trypanosomes. Antibody detection is central to the diagnosis of chronic infection in the indeterminate phase and in the presence of complications. An ELISA is commonly used, with IFAT also deployed. A rapid immunochromatographic strip test for antibody is also available.

Strongyloides serology

Antibody detection by ELISA or IFAT is available. The test is indicated for the investigation of eosinophilia or if there is a good clinical history to suggest strongyloidiasis. ELISA is more sensitive in migrants than in travelers.[5] There is cross-reaction between filaria and Strongyloides in the ELISA.

Toxocariasis

Serology is the method of choice for the diagnosis of toxocariasis. The ELISA is usually performed on serum, but can be undertaken on vitreous humor where appropriate. The Toxocara IgG antibody ELISA test against larval excretory/secretory antigen is the method most commonly used. Positive ELISA tests are confirmed using a Western blot. Negative ELISA on serum does not exclude ocular cases. Vitreous sampling may be necessary to exclude ocular toxocariasis.

Toxoplasmosis

Methods in routine use for detection of Toxoplasma gondii antibodies include ELISA, microparticle enzyme immunoassay and two-step enzyme immunoassay with paramagnetic microparticles, and chemiluminescence detection. An enzyme-linked fluorescent assay can be used to determine the avidity of IgG antibodies where it is important to know whether there has been recent infection. The toxoplasma dye test measures the total amount of antibody in serum capable of complement-mediated killing of T gondii tachyzoites. The requirement for live parasites has restricted its use to specialist reference laboratories.

Trichinosis

Early cases are diagnosed by muscle biopsy, before seroconversion occurs. Serology is valuable in later cases and for detection of exposure in epidemiologic investigation of outbreaks.

HISTOPATHOLOGY

Histopathology plays a central role in the diagnosis of amoebic colitis; cutaneous, mucosal, and visceral leishmaniasis; histoplasmosis; tuberculosis; leprosy; Whipple's disease; the deep mycoses; and the confirmation of critical viral infections (eg, Negri bodies are seen in about two-thirds of humans infected with rabies).

NEWER TECHNOLOGIC APPROACHES
Rapid Diagnostic Tests

There is a move toward faster identification of a variety of infections using RDTs. These assays, also known as lateral flow or immunochromatographic devices, are typically run on nitrocellulose or nylon membranes contained within a plastic or cardboard housing. They may not be as sensitive as more conventional methods, but are quick to perform and convenient for near-patient use. RDTs may be used for antigen or antibody detection, depending on their format, and are increasingly deployed to detect a variety of infections in many settings. Examples are dengue antigen detection, HIV antibody, *T cruzi* antibody, *Leishmania* antibody, and syphilis antibody. A major application is in the diagnosis of malaria in endemic regions where diagnosis by microscopy is not available. The World Health Organization Web site[4] should be consulted for an assessment of a variety of different malaria RDTs.

Nucleic-Acid Amplification Techniques

There are multiple methods for amplifying target, probe, or signal. These are increasingly being used for the diagnosis or specific identification of tropical infections and can be more sensitive than serologic tests in the early stages of infection before an antibody response has developed.

Nucleic acid amplification tests in common use include those for HIV; *Chlamydia trachomatis*; and gonorrhea (rectal swabs, throat swabs). They are used increasingly to diagnose parasitic infections including malaria, leishmaniasis, and microsporidiosis. Many viral infections, including rabies, may be detected by nucleic acid amplification tests. Bacterial toxin genes may be identified (eg, diphtheria toxin gene in swabs taken from nose, throat, or wounds).

Target Amplification Methods

These methods include PCR (eg, for chlamydia) and RT-PCR, which is used for HIV and other RNA viruses. Nested PCRs use two sets of amplification primers. One set is used for the first round of amplification, then the products are subjected to a second round of amplification with another set of primers specific for an internal sequence that is also amplified by the first primer pair. Nested PCR has extremely high sensitivity because of the dual amplification process. It is used as a reference assay in malaria diagnosis.

In multiplex PCRs two or more sets of primer pairs specific for different targets are used simultaneously. This can be used to detect multiple pathogens from a single specimen. Multiplex PCR is in use for the detection of *E histolytica*, *Cryptosporidium*, and *Giardia* in feces.

Loop-Mediated Isothermal Amplification

Loop-mediated isothermal amplification is a novel technique for amplification of target DNA in isothermal conditions, using a robust DNA polymerase and primer pairs that produce a specific double-hairpin DNA template, which can be amplified and concatenated with high efficiency. It can be used in basic laboratories, giving results within 90 minutes, and without requiring complex equipment. Diagnostic tests for malaria, tuberculosis, and sleeping sickness have been devised (**Fig. 8**).

Rolling Circle Amplification

This is an isothermal method that amplifies signals from proteins and DNA and RNA. Many different targets may be detected simultaneously.

Transcription Mediated Amplification

This method is isothermal and has been used for detecting the presence of *M tuberculosis* (eg, Gen-Probe), *C trachomatis*, HIV, and *Listeria* and *Salmonella* in food samples.

Nucleic Acid Sequence-Based Amplification

Nucleic acid sequence-based amplification is able selectively to amplify RNA sequences in a DNA background, which avoids false-positive signals caused by dead bacteria. Nucleic acid sequence-based amplification uses simultaneous enzymatic activity of reverse transcriptase, T7 RNA polymerase, and RNase in combination with two oligonucleotides. It has been used to achieve rapid (2 hour) HIV viral load testing and for enterovirus detection in CSF. Quantitative nucleic acid sequence-based amplification has been used for quantification of leishmania in biopsy samples.

Probe Amplification

These tests include the following:

- Ligase chain reaction can be used for detection of *Chlamydia*, *Neisseria gonorrhoeae*, and HIV.
- Strand displacement amplification after initial denaturation can be used in isothermal conditions (eg, for *Chlamydia*, gonorrhea, *M tuberculosis*, and HIV).

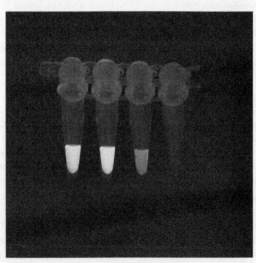

Fig. 8. The LAMP assay. (*Courtesy of* Dr Spencer Polley.)

- Qβ replicase is an RNA-dependent RNA polymerase from bacteriophage Qβ that uses reporter probes containing a promoter sequence that is recognized by Qβ replicase. It has been used for detection of HIV.

Signal Amplification

Several signal amplification tests are now available:

- Branched DNA amplification tests have been used to measure HIV viral loads.
- Hybrid capture has been deployed for detection of human papillomavirus, *C trachomatis*, *N gonorrhoeae*, CMV, and hepatitis B.
- Cleavage-based amplification is used to detect human papilloma virus.
- Cycling probes are currently used in clinical trials in assays for HIV resistance mutations.
- Immuno-PCR has been used for the detection of ultralow levels of HIV p24 antigen.

Microarrays

Microarrays have been applied to the detection of HIV mutations that confer resistance to antiretroviral drugs. They are rapid but relatively expensive to set up. DNA microarrays have been used to monitor antimalarial drug resistance mutations (eg, the dihydrofolate reductase and dihydropteroate synthetase genes dotted onto a glass slide and then hybridized to DNA from clinical isolates).[7] The European Union Fluarray project seeks to develop a point-of-care test to distinguish influenza types A and B, and A subtypes.

Mass Spectrometry

Mass spectrometry has been used in novel identification methods, such as PLEX-ID DNA mass spectrometry, which uses common primers for all organisms, and mass spectrometry of products, which is analyzed to generate an identity by comparison with that of known isolates.

Surface-enhanced laser desorption/ionization TOF mass spectrometry combines chromatography and mass spectrometry. It is similar to MALDI-TOF technology and has a role in proteomic analysis and novel biomarker discovery.

Microfluidics, Microelectromechanical Systems, and Lab-on-a-Chip

Using a combination of technologies, sample processing, amplification, and detection of product can take place in a miniature flow-through format. Novel sensor technologies will enable control of pumps, microheaters, temperature sensors, miniaturized fluorescence detectors, sample/analyte concentrators, and filters.

A lab-on-a-chip is a device that integrates laboratory functions onto a chip, which may be measured in millimeters, handling subpicoliter fluid volumes.

THE FUTURE

There is a continuous need to develop new diagnostic tests for emerging infections, and because these are frequently zoonoses, tests are likely to be shared with the veterinary world. Methods currently used in the food and water industry and pharmaceuticals can be modified for diagnostic microbiology. This is the brink of a revolution in clinical diagnostics. Imaginative use and combination of new technologies will increase ease, speed, and accuracy of organism detection. Gene transcript abundance profiles on microarrays could potentially lead to diagnosis of infection by recognition of its effect on the host. Current research is focusing on identifying a pathogen and determining its virulence and drug sensitivities, all from one chip.

REFERENCES

1. Cook GC, Zumla A, editors. Manson's tropical diseases. 22nd edition. London: Saunders Elsevier Publishing Group; 2009.
2. Johnston V, Stockley JM, Dockrell D, et al. Fever in returned travellers presenting in the United Kingdom: recommendations for investigation and initial management. J Infect 2009;59(1):1–18.
3. Zumla A, Yew WW, Hui D. Emerging respiratory infections in the 21st century. Infect Dis Clin North Am 2010;24(3):xiii–xvi.
4. The use of malaria rapid diagnostic tests. Available at: www.wpro.who.int/sites/rdt/documents/pub_9290612045.htm. Accessed May 26, 2012.
5. Checkley AM, Chiodini PL, Dockrell DH, et al. Eosinophilia in returning travellers and migrants from the tropics: UK recommendations for investigation and initial management. J Infect 2010;60(1):1–20.
6. Schmitt BH, Rosenblatt JE, Pritt BS. Laboratory diagnosis of tropical infections. Infect Dis Clin North Am 2012;26(2):513–54.
7. Crameri A, Marfut J, Mugittu K, et al. Rapid microarray-based method for monitoring of all currently known single-nucleotide polymorphisms associated with parasite resistance to antimalaria drugs. J Clin Microbiol 2007;45(11):3885–91.

Index

Note: Page numbers of article titles are in **boldface** type.

Infect Dis Clin N Am 26 (2012) 819–838
http://dx.doi.org/10.1016/S0891-5520(12)00090-6
0891-5520/12/$ – see front matter © 2012 Elsevier Inc. All rights reserved.